Get Started

Yoga

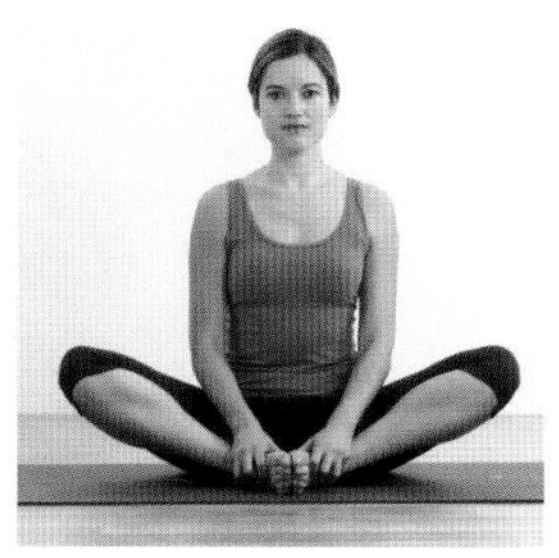

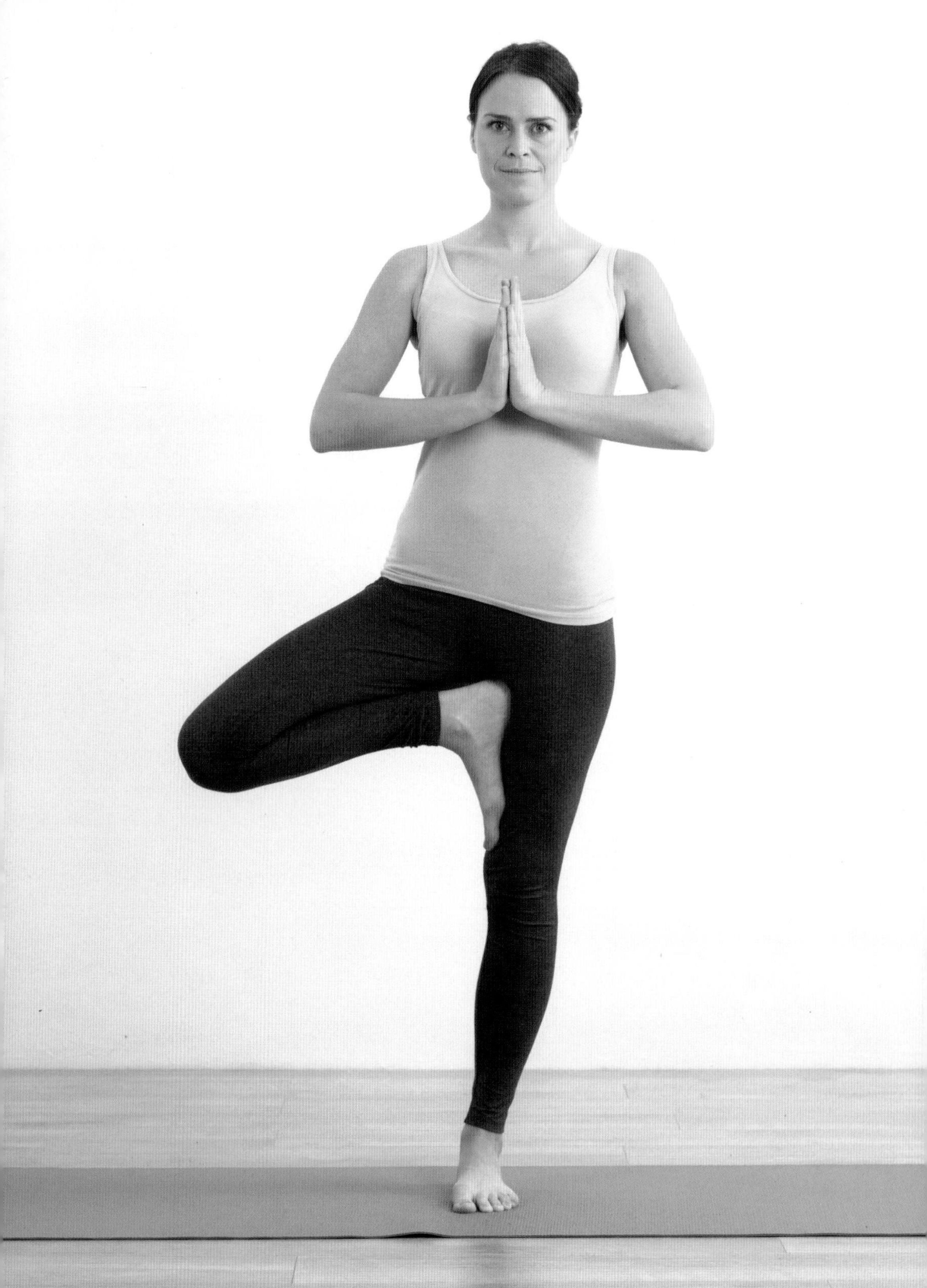

Get Started

Yoga

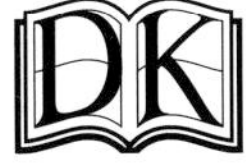

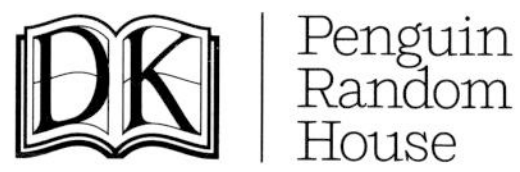

Project Editor Becky Shackleton
Project Art Editor Gemma Fletcher
Senior Editor Alastair Laing
Managing Editor Penny Warren
Managing Art Editor Alison Donovan
Senior Jacket Creative Nicola Powling
Jacket Design Assistant Rosie Levine
Preproduction Producer Sarah Isle
Senior Producers Jen Lockwood, Seyhan Esen
Art Directors Peter Luff, Jane Bull
Publisher Mary Ling

DK Publishing
Editor Jenny Siklos
Senior Editor Shannon Beatty

DK India
Senior Editor Garima Sharma
Senior Art Editor Ivy Roy
Managing Editor Alka Thakur Hazarika
Deputy Managing Art Editor Priyabrata Roy Chowdhury

Tall Tree Ltd
Editors Joe Fullman, Camilla Hallinan, Catherine Saunders, Deirdre Headon
Designer Malcolm Parchment

Written by Nita Patel
Photographer Dave King

First American Edition, 2013

Published in the United States by DK Publishing, 345 Hudson Street, New York, New York 10014

15 16 17 10 9 8 7 6 5 4 3
014—185476—Jan/2013

Published in Great Britain by Dorling Kindersley Limited.

A catalog record for this book is available from the Library of Congress.

ISBN 978-1-4654-0198-4

DK books are available at special discounts when purchased in bulk for sales promotions, premiums, fund-raising, or educational use. For details, contact: DK Publishing Special Markets, 345 Hudson Street, New York, New York 10014 or SpecialSales@dk.com.

Printed and bound in China

A WORLD OF IDEAS:
SEE ALL THERE IS TO KNOW
www.dk.com

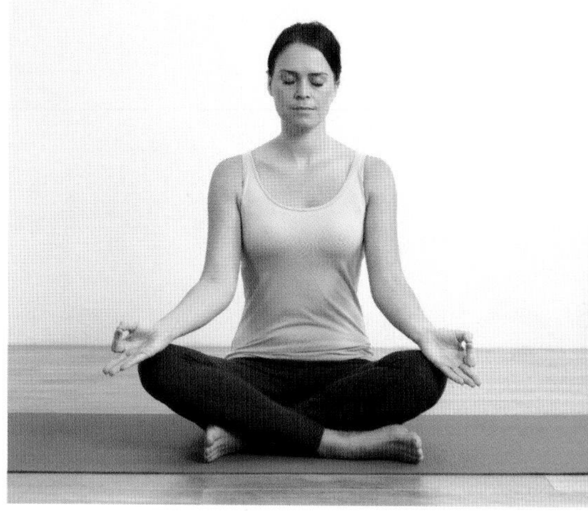

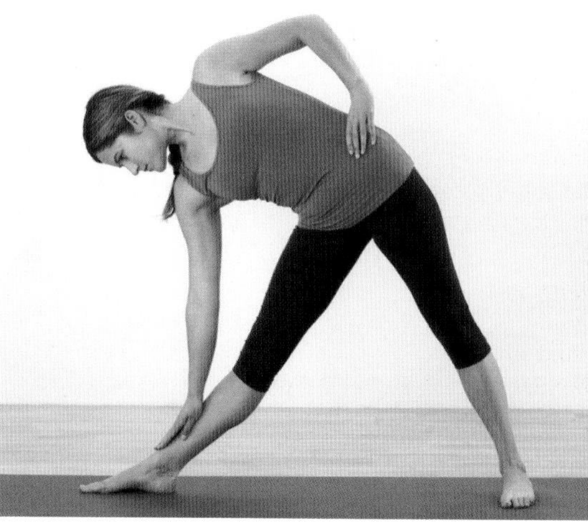

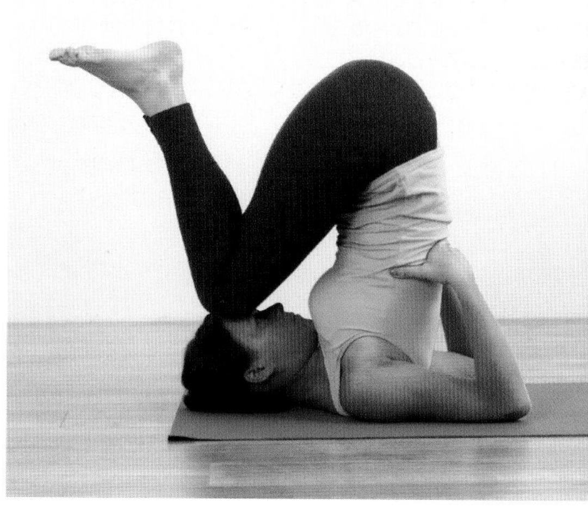

Contents

Build Your Course

This book guides you through 38 key yoga poses. It is divided into three carefully structured chapters—Start Simple, Build On It, and Take It Further—in which you will learn the core yoga positions and breathing techniques before moving on to more complex and challenging poses.

Getting Started

Learning yoga at home should be a safe, practical, and enriching experience. But before you attempt any yoga postures, it is important to understand the principles of yoga, its key benefits, and a little of the science behind the poses. In addition, you will need some yoga equipment. A nonslip yoga mat is essential, but you might also find props such as straps useful, at least at the beginning. If you're struggling to attain a pose, props can help, and this book will show you how best to use them.

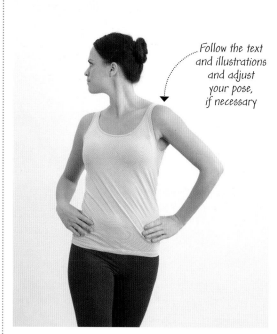
Follow the text and illustrations and adjust your pose, if necessary

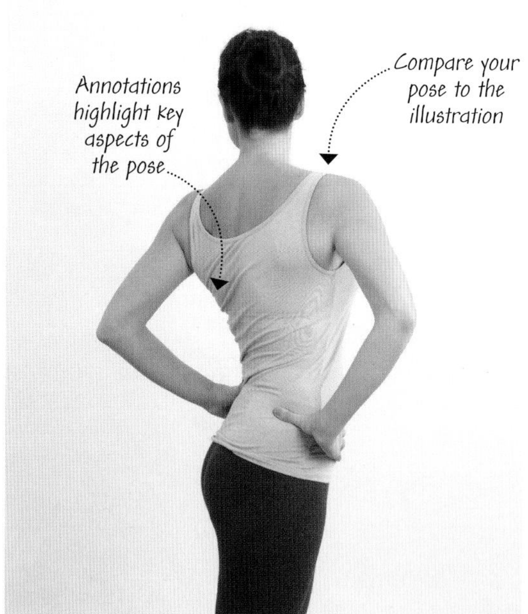
Annotations highlight key aspects of the pose
Compare your pose to the illustration

Key Techniques

To make your yoga practice both safe and effective, key techniques are explained. At the start of each section you will find information you need for the next stage of your course, from breathing techniques to developing your own sequences and improving self-awareness.

1 Illustrated step-by-step text guides you through the poses. It is important to follow the steps so that you attain correct alignment, activate the correct muscles for the desired stretch, and practice safely.

Useful tips focus on an area or suggest ways of making the pose easier.

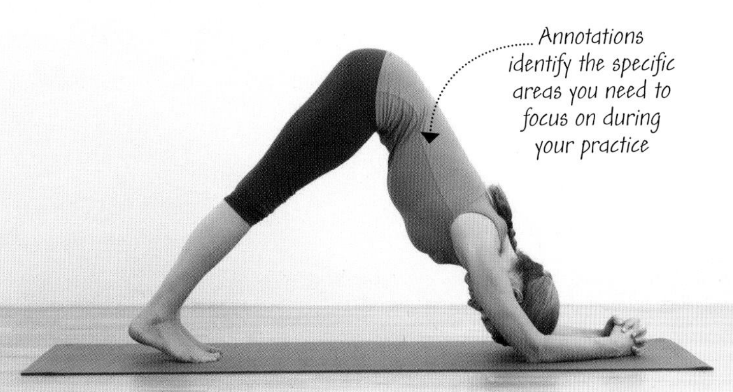
Annotations identify the specific areas you need to focus on during your practice

1 Mountain Pose
pp.44–45

You will build confidence in moving between poses

2 Warrior Lunge
pp.104–105

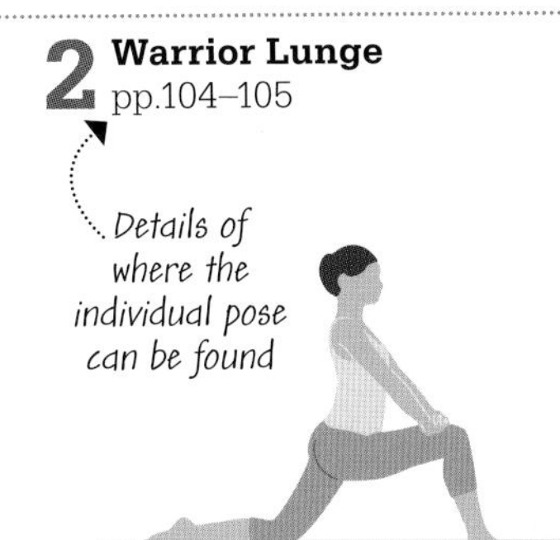
Details of where the individual pose can be found

Sequences

At the end of each section, the postures you have practiced are combined into 15-, 30-, and 45-minute sessions. The sequences become more challenging as you progress through sections of the course.

Take care...

These assessment and advice sections help you to monitor your own progress and make adjustments to your body position, if necessary. This encourages you to measure your personal yoga progress and demonstrates the importance of cultivating self-awareness to achieve this.

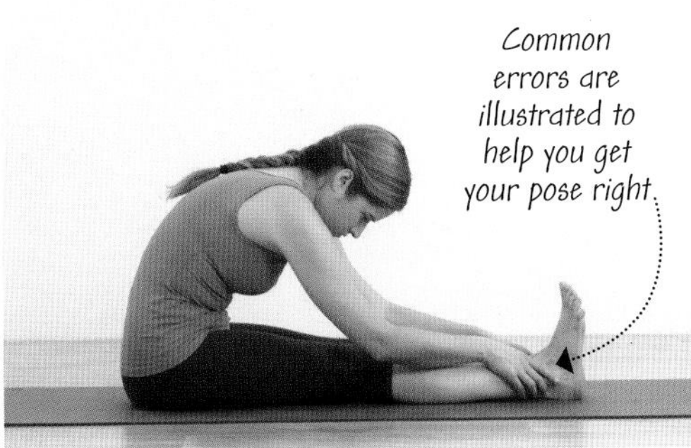
Common errors are illustrated to help you get your pose right

Make it easier

There's usually an easier way in yoga if you need it, and this book shows you how to safely adapt poses to the limits of your body. By encouraging you to assess your progress, it will also enable you to reflect on the changes to your body and you will see your limits decrease.

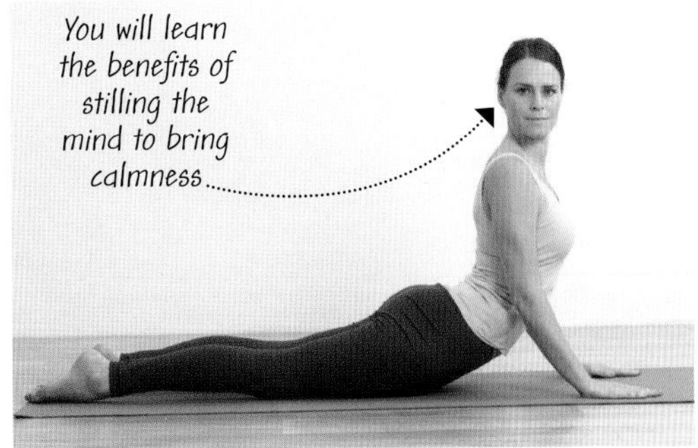
You will learn the benefits of stilling the mind to bring calmness

The 5 Principles of Yoga

As a newcomer wanting to learn yoga, you may wonder how best to approach such a diverse subject. Five basic principles underpin all forms of yoga practice and these will provide you with a starting point to understand this vast and sometimes mystical school of thought.

1. Beneficial exercise

Sometimes viewed incorrectly as undemanding forms of exercise, yoga routines can provide you with a full cardiac workout and increase your aerobic stamina.

Practicing yoga sequences will provide you with a workout that is strenuous and varied enough to be considered "real exercise." The sequences in this book also ensure that all areas of the body are worked on. Yoga achieves this by massaging the internal organs, stretching and toning the muscles and ligaments, enhancing the flexibility of the spine and joints, as well as improving blood circulation. Any worthwhile exercise regime should take into account existing levels of fitness and stamina as well as any medical conditions. In yoga, postures can be modified or aids used to enable safe practice for people of different physical abilities.

Key points

- **Poses should be held** steady for a few breathing cycles with the aim of attaining a deeper stretch to increase the strength, flexibility, and vitality of the spine.
- **Try to travel through** the different stages of a posture in a smooth and fluid fashion, working within your physical capabilities so as not to overstrain your body.

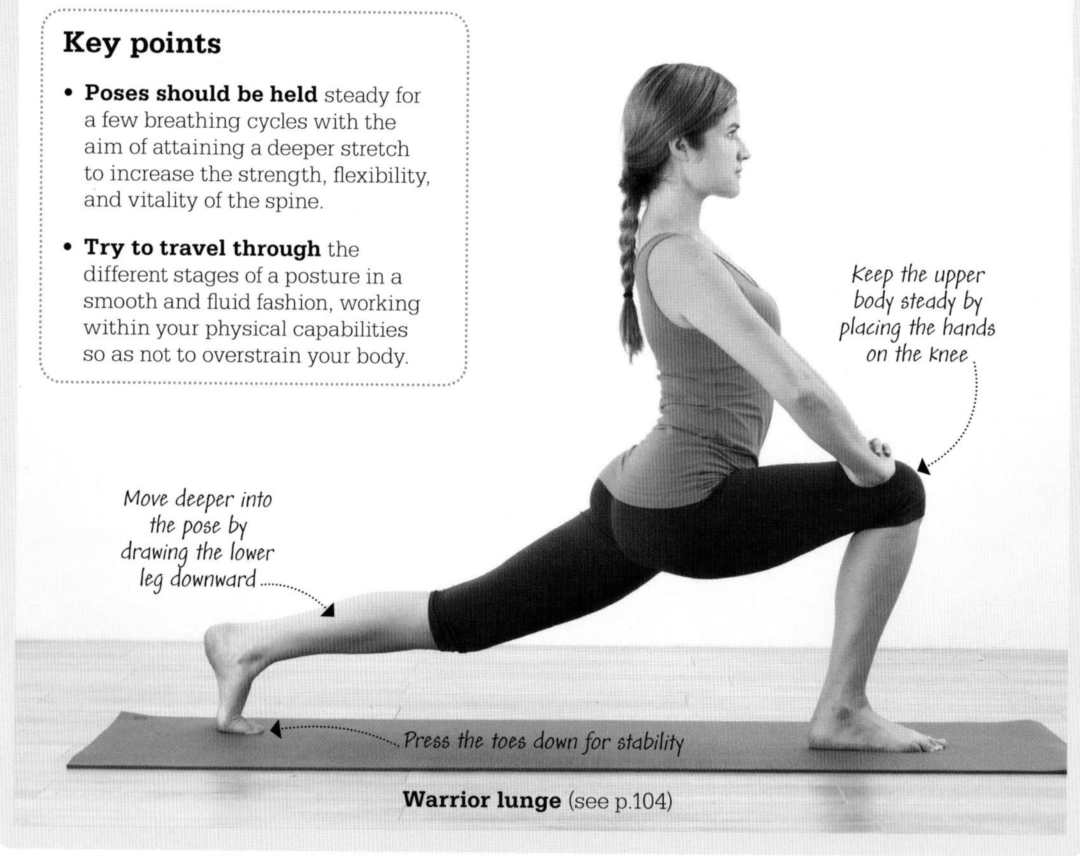
Keep the upper body steady by placing the hands on the knee
Move deeper into the pose by drawing the lower leg downward
Press the toes down for stability

Warrior lunge (see p.104)

2. Correct breathing

Yoga places great importance on the breath as it is considered to be a bridge between the mind and the physical body. Breathing correctly in yoga requires you to breathe fully and rhythmically, actively employing your entire lung capacity in order to maximize your intake of oxygen. To achieve breathing that is deep, slow, and rhythmical, you need to be able to regulate the depth and duration of not only inhalation but also exhalation of the breath. Yoga encourages breathing in and out through the nose.

Yoga breathing techniques reinvigorate your body by maximizing oxygen levels in the blood. Proper execution of the postures is needed to ensure that you breathe correctly. When adopting the poses, be aware of the position of the upper torso, ensuring that the ribs can be lifted up and outward, the chest is open, and you are connecting to the movements of the diaphragm. Deepening the breath also helps remove the stale air from the lungs. In addition to increasing energy levels, control of the breath also influences your mental state, helping you to achieve a calmer and more focused mind.

Familiarity with the concept of *prana*, or vital energy, will help you to understand why such importance is attached to breathing in yoga theory and practice. Put simply, *prana* is the energy that animates matter and is present in all living things, including ourselves. By teaching how to control our breath, yoga enables us to ingest, distribute, and store *prana* more effectively.

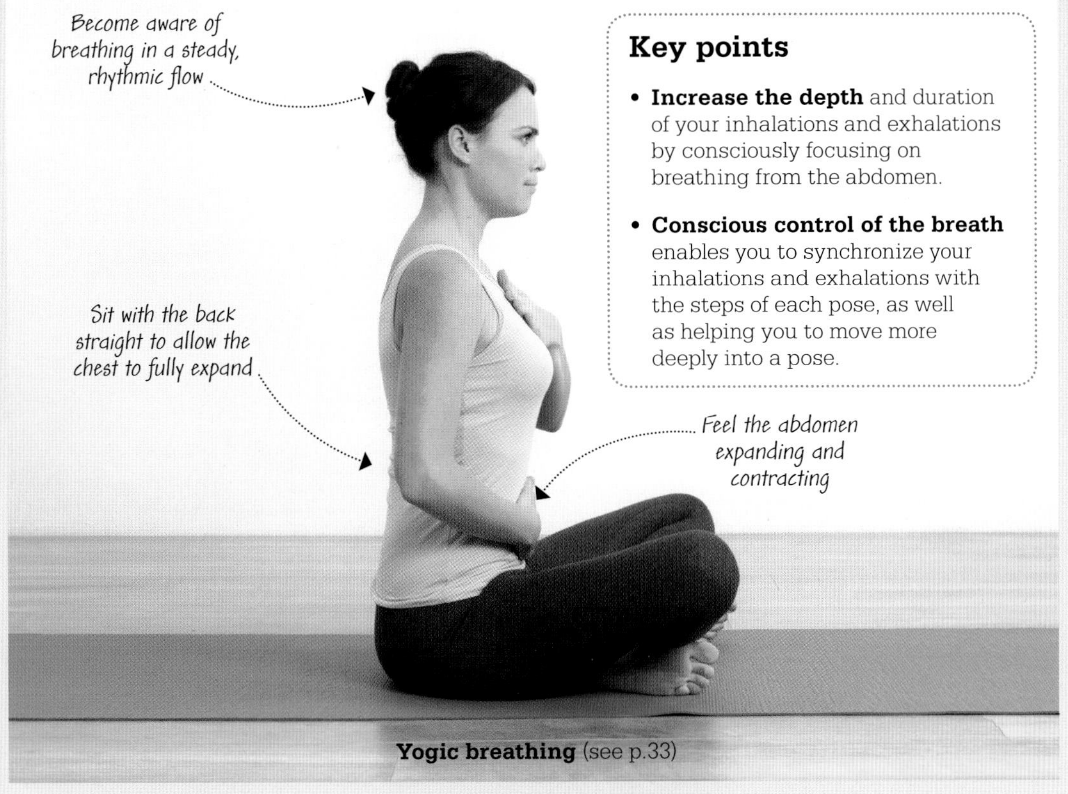
Become aware of breathing in a steady, rhythmic flow
Sit with the back straight to allow the chest to fully expand
Feel the abdomen expanding and contracting

Yogic breathing (see p.33)

Key points

- **Increase the depth** and duration of your inhalations and exhalations by consciously focusing on breathing from the abdomen.
- **Conscious control of the breath** enables you to synchronize your inhalations and exhalations with the steps of each pose, as well as helping you to move more deeply into a pose.

3. Complete relaxation

Yoga defines a state of true relaxation as existing when the body consumes the minimum amount of energy required to exist. Yoga distinguishes between physical, mental, and spiritual relaxation, each of which may be accomplished in a different way. Physical relaxation, for example, involves using movements to loosen and eventually disperse areas of tension created by trapped negative energies. Relaxation sequences are designed to focus on these areas, applying pressure and massaging them to release tension in a similar way to acupressure.

Key points

- **Mental relaxation** involves minimizing brain activity and quieting the mind by using breathing techniques. Yoga teaches that mental processes consume vital energy.
- **Spiritual relaxation** is an attempt, through the techniques of visualization and meditation, to connect the individual to the larger universe, which the individual is not separate from, but part of.

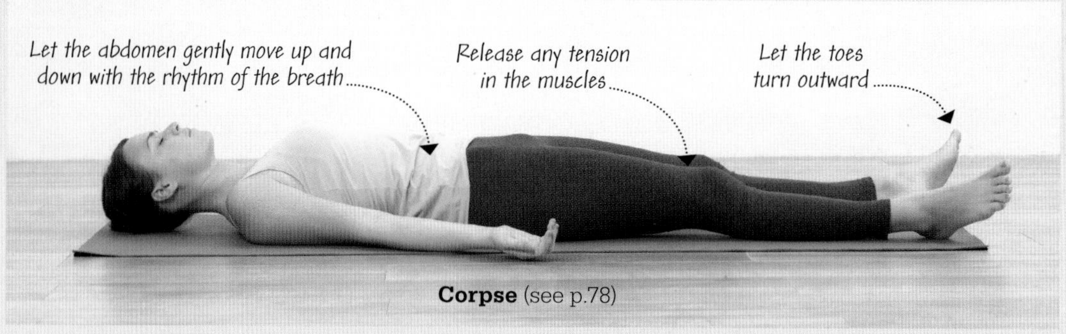
Let the abdomen gently move up and down with the rhythm of the breath
Release any tension in the muscles
Let the toes turn outward

Corpse (see p.78)

4. Balanced diet

The yogic approach to food and diet has much in common with modern ideas about healthy eating. Yoga teachings advocate a diet of fresh fruits and vegetables, dairy products, and nuts and pulses. Great importance is placed on the way in which we consume food as this will impact upon the body's ability to digest and absorb nutrients. The general rules are to eat in moderation only when hungry, take time to chew food properly, eat at set times each day, minimize fluid intake at meals, and generally have a positive attitude to food and its preparation.

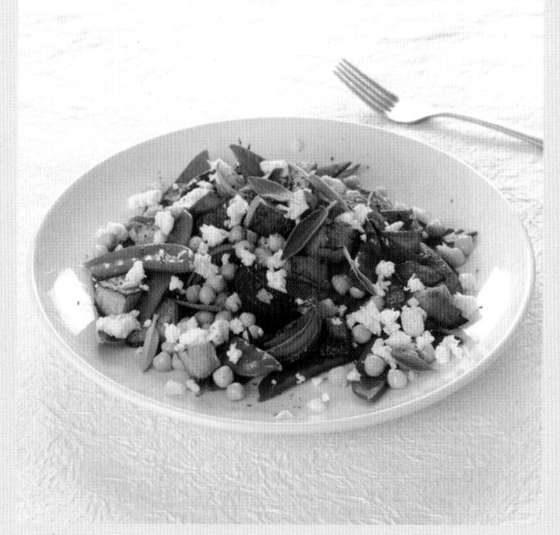

5. Positive thinking

Yoga places great importance on positive thinking for sustaining mental wellbeing. Yoga uses meditation and relaxation techniques to consciously clear the mind of negative thoughts and emotions, and employs positive affirmations to bolster self-esteem. Having put your negative thinking and emotions to one side, you will be able to see your strengths and weaknesses more realistically. Shedding your previous mindset may be no easy task, but by choosing to practice yoga, you are beginning a discipline that will eventually bring you to a state of psychological harmony and serenity.

Key points

- **Stilling the mind** and focusing inward develops self-awareness, opening the door to new insights and possibilities.
- **Channeling your thoughts** positively will enable you to unleash your creative potential.
- **Opens the connection** to the inherent stillness that is within, bringing clarity and focus to the mind.

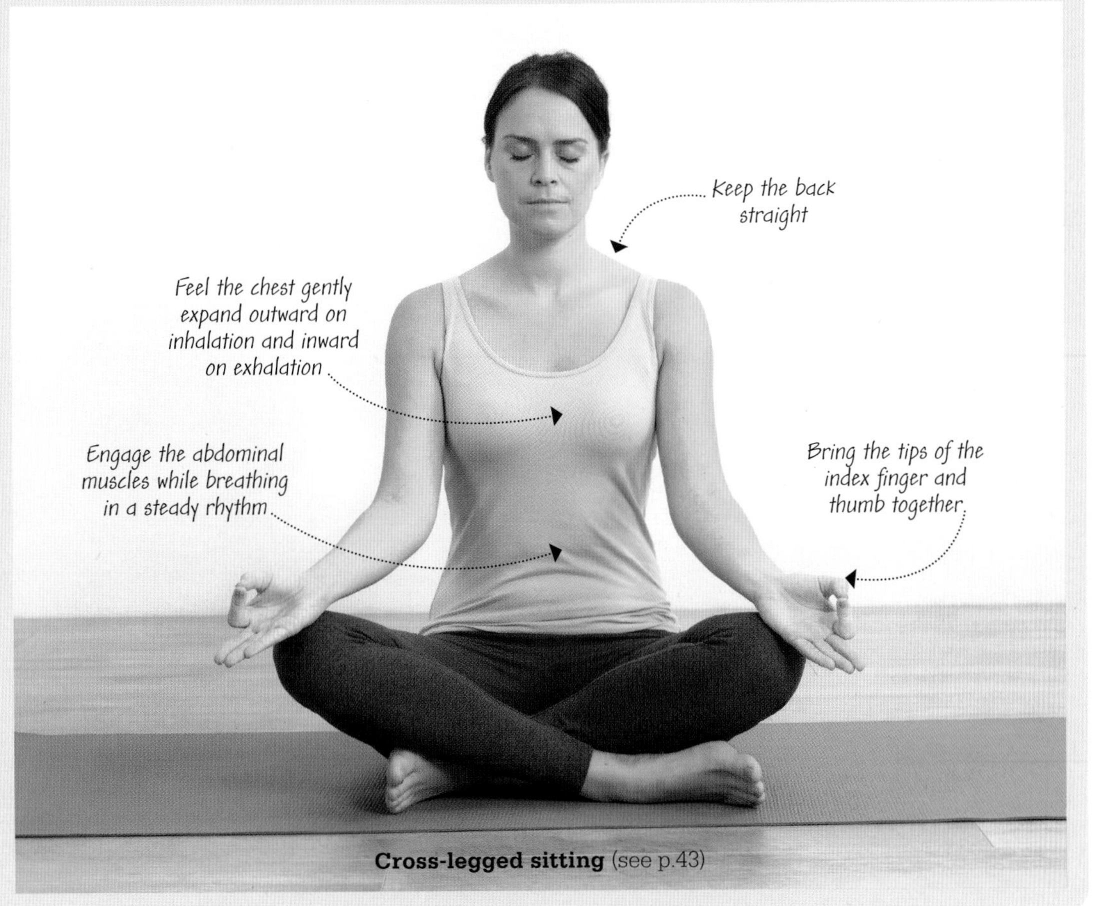
Keep the back straight
Feel the chest gently expand outward on inhalation and inward on exhalation
Engage the abdominal muscles while breathing in a steady rhythm
Bring the tips of the index finger and thumb together

Cross-legged sitting (see p.43)

The 3 Key Benefits of Yoga

Yoga creates a state where the mind, body, and spirit are in harmony with each other. This differentiates it from other physical activities and forms its unique character. Yoga creates a flexible body and a serene, sharply focused mind able to unleash the potential that is locked within.

1. Enhance your health and fitness

Modern living with its increased stresses has coincided with an increase in health problems. Yoga offers great health benefits by developing not only your overall fitness, but also your flexibility, posture, balance, and muscle tone. Yoga's restorative powers can help to alleviate existing medical conditions and to maintain your health, by slowing down physical degeneration in many ways.

Key points

- **Yoga keeps joints flexible and healthy** by stretching and toning muscles and ligaments, and increasing their flexibility.
- **Breathing techniques** keep lungs fully exercised and filled with oxygen, which is then carried to the rest of the body.
- **Yoga sequences** strengthen the body's respiratory, circulatory, digestive, and nervous systems.

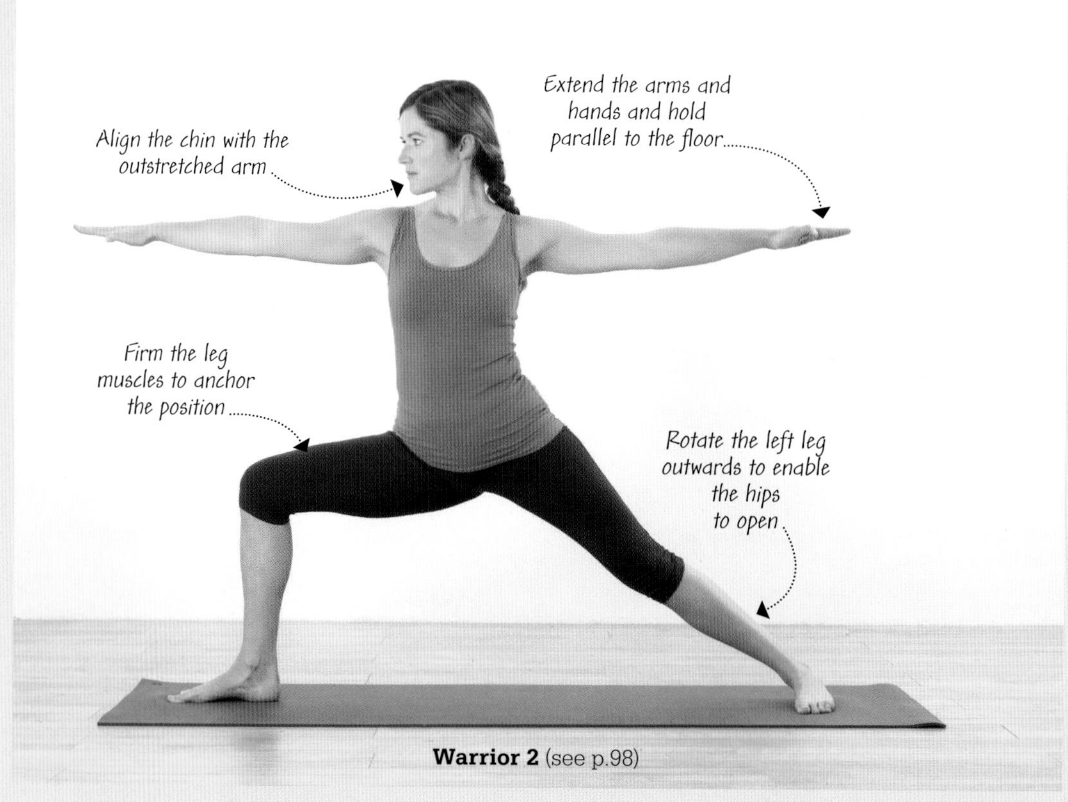
Align the chin with the outstretched arm
Extend the arms and hands and hold parallel to the floor
Firm the leg muscles to anchor the position
Rotate the left leg outwards to enable the hips to open

Warrior 2 (see p.98)

2. Increase your vitality

Accumulated toxins in the body, combined with a sedentary lifestyle, can result in lethargy that affects concentration at work as well as enthusiasm for physical activity. Regular yoga practice will gradually improve your level of vitality by making your body function much more efficiently.

Many yoga postures stimulate and massage the internal organs involved in the elimination of waste products. By increasing the blood supply to these organs, toxins are flushed out throughout the body, increasing vital nourishment to the organs.

Key points

- **Yoga inversions** provide a genuine cardiac workout, benefiting not only the heart but the whole circulatory system.
- **Combined with correct breathing** techniques, inversions also increase oxygen in the blood, nourishing and detoxifying the organs and glands.
- **Optimizing your breathing** increases your lung capacity, sending oxygen-rich and restorative blood to the brain, heart, lungs, and digestive organs.

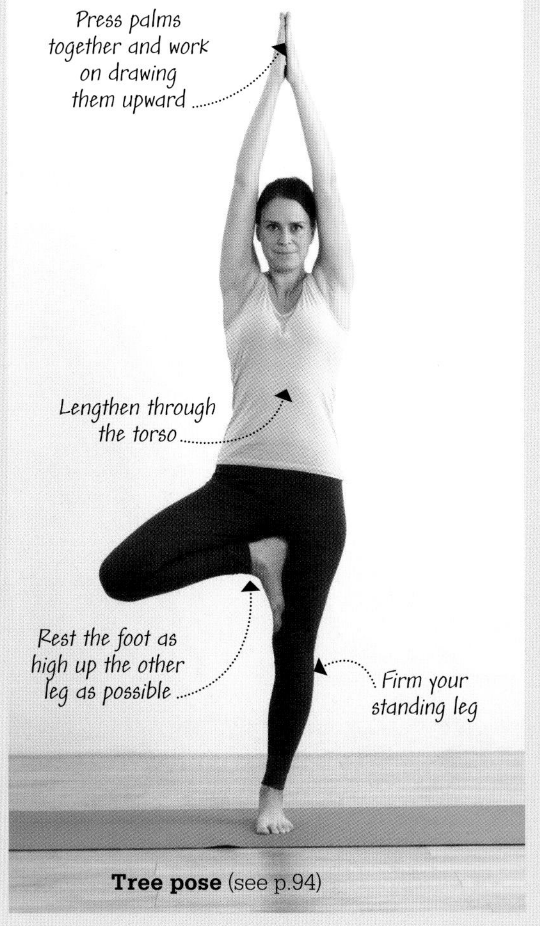
Press palms together and work on drawing them upward
Lengthen through the torso
Rest the foot as high up the other leg as possible
Firm your standing leg

Tree pose (see p.94)

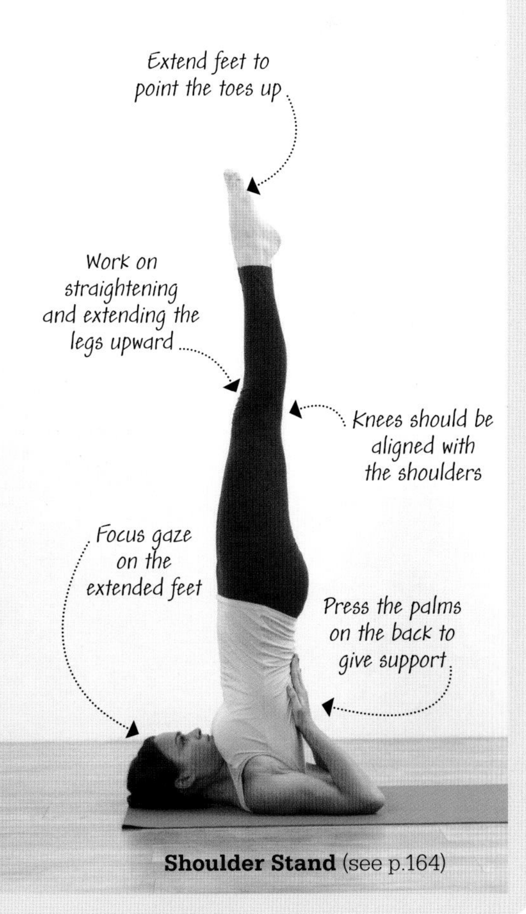
Extend feet to point the toes up
Work on straightening and extending the legs upward
Knees should be aligned with the shoulders
Focus gaze on the extended feet
Press the palms on the back to give support

Shoulder Stand (see p.164)

3. Nurture the nervous system

The nervous system is made up not only of nerves, but also the glands that secrete hormones affecting our emotions. These glands also control other organs, secreting hormones that control how they function.

Our nervous system has two modes of operation: sympathetic and parasympathetic. The first increases our chances of survival when we are faced with danger. The other helps the body to heal itself. The stresses of everyday life often cause the nervous system to lock into the sympathetic mode, preventing the body from entering its restorative mode and leading to many health problems. Practicing yoga can influence the nervous system to release blocked energy channels and activate healing.

Key points

- **Forward and back bends** release any blockage in the energy channels to allow nervous energy to flow freely, reducing symptoms of stress.
- **Yoga postures**, especially those that twist or bend the neck, are very effective in bringing the body into its restorative, or parasympathetic, mode.
- **Yoga breathing techniques** used for postures induce a state of relaxation, during which the nervous system switches into its restorative mode.

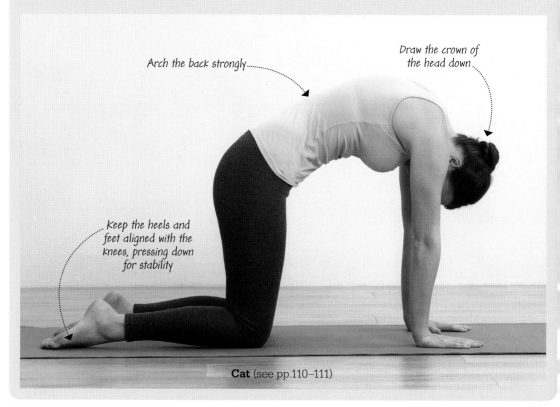
Arch the back strongly
Draw the crown of the head down
Keep the heels and feet aligned with the knees, pressing down for stability

Cat (see pp.110–111)

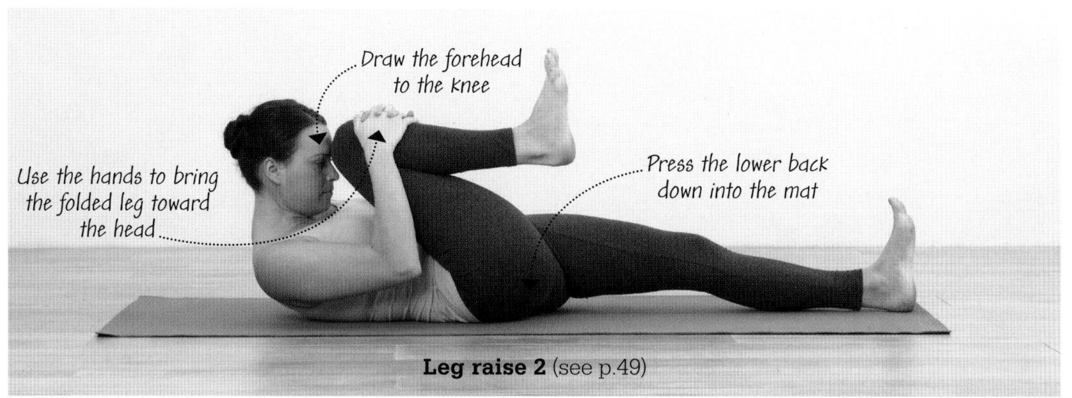
Draw the forehead to the knee
Use the hands to bring the folded leg toward the head
Press the lower back down into the mat

Leg raise 2 (see p.49)

Stretching pose

This pose involves working with your breathing to compress part of the abdomen as your folded leg is pressed down. The resulting stretch provides a gentle massage to the abdominal organs and improves digestion. The pose is a good counter-stretch to the back bend poses as the spine is lengthened in the opposite direction. The pose gives a soothing stretch to the spinal cord and eases any tension in the thighs and lower back. If you find the back bends difficult, practice this stretch for longer periods. Avoid this pose if you are recovering from recent hernia or abdominal surgery.

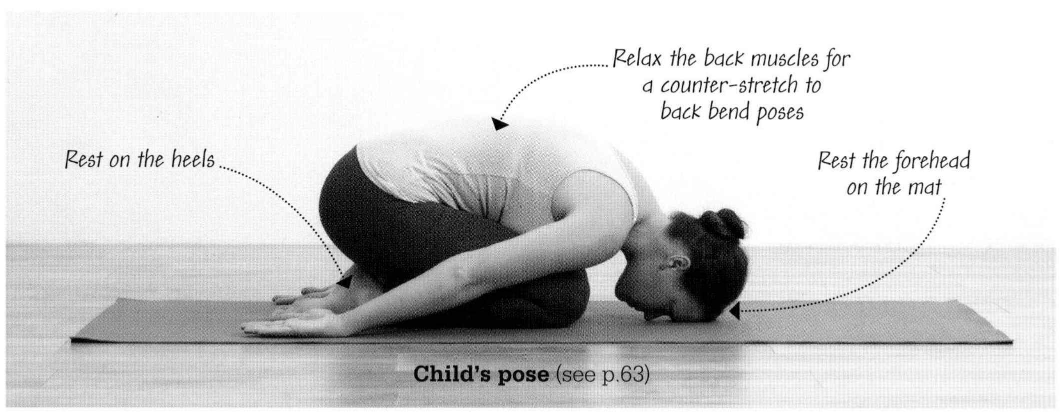
Relax the back muscles for a counter-stretch to back bend poses
Rest on the heels
Rest the forehead on the mat

Child's pose (see p.63)

Relaxing pose

The child's pose is a resting pose and is usually practiced between poses, particularly after strenuous back bend postures, because of its ability to restore and rejuvenate the body. This folded, almost fetal position allows all the muscles of the back, neck, shoulders, legs, and arms to be relaxed. The whole length of the spine is also counter-stretched to any preceding back bend poses and allowed to relax and to soothe the nervous system. This pose's deeply relaxed state activates the parasympathetic nervous system to release tension and activates the body's inherent healing abilities.

When and Where to Practice

To establish yoga as an integral and enjoyable part of your daily routine, you'll need to think about where you'll practice and for how long. You should also try to figure out what the best time of day is for you, so that yoga practice fits in with your other daily commitments.

The right time of day

Because yoga practice should be done on an empty stomach, early mornings or evenings tend to be the best times for practice. You are also less likely to be disturbed at these times of day. When you're deciding the best time to practice, think about what would suit you best.

Morning practice awakens the body and eases stiffness by lubricating the joints and energizing the muscles. Digestion is stimulated and mental alertness is increased, ready for a productive day. Conversely, yoga practiced in the evening can be used to dissipate stress accumulated during the day, and the quality of your sleep will improve dramatically.

How often you practice is really up to you. Ideally practice should to be carried out daily, but it is not necessary to set yourself a strict timetable. Setting aside a regular time is good for establishing a routine. Don't worry if you stop for a period of time; you can always start again. As you practice more, it will become second nature to you and a pleasurable part of your daily routine.

A pleasant environment

A specialized environment and high-tech equipment are not prerequisites when practicing yoga. There are, however, some desirable features to look for when choosing your practice area. Your primary consideration is to choose a private area where you are less likely to be distracted by unwanted intrusions. If that area is spacious, all the better as this can have a positive effect on the mind—encouraging you to take the deep breaths that are conducive to total relaxation. If you are not lucky enough to have a large area at your disposal, you can still create your own oasis of calm by adorning your space with tranquil pictures or objects that have a calming and positive effect on your mood.

Ideally your space should to be lit by diffuse natural light that is soft, gentle, and relaxing. There should also be some form of ventilation so the air you are inhaling does not become stale. The floor should be level, firm, and nonslip. Most people find it better to use a yoga mat as this provides good grip and a clean surface to practice on. A personalized space and pleasant atmosphere will help to calm the mind, enabling you to derive maximum benefit from your practice.

Key points

- **Poses should ideally be** practiced at sunrise or sunset, but if this isn't possible, then practice at another time that fits in with your routine.
- **Practice in a well-ventilated** and warm room suffused with soft, natural light.
- **Create a calm and serene place** in which to practice, where you will not be distracted.

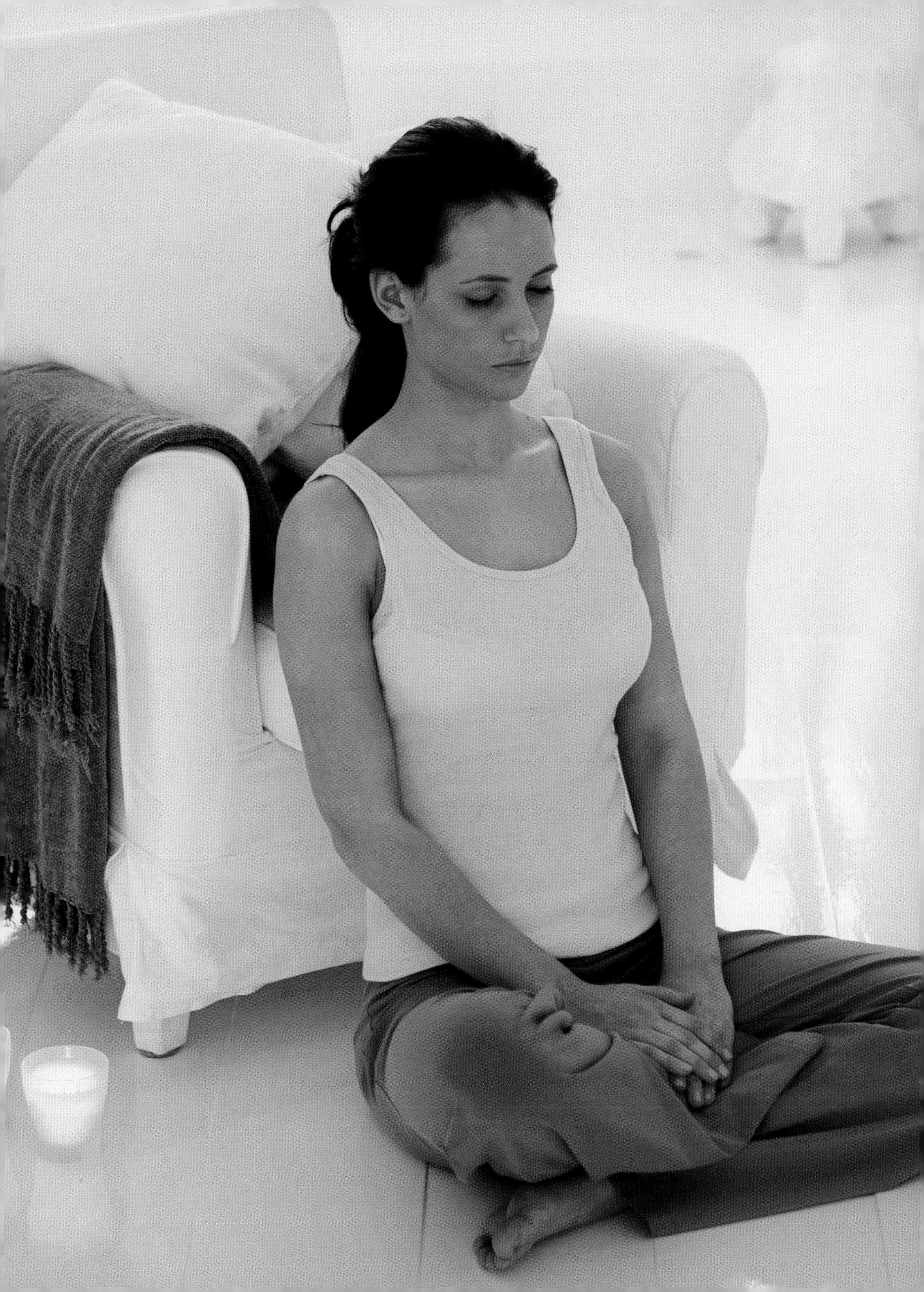

Essential **Equipment**

Key items of equipment

Yoga equipment will bring safety and comfort to your practice at home. Equipment can also be used to make the more challenging poses more achievable than may otherwise be the case, as you continue to work on expanding your level of flexibility. Props and supports can also extend the time you can spend in a particular posture, ensuring proper body alignment at the same time.

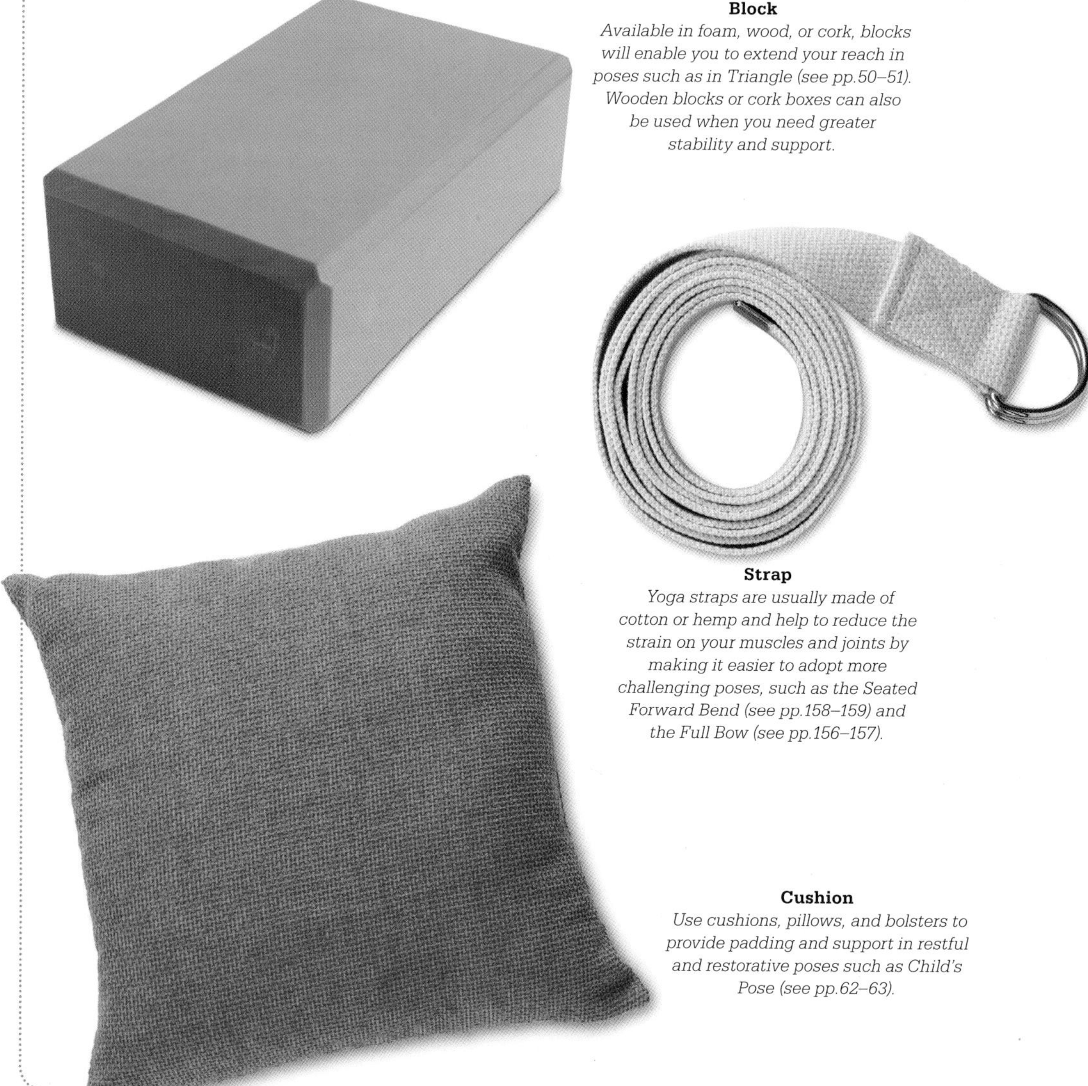

Block

Available in foam, wood, or cork, blocks will enable you to extend your reach in poses such as in Triangle (see pp.50–51). Wooden blocks or cork boxes can also be used when you need greater stability and support.

Strap

Yoga straps are usually made of cotton or hemp and help to reduce the strain on your muscles and joints by making it easier to adopt more challenging poses, such as the Seated Forward Bend (see pp.158–159) and the Full Bow (see pp.156–157).

Cushion

Use cushions, pillows, and bolsters to provide padding and support in restful and restorative poses such as Child's Pose (see pp.62–63).

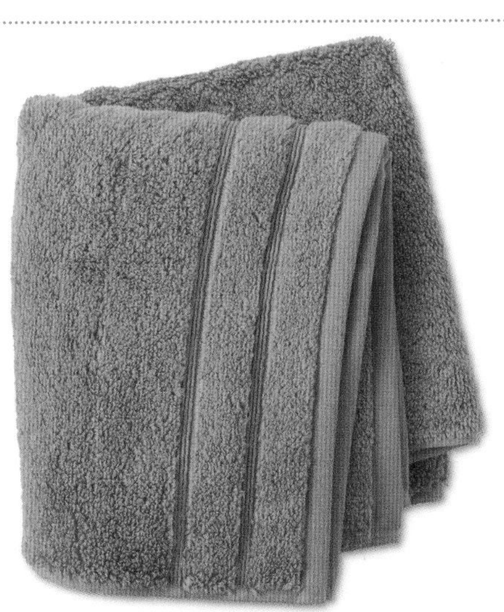

Towel
Having a towel to hand is useful for absorbing sweat, particularly from the hands and feet, when you're moving on to your next pose and will help to prevent you from slipping on the mat.

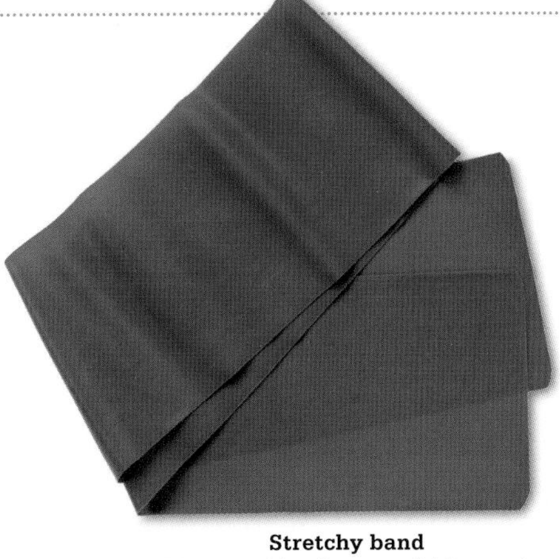

Stretchy band
Elasticated bands are useful for people who experience stiffness and find it difficult to sustain some poses. The elasticity of the band gives light resistance, allowing the muscles to be stretched gently. Use a band for binding poses, such as Cow Arms (see pp.108–109).

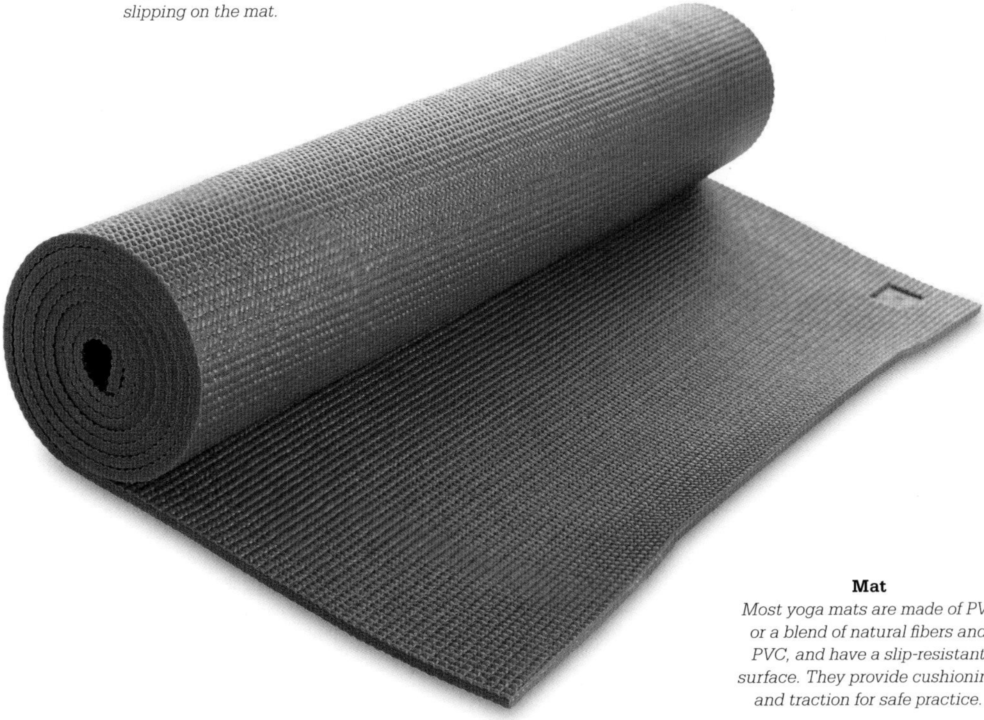

Mat
Most yoga mats are made of PVC or a blend of natural fibers and PVC, and have a slip-resistant surface. They provide cushioning and traction for safe practice.

The Spine

The spine, or vertebral column, supports the body and protects the spinal cord. Its natural curves allow a range of movement. Yoga helps to keep the spine flexible, which is vital for good health and fitness.

The spine is the central axis of the body, combining with the joints and muscles to make a supportive frame for the trunk and limbs. Its 33 vertebrae house the spinal cord, a complex bundle of nerves that carries messages from the brain to other parts of the body.

The spine's flexibility is remarkable. It lets us twist, flex, and extend the body; these movements are possible because of the spine's segmented structure, consisting of a stack of spinal bones called vertebrae.

A basic vertebra consists of a bony block and a bony ring, and sandwiched in between each vertebra is a disk made of cartilage. These disks keep the vertebrae from rubbing against one another and act as the spine's natural shock absorbers. When you jump or sprint, for example, the disks give the vertebrae all the cushioning they need.

Each vertebra has four joints or facets. The angle of the facets changes with each level of the vertebrae, creating the four natural curves of the spine known as the cervical, thoracic, lumbar, and sacral curves. As we grow, some of the spinal vertebrae fuse and there is a natural reduction in the spine's flexibility.

The adult spine develops natural convex and concave curves to form an elongated S-shape. Working like a coiled spring, it absorbs shock, maintains balance, and allows a full range of movement throughout the spinal column.

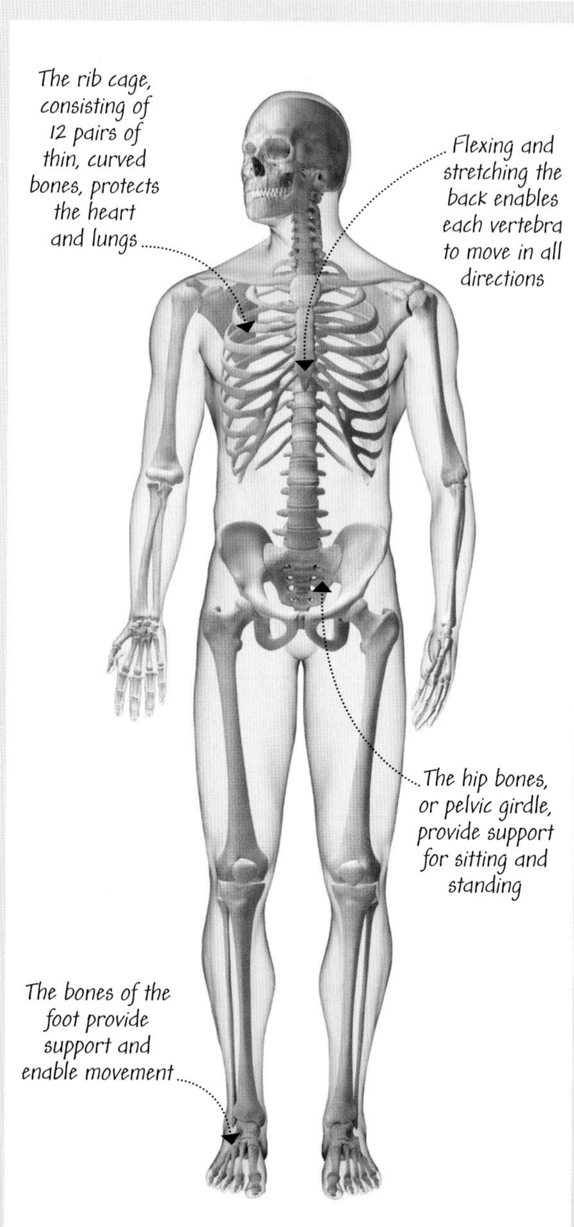
The rib cage, consisting of 12 pairs of thin, curved bones, protects the heart and lungs
Flexing and stretching the back enables each vertebra to move in all directions
The hip bones, or pelvic girdle, provide support for sitting and standing
The bones of the foot provide support and enable movement

Protected by the bones of the spine, the spinal cord transmits impulses from the brain to the body. Cerebrospinal fluid surrounds the brain and spinal cord, providing protection and acting as a medium through which energy flows.

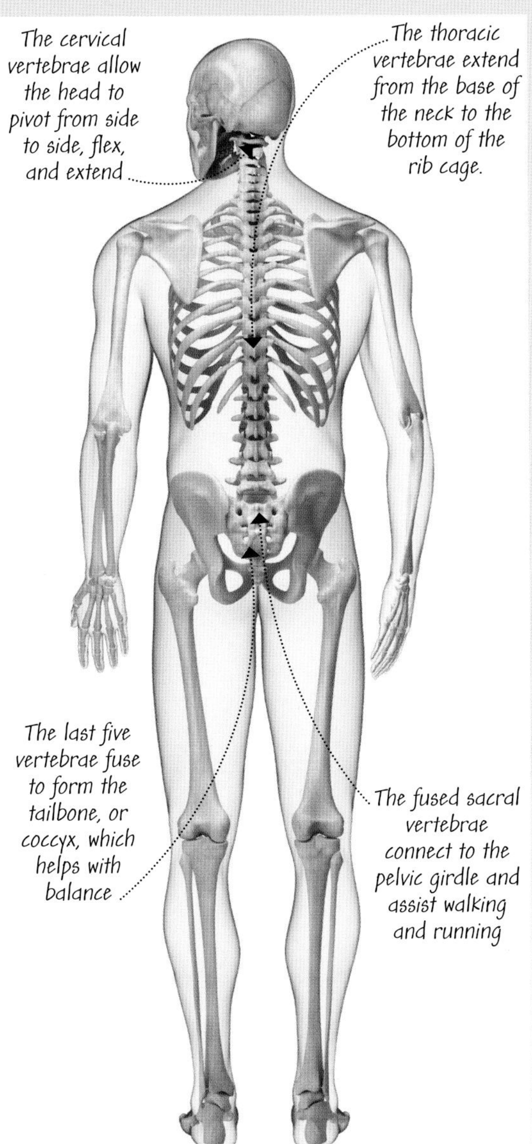
The cervical vertebrae allow the head to pivot from side to side, flex, and extend
The thoracic vertebrae extend from the base of the neck to the bottom of the rib cage.
The last five vertebrae fuse to form the tailbone, or coccyx, which helps with balance
The fused sacral vertebrae connect to the pelvic girdle and assist walking and running

Energizing the spine

Yoga poses flex and extend different sections of the spine to varying degrees to develop spinal flexibility. The postures with the most obvious benefits for the spine include back-and-forth bends and twists. These poses maintain and restore the structures that support the spine, such as ligaments that bind the vertebrae together, spinal joints, and the disks in between the vertebrae, as well as the surrounding muscles. Yoga poses also help to correct any abnormal curvatures of the spine that may have developed through poor posture.

A flexible spine also nourishes the cerebrospinal fluid surrounding the spinal cord and allows *prana* to flow freely through the seven energy centers in the body.

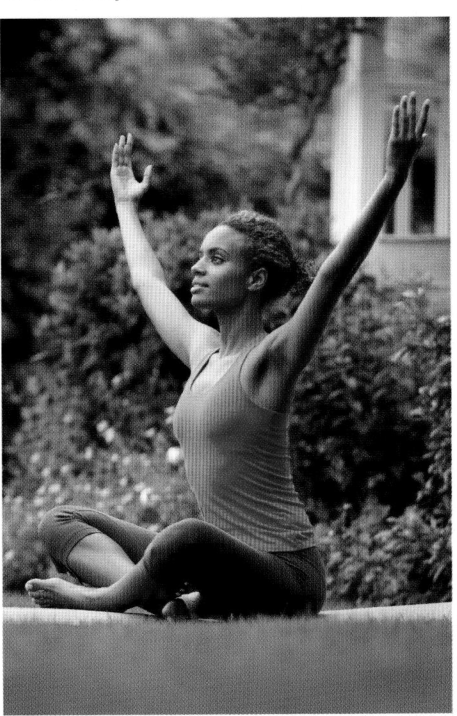

Caring for Your Back

Yoga postures give the back a unique and thorough workout, increasing spinal flexibility and strengthening the back muscles to help counteract the stresses of busy everyday lives, which can lead to back problems.

Building a strong, fluid back

In modern life, the mechanical stress of prolonged chair-sitting tightens our hips and tenses our neck and shoulder muscles, resulting in poor postures, rounded shoulders, and exaggerated spinal curvatures. The consequences can be back problems, headaches, and poor breathing patterns, impacting negatively on the quality of our everyday lives. Yoga postures give the spine a workout. The postures flex and extend each section of the spine to help it regain its inherent flexibility. Each vertebra goes through the full range of movement in all directions, although to varying degrees. The increased mobility of the intervertebral disks reduces injuries as there is less strain on movement. The postures work on toning and strengthening the muscles that support the back, giving additional support to the spine.

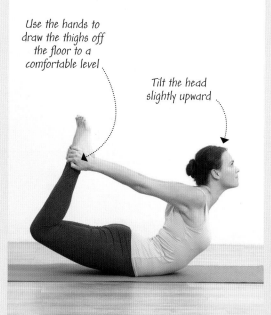
Use the hands to draw the thighs off the floor to a comfortable level
Tilt the head slightly upward

Full Bow

Particularly effective in redressing the hours spent in front a computer, this pose (see pp.156–157) opens up the rib cage to allow the chest to expand and mobilizes the entire length of the spinal column.

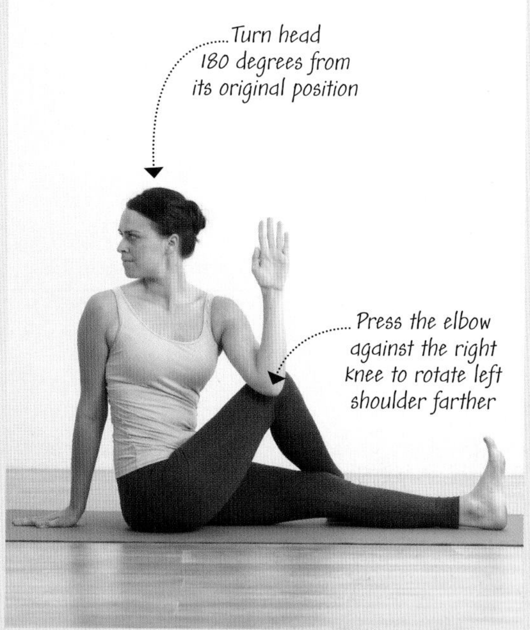
Turn head 180 degrees from its original position
Press the elbow against the right knee to rotate left shoulder farther

Half Spinal Twist

This pose (see pp.120–121) twists the entire spine. The back muscles are contracted on one side and simultaneously stretched on the opposite side. The pose promotes spinal flexibility and tones the back muscles to make twisting movements safer.

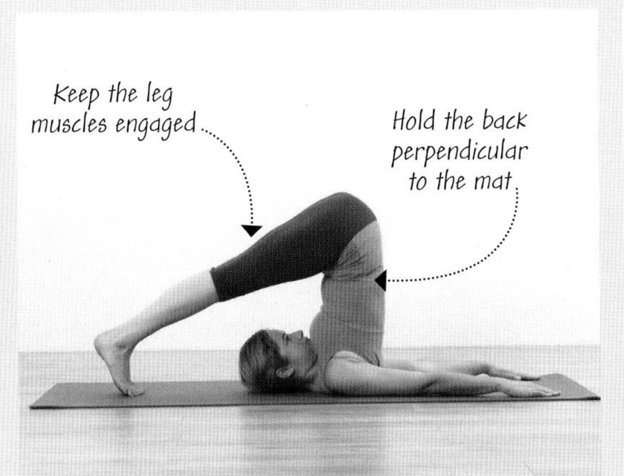
Keep the leg muscles engaged
Hold the back perpendicular to the mat

Plow

This pose (see pp.168–169) stretches the neck and shoulder muscles, stimulates the spinal cord, and increases flexibility of the spine. The strong flexion at the neck strengthens the cervical vertebrae and releases any accumulated tension.

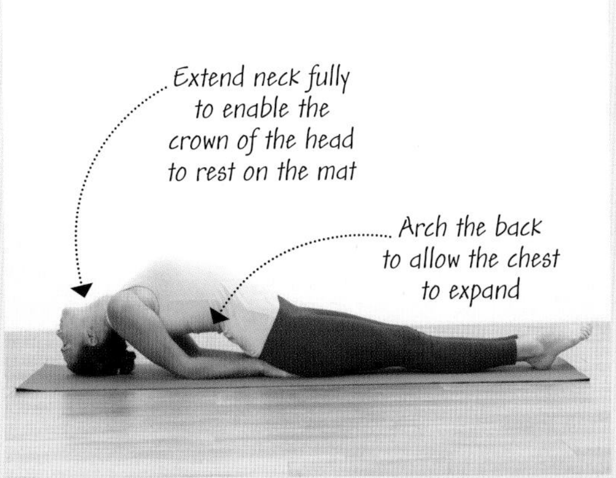
Extend neck fully to enable the crown of the head to rest on the mat
Arch the back to allow the chest to expand

Fish

In this pose (see pp.172–173), the neck is fully extended and the shoulder blades move upward and outward. The thoracic part of the spine is stretched, allowing the ribs to expand and opening the chest. Avoid, however, if you have neck problems.

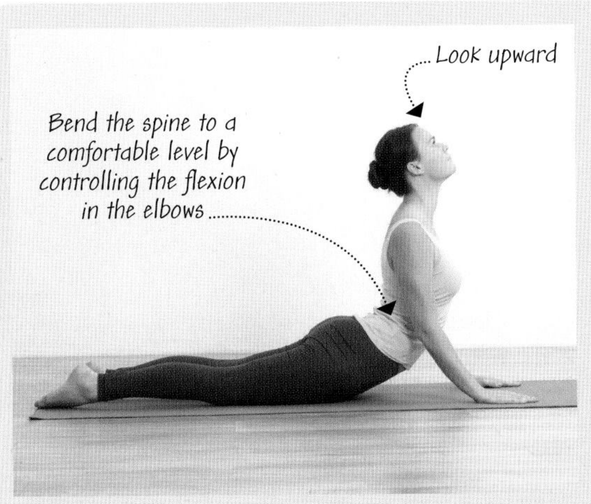
Look upward
Bend the spine to a comfortable level by controlling the flexion in the elbows

Cobra

This pose (see pp.60–61) strengthens the abdominal and lower back muscles. Because you can control the bend by the degree of flexion in the arms, the cobra is an excellent pose for beginners to start with, in order to develop spinal flexibility.

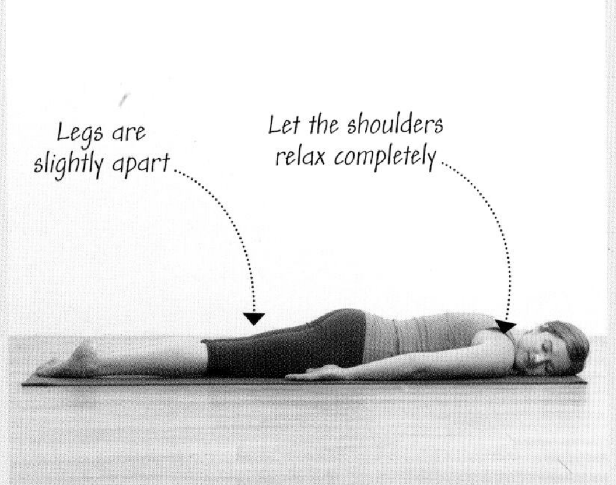
Legs are slightly apart
Let the shoulders relax completely

Diagonal Stretch

Lying in a prone position on the floor allows the weight of the body to be fully supported, releasing tension and allowing the muscles to relax. This position (see pp.58–59) encourages the spine to be centered and aligned in its natural position.

Aligning your body

Learning to hold your body in line is the foundation of yoga. Think of the body as divided into eight segments—from the head, trunk, arms, forearms, hands, thighs, legs, to the feet—and remember the straight line can be horizontal, vertical, or angled, depending on the pose.

Achieving alignment safely can be challenging. One of the most common mistakes is to stretch from more flexible areas of your body using your better-developed muscles to compensate for your weaker ones. Also restoring your spine's natural alignment will be a gradual process. Its vertebrae should only be stretched or compressed to a comfortable level.

The term alignment has become synonymous with the Indian yoga guru B. K. S. Iyengar, who describes postures as "aligning the body, the mind, the fibers, the joints, the muscles" and in doing so, "the mind can be aligned with the movement."

Using your "internal mirror"

Through regular practice you can create a mind-map or an "internal mirror" of the body. Use this mind-map to realign the body by working slowly upward: from the toes through to the head. Make tiny corrective adjustments until you feel grounded and centered. Become aware of the steady rhythm of your breath as you ease your body into correct alignment.

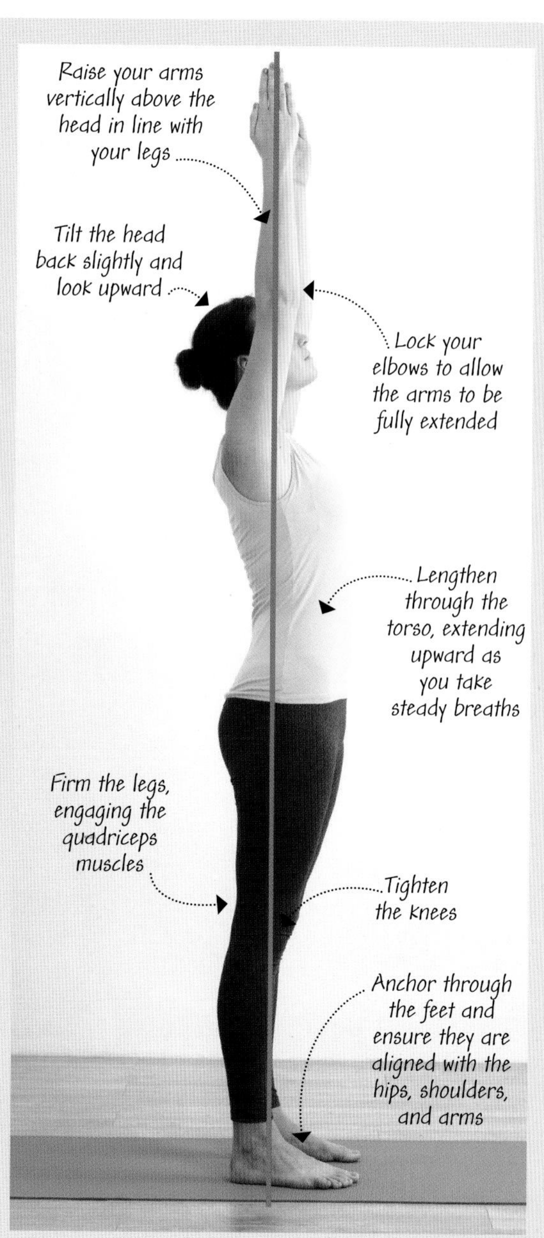
Raise your arms vertically above the head in line with your legs
Tilt the head back slightly and look upward
Lock your elbows to allow the arms to be fully extended
Lengthen through the torso, extending upward as you take steady breaths
Firm the legs, engaging the quadriceps muscles
Tighten the knees
Anchor through the feet and ensure they are aligned with the hips, shoulders, and arms

The mountain pose (right) provides a good starting point for alignment. Viewed from the side in an aligned standing position, a straight line passes through the middle of the hand, elbow, and shoulder, descending through the center of the hip, back of the kneecap, and in front of the ankle bone.

What to remember when you are aligning your body

- Ensure you have a firm base by rooting down through the feet and hands and contracting the appropriate muscles to the correct degree.
- Stabilize the body core by pulling in the navel to bring the abdominal muscles into action, helping to support the spine and to deepen the breath.
- Align the spine by making sure that the head is in line with the neck and follows the movement of the spine. Draw the shoulders down and engage the muscles of the trunk to keep the natural curvature of the spine.
- Bend at the hip when moving into a forward bend pose. Use the natural pulley system of the ball and socket hip joint to control the forward movement. This helps to keep your back straight.

Key points

- Stack the joints vertically, adjusting their position where necessary, and ensure that your body weight is evenly distributed and that you are using the natural force of gravity.
- Move in a controlled manner, slowly and purposefully, ensuring your alignment does not strain your muscles, ligaments, and joints.
- Be aware of the body segments and what their position should be in relation to each other.
- Use your breath to help you refine your position in a pose.

Warrior 2 is a good pose for horizontal alignment. The pose also engages the leg muscles and the feet fully to give stability, allowing the hips to be drawn downward.

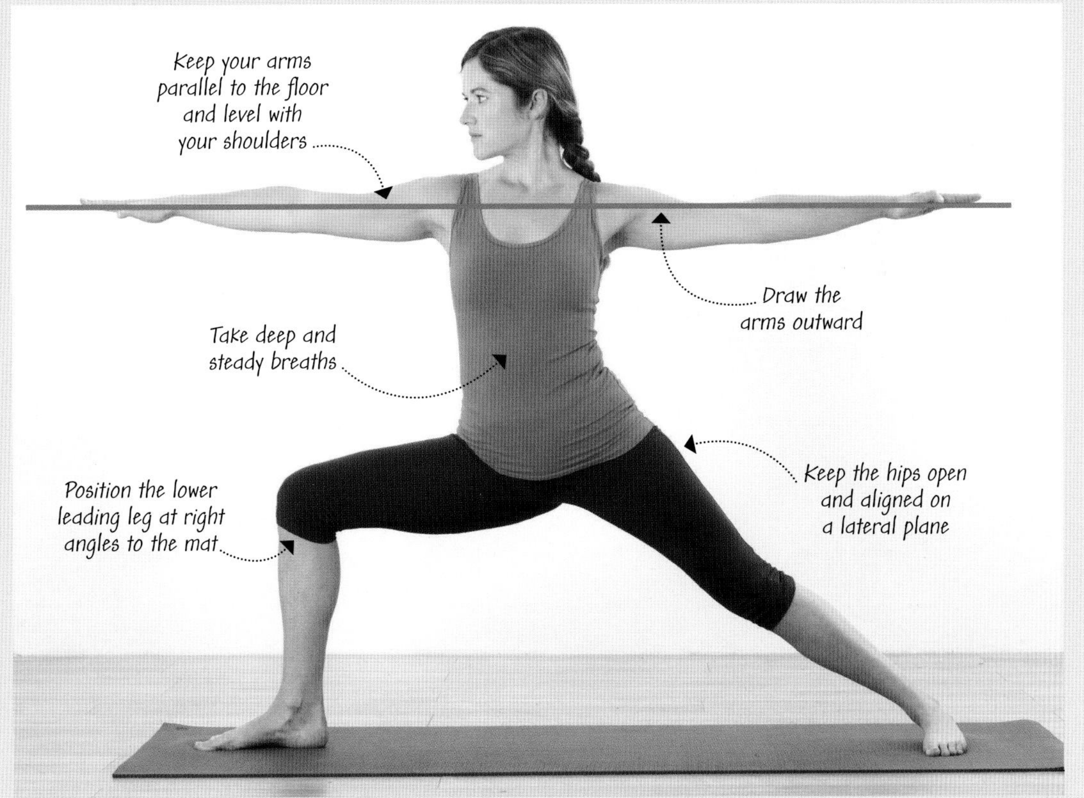
Keep your arms parallel to the floor and level with your shoulders
Draw the arms outward
Take deep and steady breaths
Keep the hips open and aligned on a lateral plane
Position the lower leading leg at right angles to the mat

Muscles

When the muscles contract, we move. Ligaments keep the joints stable by holding the bones together. Practicing yoga works on your muscles, increasing their tone, strength, and joint flexibility.

As you hold a yoga posture, your muscles engage actively and pull on the bones. As you deepen your breathing, the supply of oxygen and blood to the muscles is boosted, resulting in an increase in their strength and elasticity.

Depending on the action performed, each muscle acts either as an agonist or antagonist. The agonist, or prime mover, is the muscle initiating the movement; while the muscle controlling the speed and extent of the movement is called the antagonist. Muscles such as these are usually found on opposite sides of a joint. For example, when extending at the knee, the quadriceps muscles act as the agonists and the hamstring muscles as the antagonists. Conversely, when the knee flexes, the hamstrings initiate and the quadriceps control the movement.

Elasticity of the muscles, in turn, aids greater joint mobility and spinal flexibility. Yoga postures involve the mind as well as the body: Engaging the muscles to hold the limbs, or body, in a single position, against gravity, requires effort, focus, and concentration. Yoga enables postures to be maintained in different positions by using the body's own mass as a balancing counterweight.

Muscle is made up of fibrous and connective tissues arranged in layers so that movement can be controlled through opposing muscle forces.

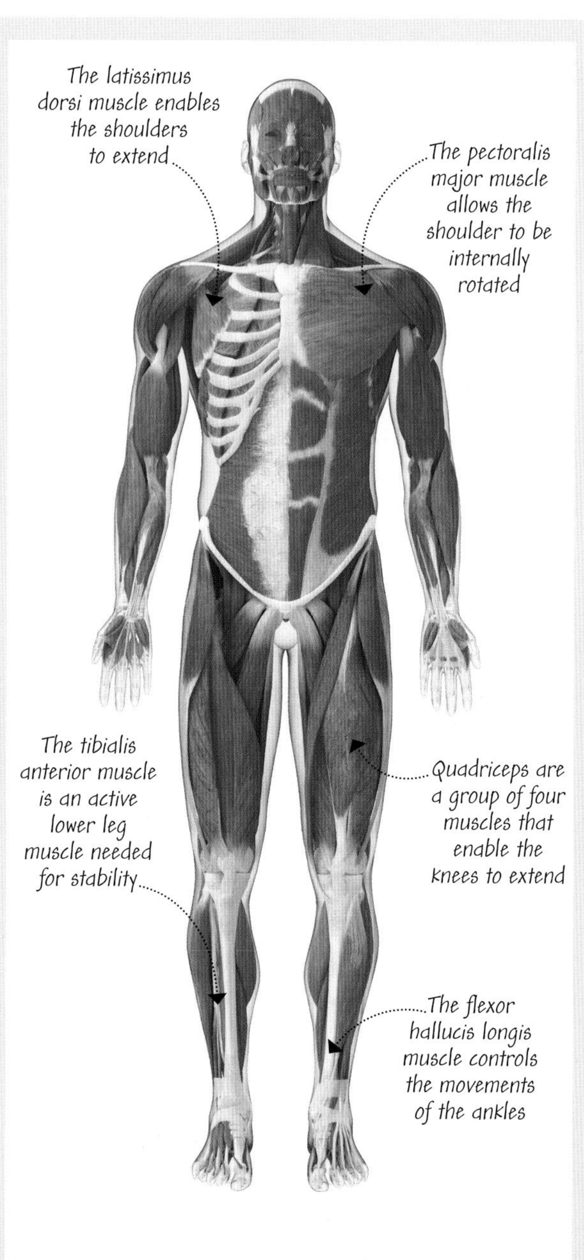
The latissimus dorsi muscle enables the shoulders to extend
The pectoralis major muscle allows the shoulder to be internally rotated
The tibialis anterior muscle is an active lower leg muscle needed for stability
Quadriceps are a group of four muscles that enable the knees to extend
The flexor hallucis longis muscle controls the movements of the ankles

Counterbalancing and complementing each other, many muscles act in pairs. For example, the biceps muscles are opposed to the triceps, and the back extensor muscles are opposed to flexors.

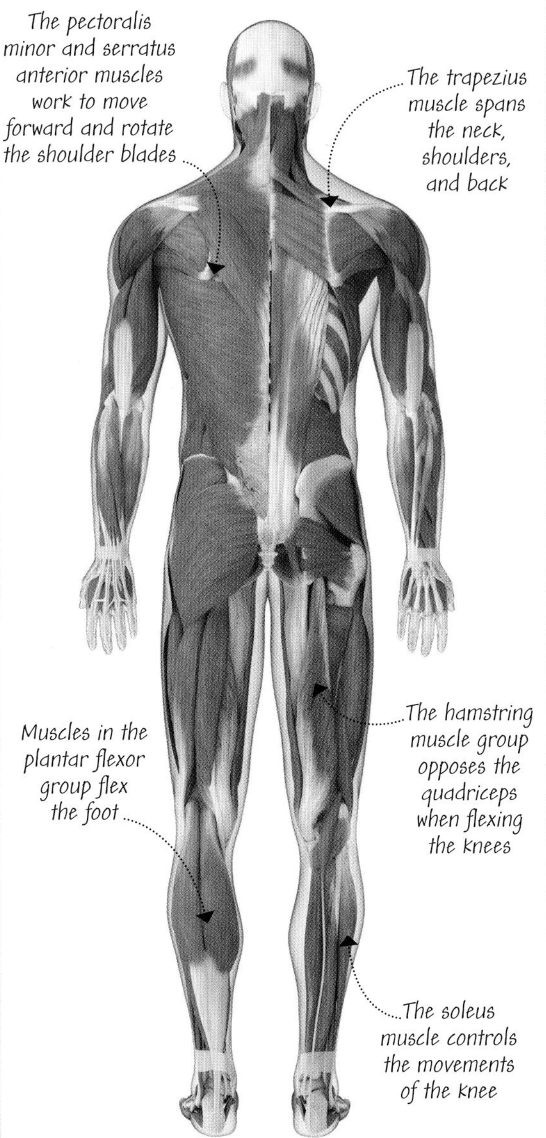
The pectoralis minor and serratus anterior muscles work to move forward and rotate the shoulder blades
The trapezius muscle spans the neck, shoulders, and back
Muscles in the plantar flexor group flex the foot
The hamstring muscle group opposes the quadriceps when flexing the knees
The soleus muscle controls the movements of the knee

Standing forward bend

In this pose (see pp.52–53) the quadriceps muscles act as the agonists and the hamstring muscles as the antagonists. The breath is crucial in holding this posture. With each breath, you can consciously move deeper into the pose. Concentration enables you to engage the quadriceps just a fraction more, sending a neural signal for the hamstrings to relax a fraction more. The erector spinae muscles in the back also participate in this gentle elongation, as the whole back is stretched. Because both limbs are worked equally, correct muscular balance is restored.

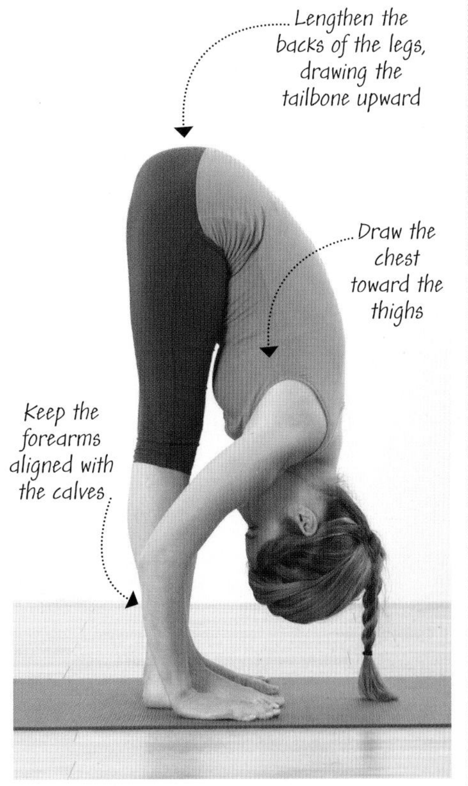
Lengthen the backs of the legs, drawing the tailbone upward
Draw the chest toward the thighs
Keep the forearms aligned with the calves

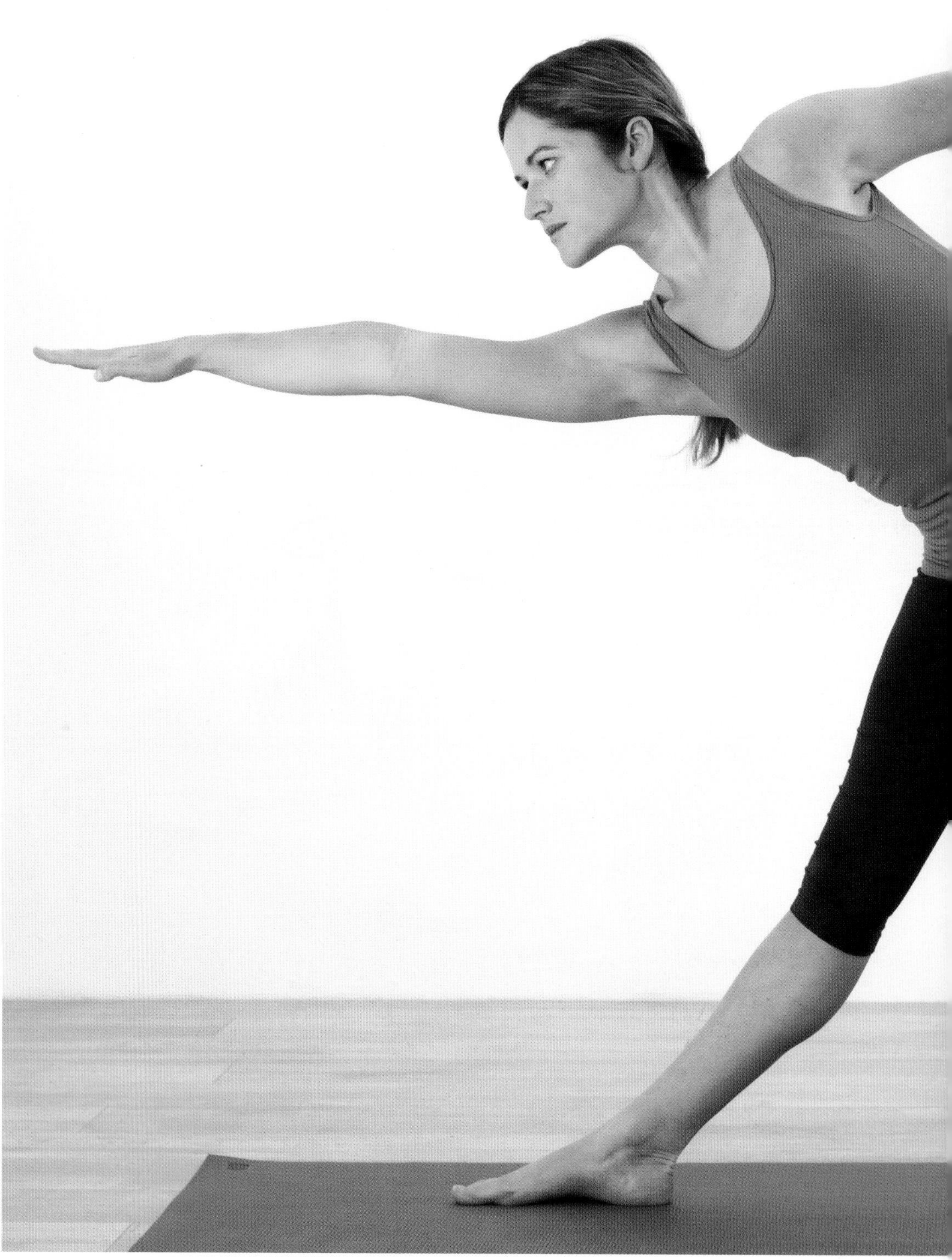

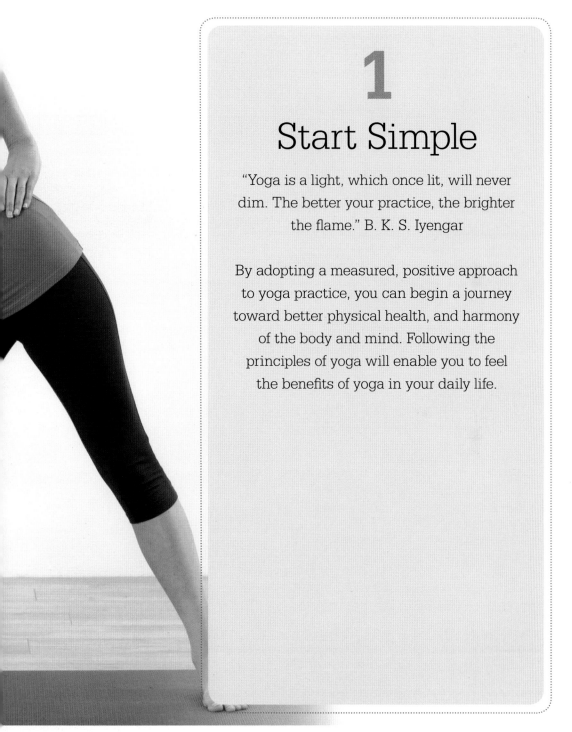

1 Start Simple

"Yoga is a light, which once lit, will never dim. The better your practice, the brighter the flame." B. K. S. Iyengar

By adopting a measured, positive approach to yoga practice, you can begin a journey toward better physical health, and harmony of the body and mind. Following the principles of yoga will enable you to feel the benefits of yoga in your daily life.

Plan Your Course

The five principles of yoga (see pp.8–11) are a good foundation and give you a solid starting point from which to begin practicing yoga regularly. Once you have absorbed the concepts behind these principles, you can begin to apply elements of them to your daily life, which will build and maintain momentum on your journey.

1. Planning your course

Before starting, give some thought to how, when, and where you'll practice yoga. To do this, it is necessary to make some decisions about your practice. Take time to think about what existing commitments you already have, and when you'll be able to practice. By planning your course carefully, you'll be able to anticipate difficulties that might otherwise stop you from being able to practice effectively.

Affirming what you want to achieve in your yoga practice will motivate and focus your mind. It's important to put your goals in writing, and to keep referring back to them.

Keeping a written record of your yoga practice will be a valuable aid in the long term. Include not only a record of physical feelings, but also a description of your emotional states both before and after practice. By comparing thoughts and feelings at different stages of your practice you will provide yourself with a yardstick with which to measure your progress.

2. Assessing your progress

Assessing oneself can sometimes be difficult, particularly when practicing alone, so we have included some advice (see pp.88–89) on how effective self-assessment can be carried out. It's important for anyone practicing a discipline to have an effective means of measuring their progress.

Listening to your body, or self-awareness, is one of the keys to effective self-assessment. But this requires careful practice and intense concentration. By tuning in to the rhythms of your body, you will be in a better position to know if you are reaping the full benefits of correct practice.

Written goals help you track your progress, make your accomplishments more obvious, and help you to identify problem areas needing more attention.

Reviewing your yoga goals periodically will enable you to make sure that you are on track with what you want to achieve within a set time frame.

Checklist: have you...

- **Set out your goals** of exactly what you want to achieve?
- **Decided where and when** to practice?
- **Made sure that you have the correct equipment** for your practice?
- **Decided how to plan** your practice around existing commitments?
- **Paid heed** to your medical needs?
- **Set a time frame** to review your goals?

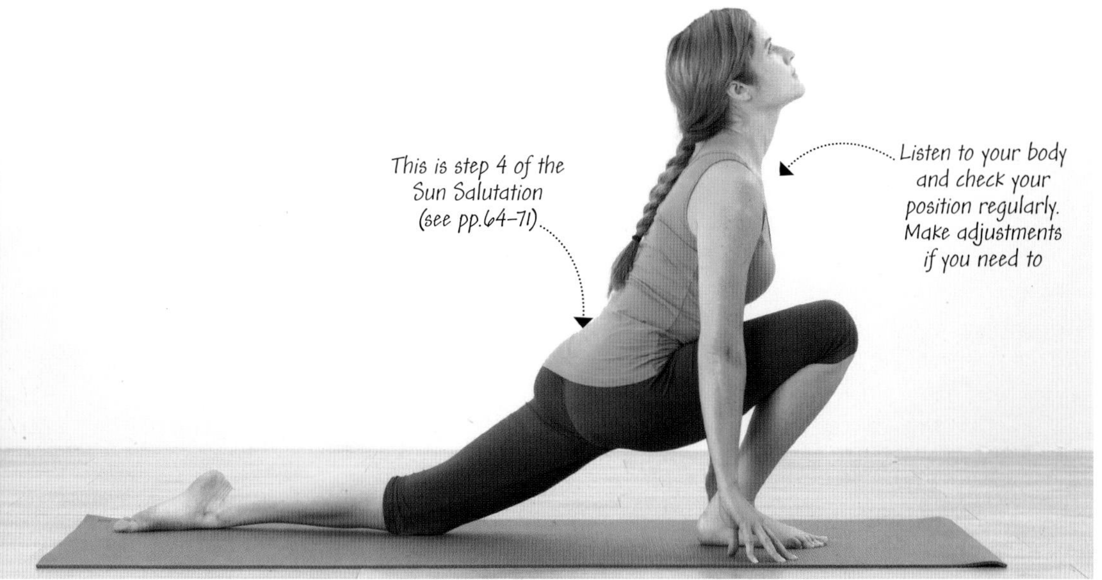
This is step 4 of the Sun Salutation (see pp.64–71)
Listen to your body and check your position regularly. Make adjustments if you need to

3. Building up to a sequence

A sequence consists of several different postures, which are performed in such a way that one posture flows naturally into the next. Because sequences can be long and somewhat complex, they may present a daunting challenge to the beginner.

There are things you can do to help you prepare yourself before practicing a sequence. Taking some time to undertake a little background research on individual postures, and getting to understand the role they play in the sequence, will make it a lot easier to memorize and practice the different moves involved.

An understanding of the importance of breath and practicing breathing techniques is fundamental to the successful practice of yoga. You should pay particular attention to breathing practice.

Break down individual postures into stages, then modify them in a way that suits you. By doing this, you can get to know your own strengths and weaknesses better, and use the correct aids when appropriate.

4. What to aim for

At this point it is wise to set yourself aims of a general nature, which you feel are going to be genuinely achievable.

Aim to establish a regular practice schedule and stick to it. Setting specific times aside for yoga provides a structure that supports regular practice and allows your future commitments to be scheduled accordingly. This helps to minimize the disruption to you and those around you. Penciling the session into your calendar also allows you to track how successful you are at adhering to the schedule.

Try to improve your general health by paying more attention to your body and the things that affect it. This could involve getting more exercise, eating healthily, and being more particular about what you put into your body.

By simply aiming to have a positive attitude toward promoting your own wellbeing, you are already creating solid foundations for your future practice. It's important to approach yoga positively.

Key Techniques for **Warming Up**

It's important to make sure you are warmed up properly before practicing yoga. You should also take time to practice breathing techniques. Mastering breath control through yoga, so you can breathe more deeply will not only enable you to position yourself correctly in the yoga poses but will also help you hold the poses.

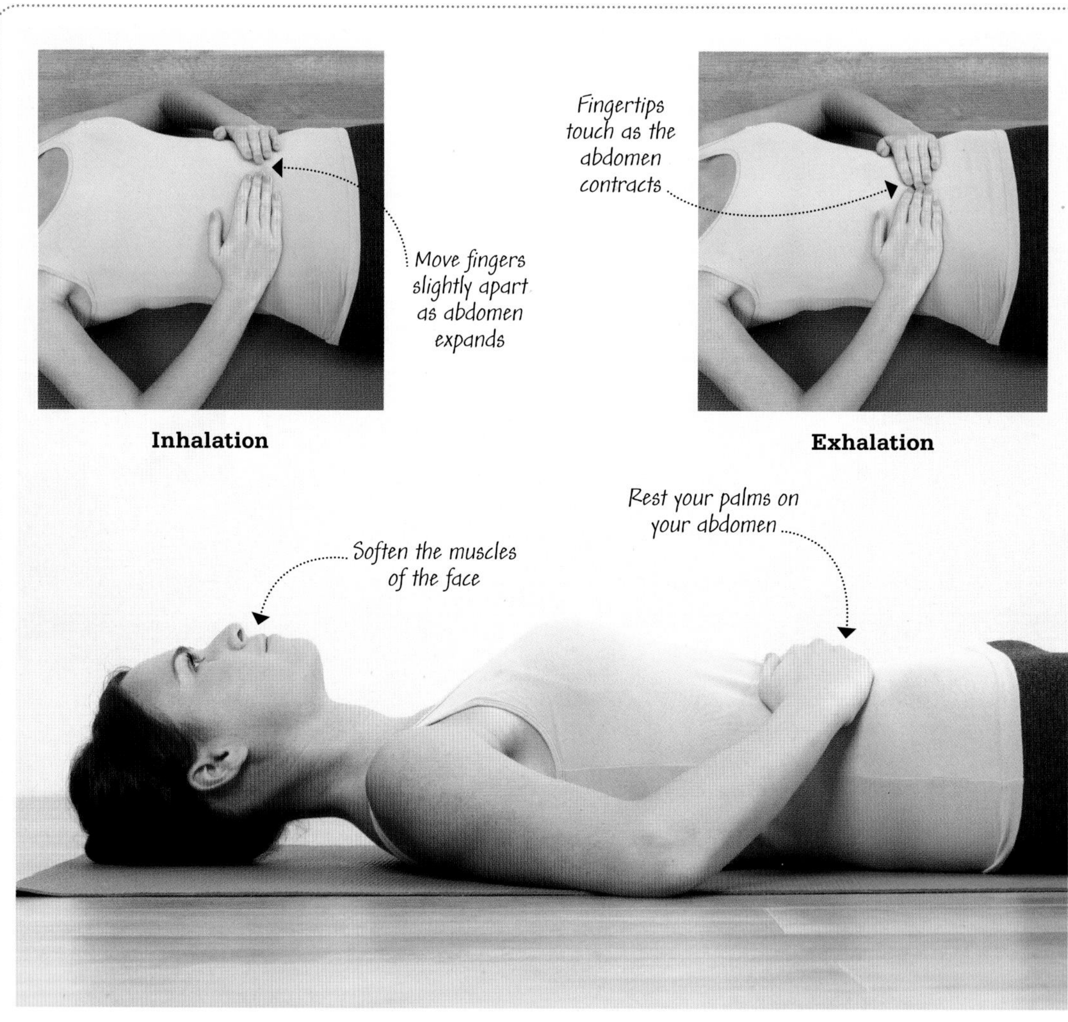
Fingertips touch as the abdomen contracts
Move fingers slightly apart as abdomen expands
Inhalation
Exhalation
Rest your palms on your abdomen
Soften the muscles of the face

Abdominal breathing

Lie on your back and place your hands on either side of your navel. The abdomen should expand outward as you inhale, your fingertips drawing apart. As you exhale, feel the abdomen contract and your fingers coming together. Try taking your hands slightly higher to feel the movements of the diaphragm. Inhale and exhale for two minutes.

Inhalation

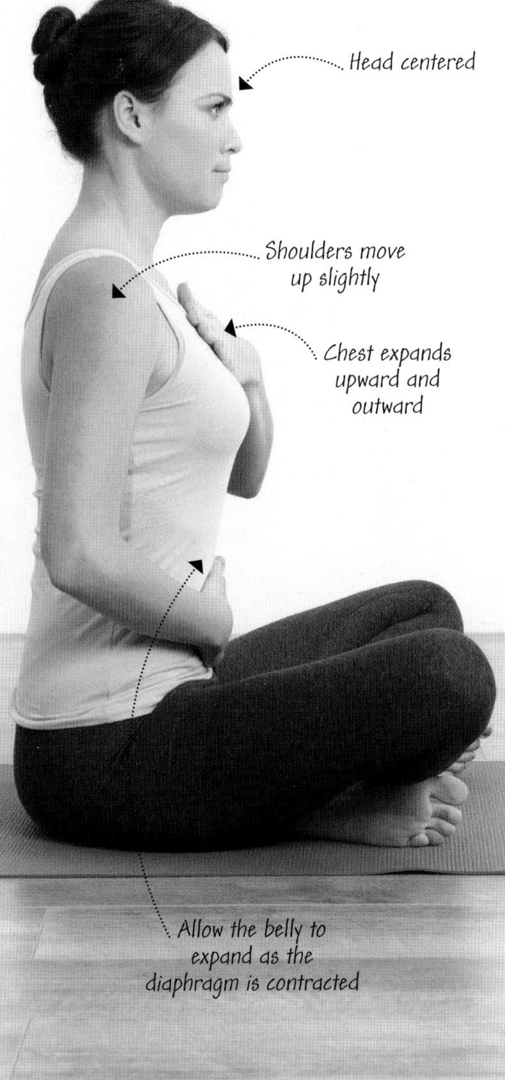
Head centered
Shoulders move up slightly
Chest expands upward and outward
Allow the belly to expand as the diaphragm is contracted

Exhalation

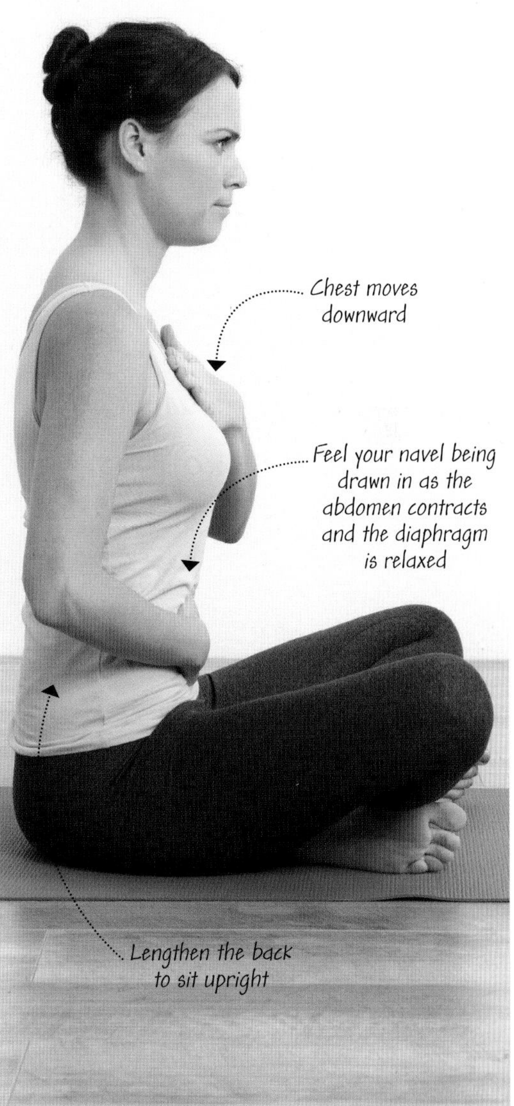
Chest moves downward
Feel your navel being drawn in as the abdomen contracts and the diaphragm is relaxed
Lengthen the back to sit upright

Yogic breathing

Inhale slowly, expanding the abdomen, rib cage, and chest area close to the collar bone. Pause momentarily. As you exhale, feel air leaving your abdomen first, then the middle of the chest, and finally the top of the chest and neck. Pause momentarily. Repeat the inhalations and exhalations in this way for about two minutes.

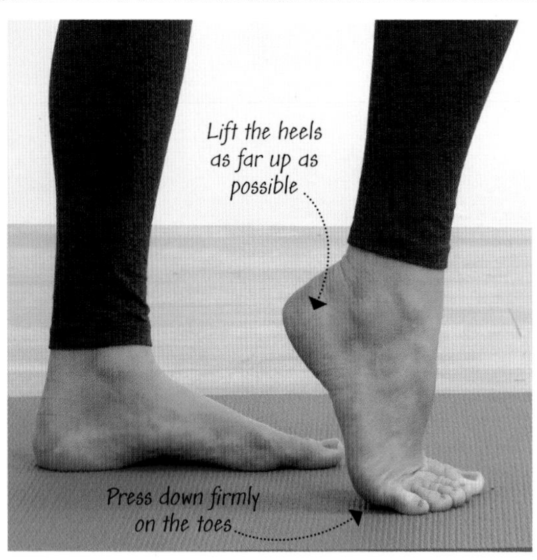
Lift the heels
as far up as
possible
Press down firmly
on the toes

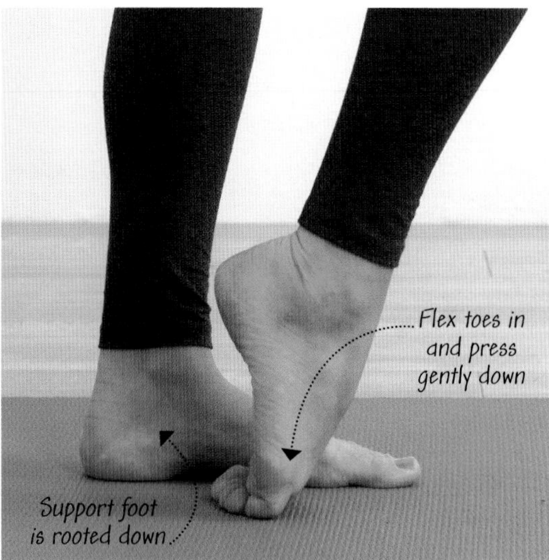
Flex toes in
and press
gently down
Support foot
is rooted down

Warming up the feet

Stretch the heel of each foot a few times, lifting the heels up as far as possible and down (left). Follow this with rolling onto the front of the toes, so they are curled and gently pressed down under the foot (right). Hold for 2–3 breaths. Repeat on the other foot.

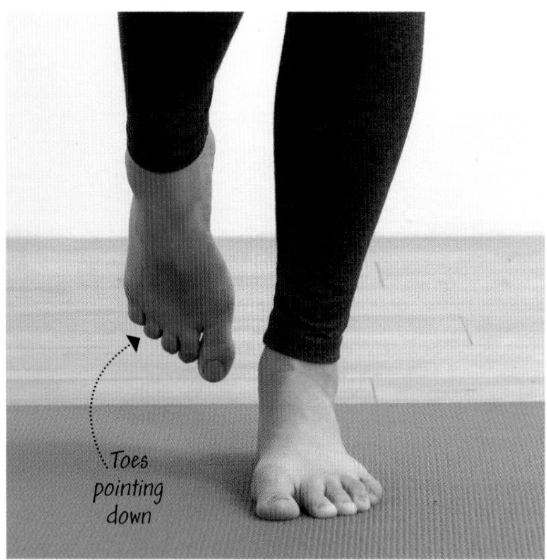
Toes
pointing
down

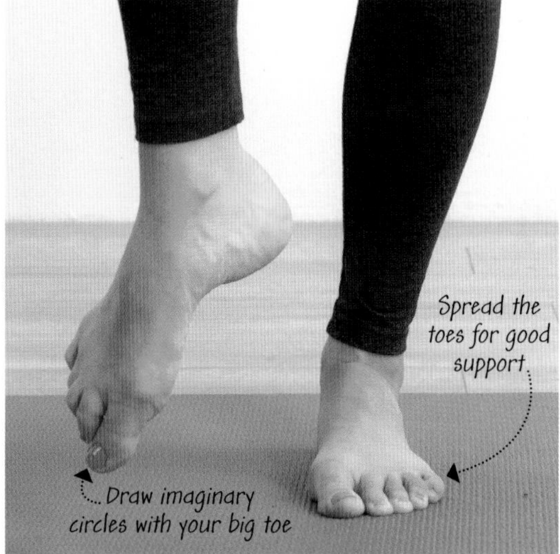
Spread the
toes for good
support
Draw imaginary
circles with your big toe

Warming up the ankles

Keeping the left leg firm, swing the right leg back off the floor, toes pointing down (left). Hold for a few breaths and swap legs. Follow this by gently rotating the right foot at the ankles first in one direction and then the other (right). Repeat on the other leg.

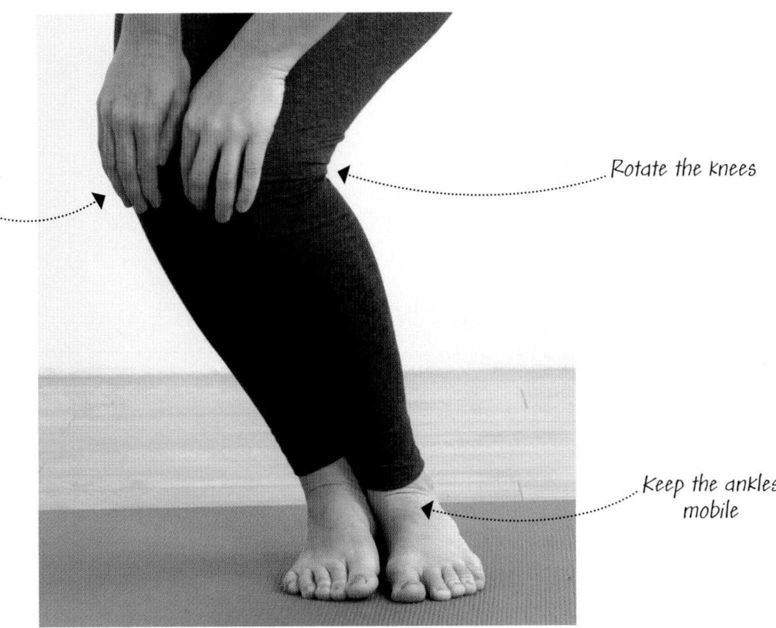
Point fingers down
Rotate the knees
Keep the ankles mobile

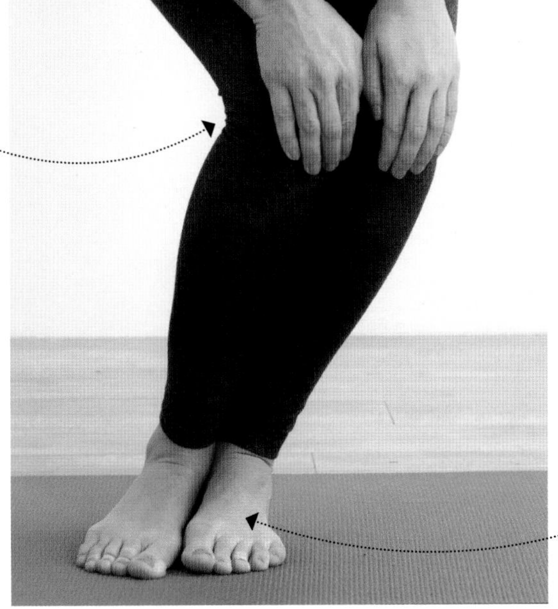
Change direction of the knee roll
Anchor the feet

Warming up the knees

Stand with your feet together, bend slightly at the knees, and allow your hands to rest on the kneecaps, fingers pointing down.

Gently move the knees in a circular motion, ten times in each direction, with the feet firmly anchored to the floor.

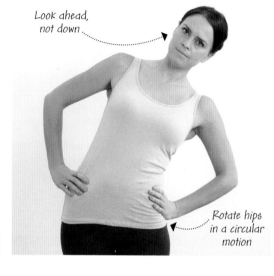

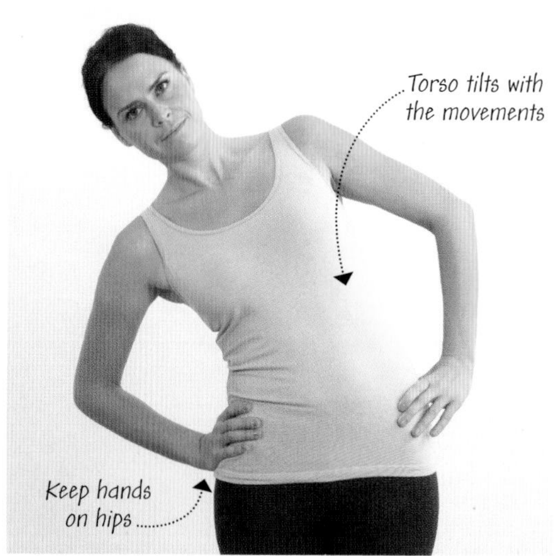
Torso tilts with the movements
Keep hands on hips

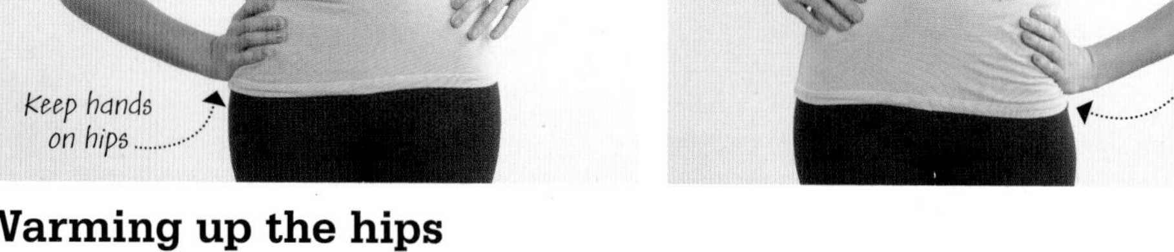
Look ahead, not down
Rotate hips in a circular motion

Warming up the hips

Stand with the feet hip-width apart and hands placed on your hips. Rotate the hips in a circular plane, ten times clockwise and ten times counterclockwise. Keep the legs straight and kneecaps pulled up, engaging the hips and upper body in the roll.

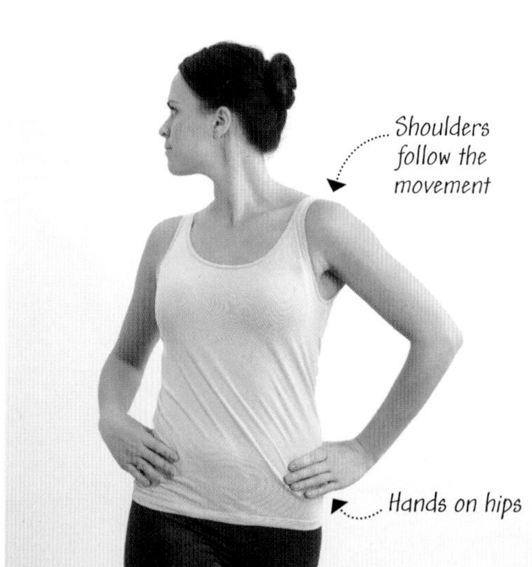
Shoulders follow the movement
Hands on hips

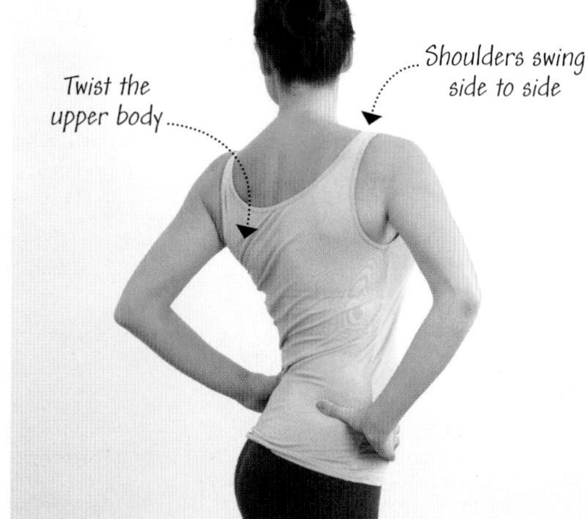
Twist the upper body
Shoulders swing side to side

Warming up the torso

Stand with the feet hip-width apart and with your palms resting on the hips. Rotate the upper body side to side in a gentle rhythm, twisting at the hips, waist, and spine. Rotate ten times to either side. Your head and shoulders should follow the movement.

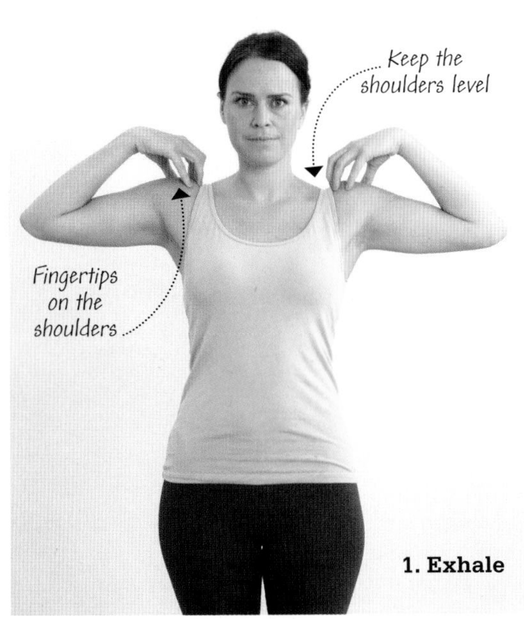
Keep the shoulders level
Fingertips on the shoulders
1. Exhale

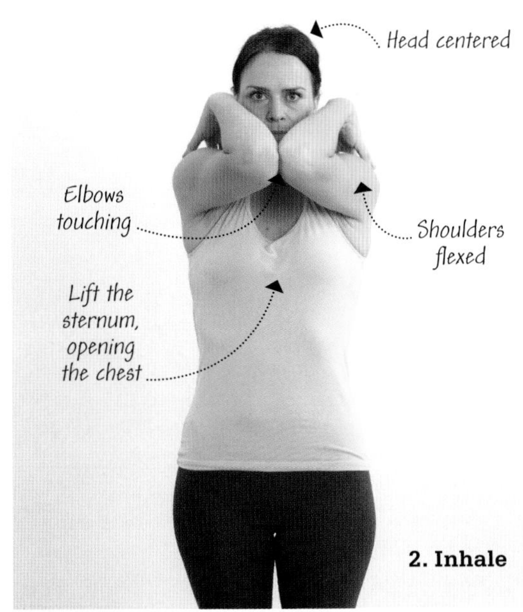
Head centered
Elbows touching
Shoulders flexed
Lift the sternum, opening the chest
2. Inhale

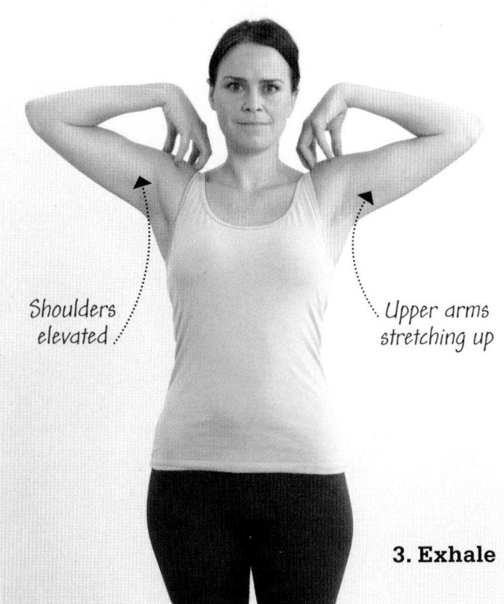
Shoulders elevated
Upper arms stretching up
3. Exhale

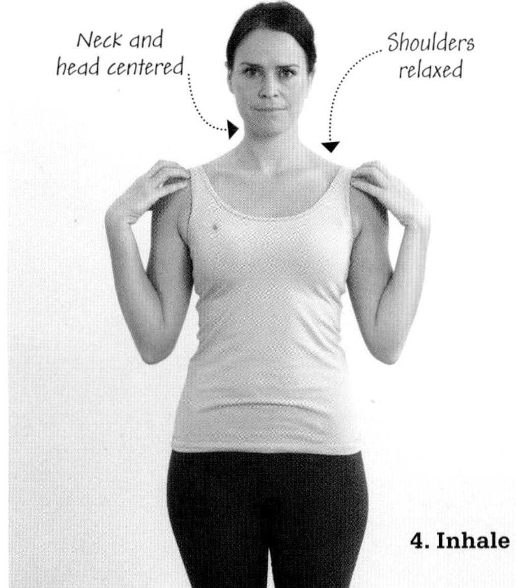
Neck and head centered
Shoulders relaxed
4. Inhale

Warming up the shoulders

Stand with your fingertips placed on the shoulders. Inhale, bringing the elbows together in front so they touch. Exhale to lift the elbows up and apart, stretching the elbows upward. Complete the motion by lowering the elbows down. Repeat ten times.

1 2 3

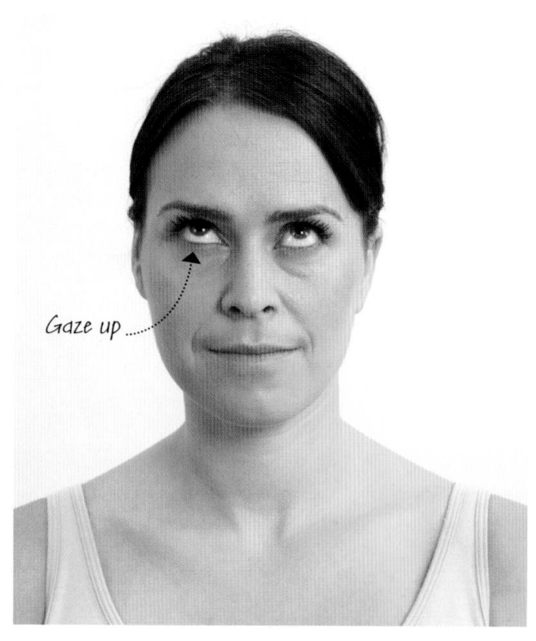
Gaze up

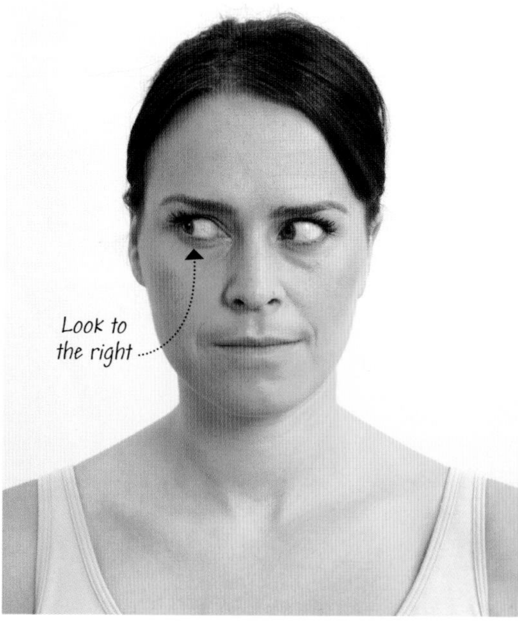
Look to
the right

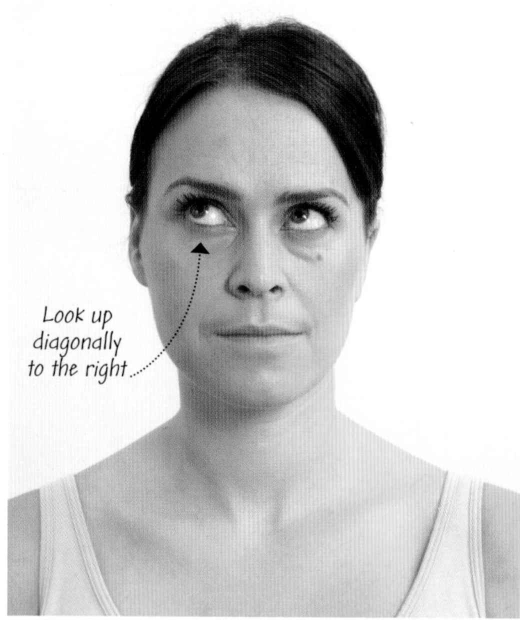
Look up
diagonally
to the right

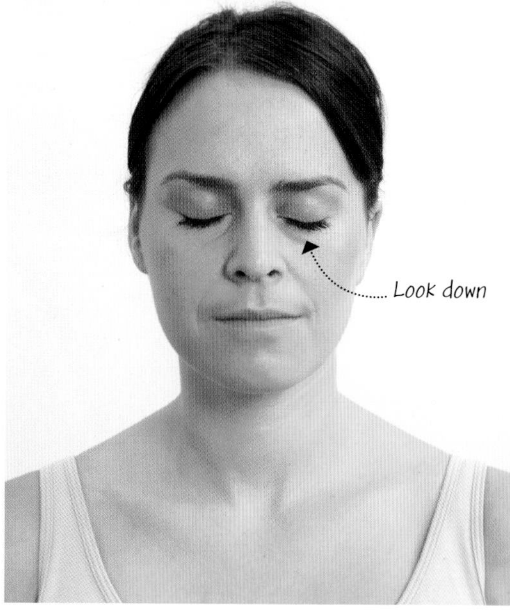
Look down

Warming up the eyes

Do not move the head or neck in the following eye exercises. Look up (top left). Look right (top right). Look up diagonally to the right (above left). Look down (above right). Repeat, looking to the left side and up diagonally to the left. Hold each position for a few seconds.

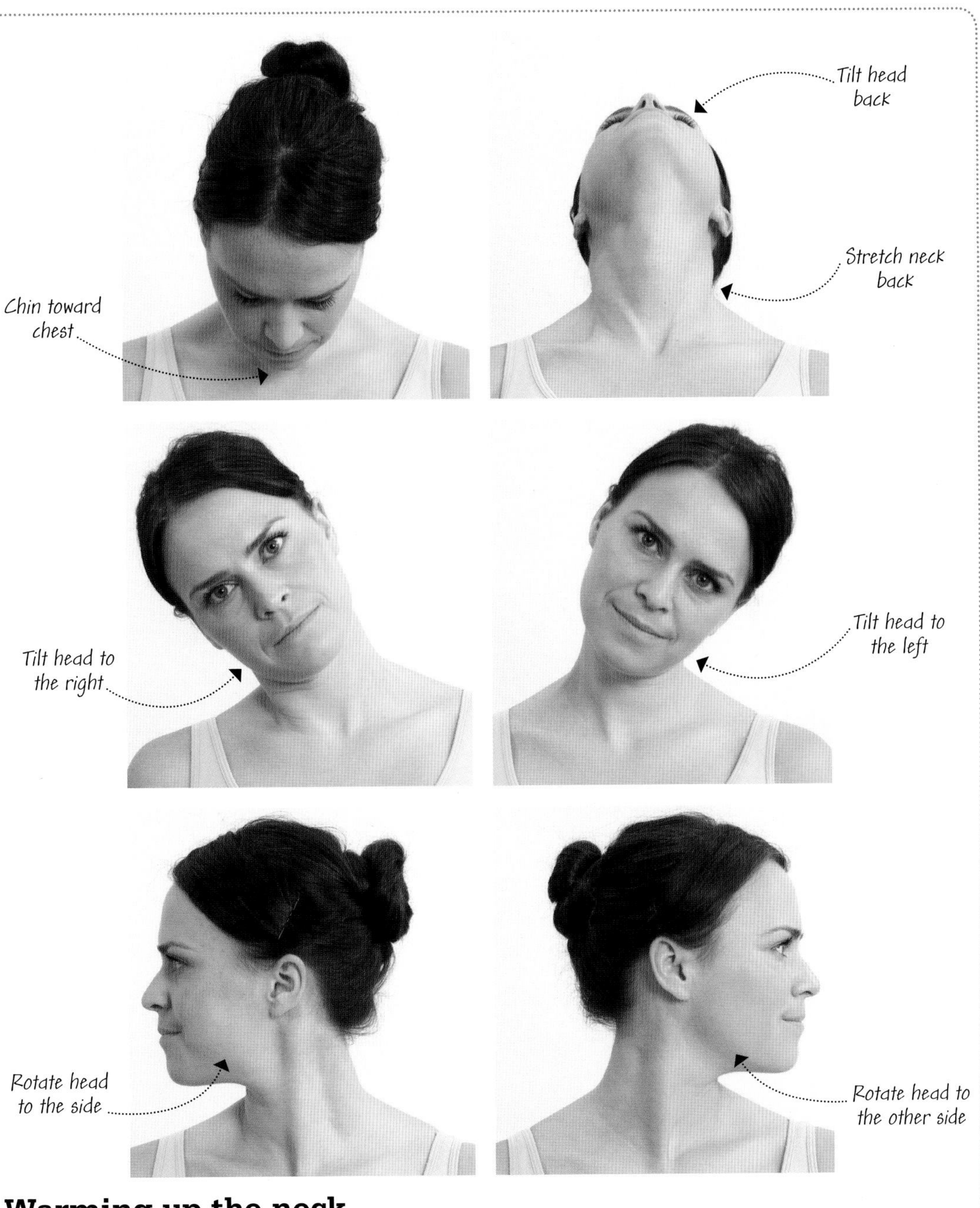

Chin toward chest
Tilt head back
Stretch neck back
Tilt head to the right
Tilt head to the left
Rotate head to the side
Rotate head to the other side

Warming up the neck

Sit with your back straight. Slowly tilt the head forward and then backward. Then tilt your head to the right and then over to the left. Finally, rotate your head 90 degrees to the right and again to the left side. Hold each position for a few seconds.

Practicing Safely

Practicing yoga involves respecting your body's physical limitations and understanding how and when to use equipment to support practice. As a note of caution, if your practice causes negative sensations, such as giddiness or pain, then consult a medical practitioner—there may be an underlying health problem for which your practice is inappropriate.

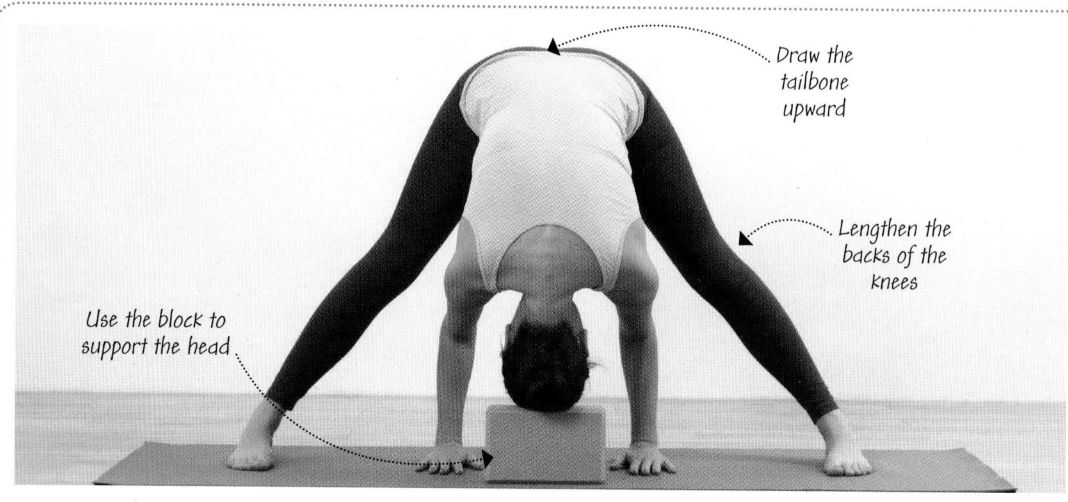
Draw the tailbone upward
Lengthen the backs of the knees
Use the block to support the head

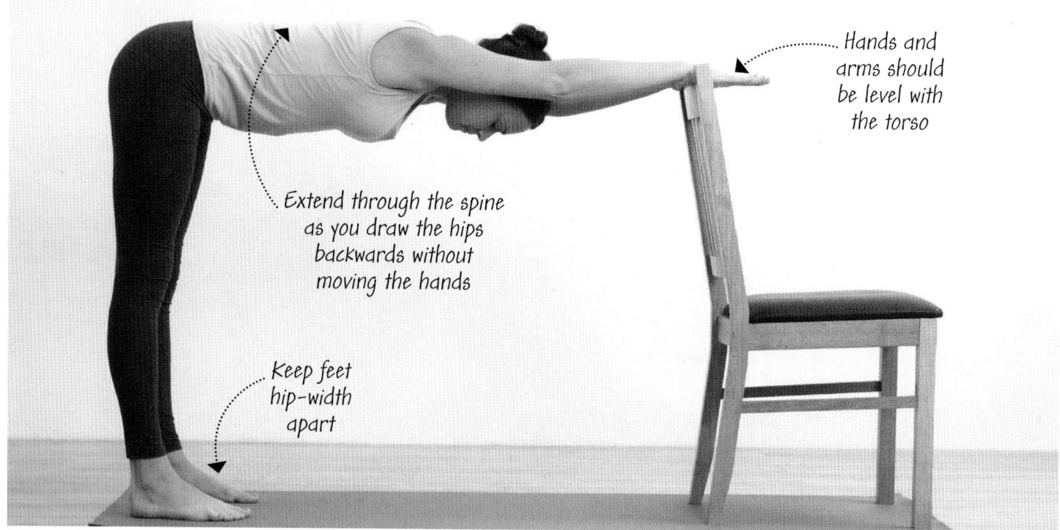
Hands and arms should be level with the torso
Extend through the spine as you draw the hips backwards without moving the hands
Keep feet hip-width apart

Props for standing poses

Postures such as forward bends may prove impossible to do correctly when you first attempt them. Blocks, or other means of support such as a chair, can be used to modify the posture so that flexibility can be gradually attained without injury.

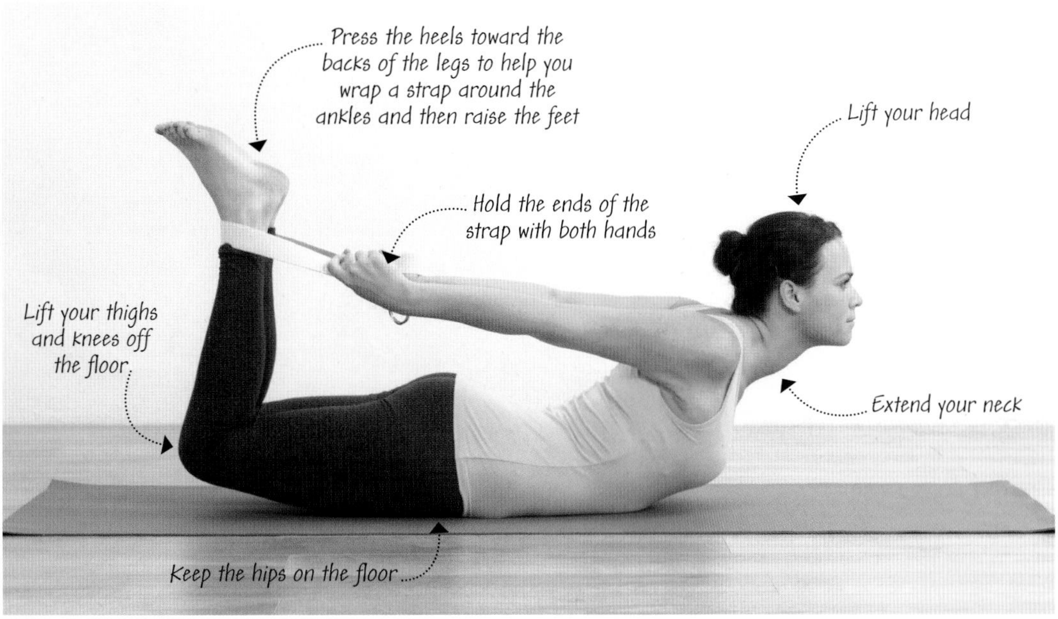

Press the heels toward the backs of the legs to help you wrap a strap around the ankles and then raise the feet

Lift your head

Hold the ends of the strap with both hands

Lift your thighs and knees off the floor

Extend your neck

Keep the hips on the floor

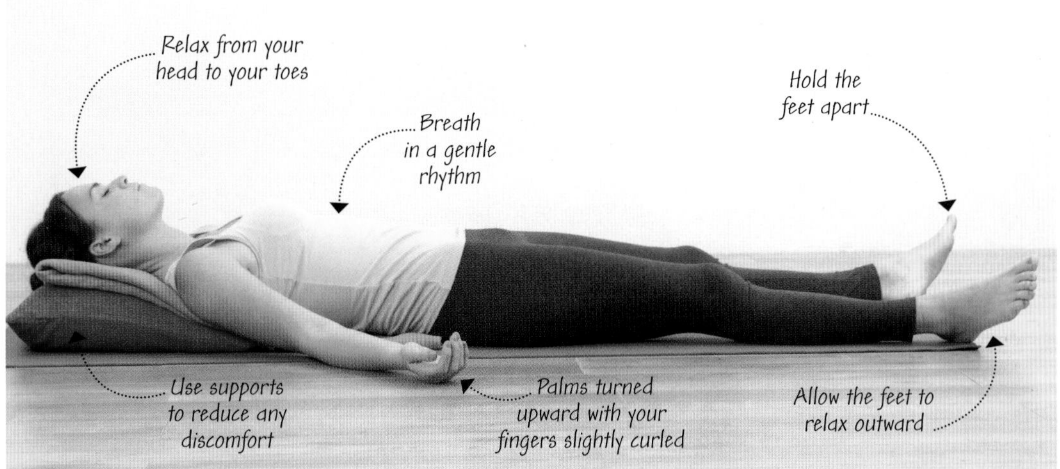
Relax from your head to your toes
Breath in a gentle rhythm
Hold the feet apart
Use supports to reduce any discomfort
Palms turned upward with your fingers slightly curled
Allow the feet to relax outward

Props for floor poses

Using a strap or belt can help you to work toward achieving a posture that you may not be able to fully achieve when you first begin to practice. Towels or bolsters can be helpful in providing the comfort you need to enable you to relax fully.

Key Techniques for **Relaxation**

In yoga, relaxation involves undertaking a conscious exploration of your inner self. Learning relaxation techniques makes this possible by creating a state of calm in which the mind and body are able to connect with each other. A key component of relaxation is breathing consciously in a gentle, wave-like pattern to deepen your sense of peace and ease.

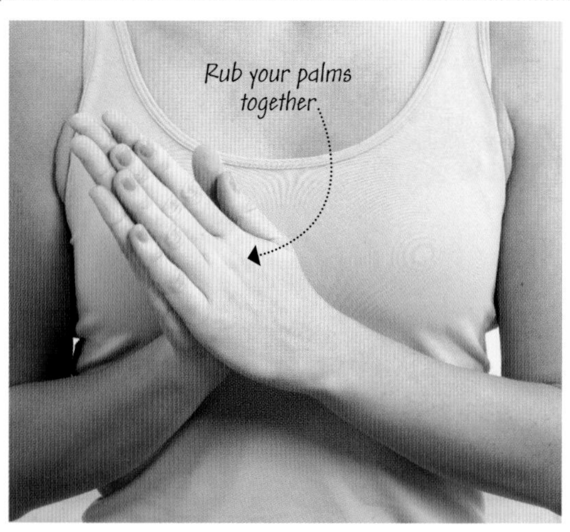
Rub your palms together

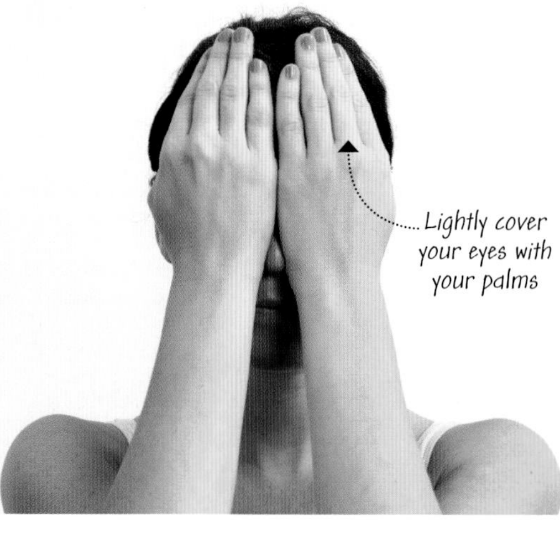
Lightly cover your eyes with your palms

Relax the eyes

Sitting comfortably with a straight back, rub your hands together until your palms feel warm. Breathing evenly, close your eyes and cover them gently with the palms of your hands so that all you experience is blackness. Hold for several minutes.

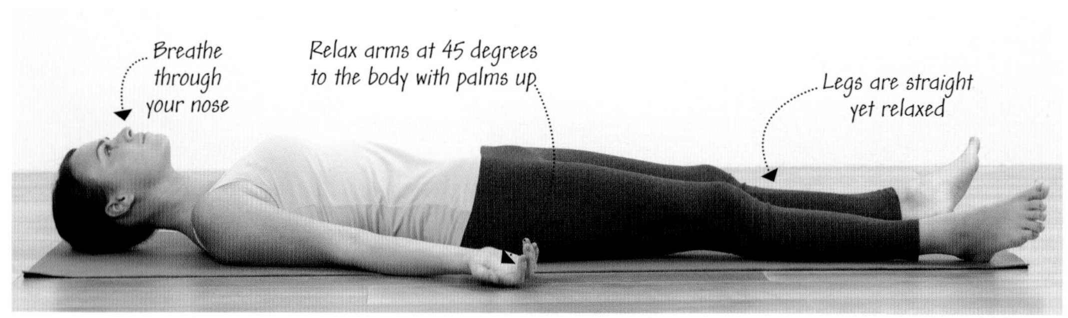
Breathe through your nose
Relax arms at 45 degrees to the body with palms up
Legs are straight yet relaxed

Corpse

Lie on your back, keeping the feet at least 2ft (60cm) apart. Relax, letting the feet roll outward. Arms should be at an angle of 45 degrees to the body, with the palms facing upward. Feel your abdomen rise and fall gently as you breathe in and out. Let the tension float out with each exhalation. Stay in this pose for at least five minutes.

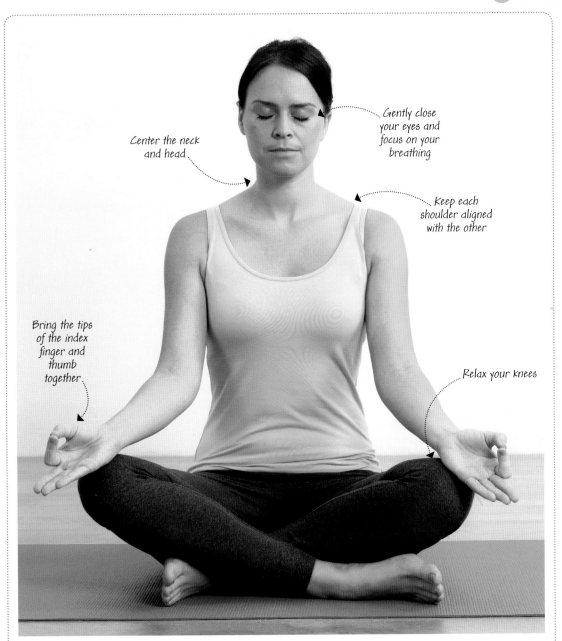
Gently close
your eyes and
focus on your
breathing
Center the neck
and head
Keep each
shoulder aligned
with the other
Bring the tips
of the index
finger and
thumb
together
Relax your knees

Cross-legged sitting

Sit on a mat or cushion for comfort and cross your legs. If necessary, avoid tension in your knees by using cushions for support. Lean slightly forward, keeping your spine erect.

Rest your hands on your knees, with your palms facing outward. Feel your chest gently rise and fall as you breathe. Like a lotus in a pond, embrace the stillness.

Mountain Pose

Develop Posture • **Promote** Spinal Alignment

The Mountain Pose enables you to use your internal mirror to correct spinal alignment. The internal focus and awareness of alignment that this pose gives will help you with other postures.

1 Stand with your feet hip-width apart, the sides of the legs parallel, and the toes pointing forward. Lift up your toes, spread them apart, then press them into the ground. Place your arms by your side. Realign your body by working slowly upward: from the toes to the ankles, knees, pelvis, chest, shoulders, neck, and head.

Useful tip Spread your body's weight evenly across your feet. Imagine your feet are growing roots into the floor, enabling you to stand strong and firm.

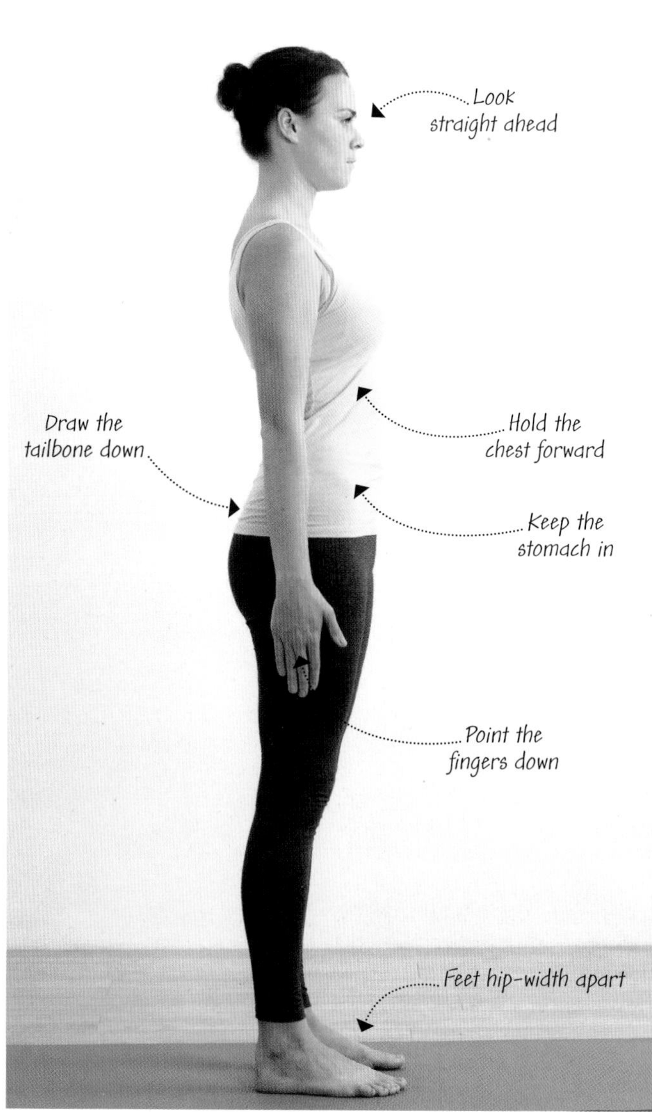
Look straight ahead
Draw the tailbone down
Hold the chest forward
Keep the stomach in
Point the fingers down
Feet hip-width apart

Take care...

Neck and head tilting forward
Stiff shoulders or a rounded upper spine (kyphosis) may cause your neck to stretch forward. Over time, this can be reduced by opening the chest, lengthening the neck, and keeping the chin at 90 degrees to the floor.

Torso leaning back When your legs are in position, the pelvis may tend to tilt forward, which causes the upper body to lean back slightly. Focus on reducing the pelvic tilt by drawing your pubic bone inward and allowing your tailbone to elongate.

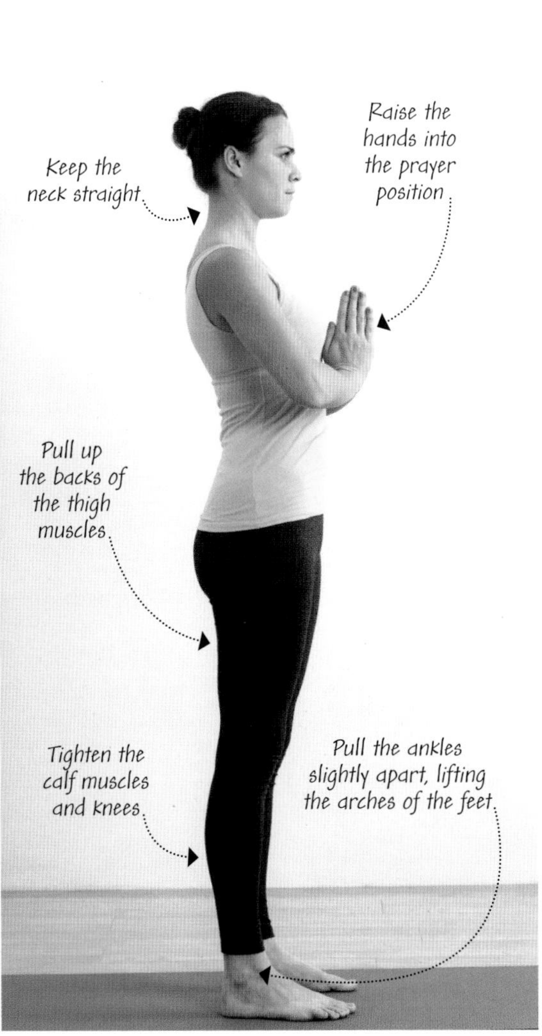
Keep the neck straight
Raise the hands into the prayer position
Pull up the backs of the thigh muscles
Tighten the calf muscles and knees
Pull the ankles slightly apart, lifting the arches of the feet

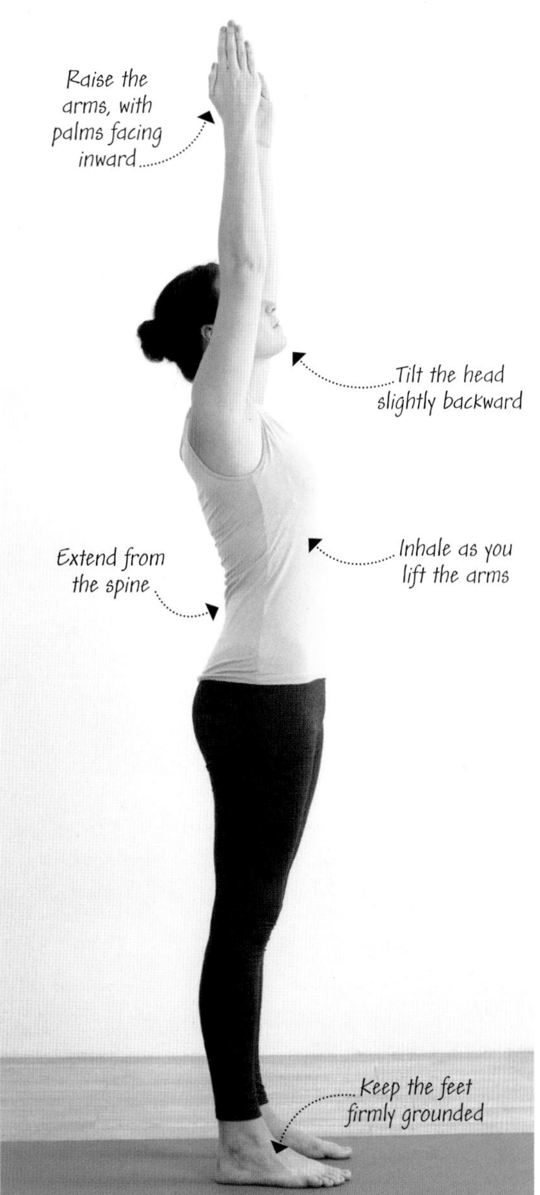
Raise the arms, with palms facing inward
Tilt the head slightly backward
Extend from the spine
Inhale as you lift the arms
Keep the feet firmly grounded

2 Bend the elbows, bringing your hands together in front of the chest in prayer position. Be aware of your spinal alignment and hold your neck and head straight, looking forward. Become aware of the steady rhythm of your breath.

3 Breathe in to stretch the arms upward with the palms facing inward, and tilt the neck so that you are looking slightly upward. Engage your back muscles to lengthen the spine. Make tiny, corrective adjustments until you feel grounded.

Standing Arm Stretches

Harmonize Breath • **Extend** Spine

These are good postures for practicing synchronized breathing and movement. They also provide a good stretch for the shoulders and the spine.

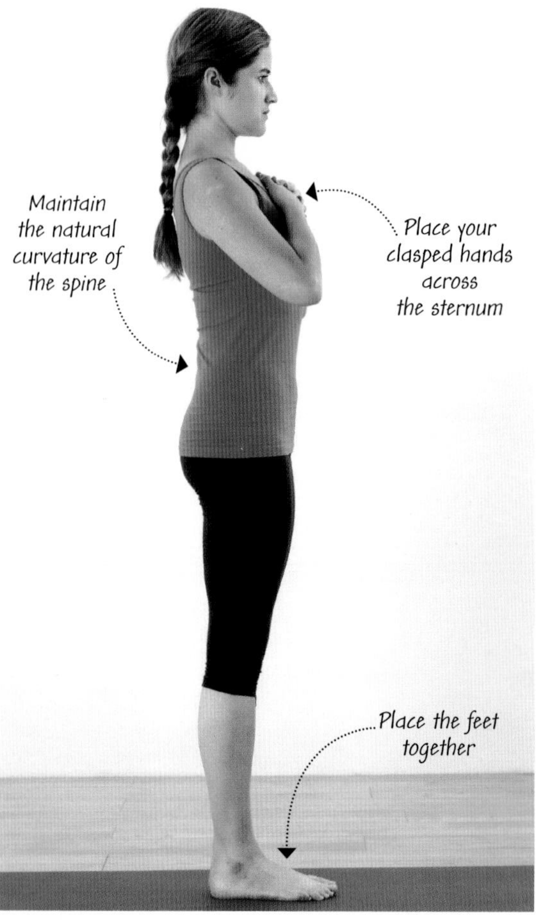

Maintain the natural curvature of the spine
Place your clasped hands across the sternum
Place the feet together

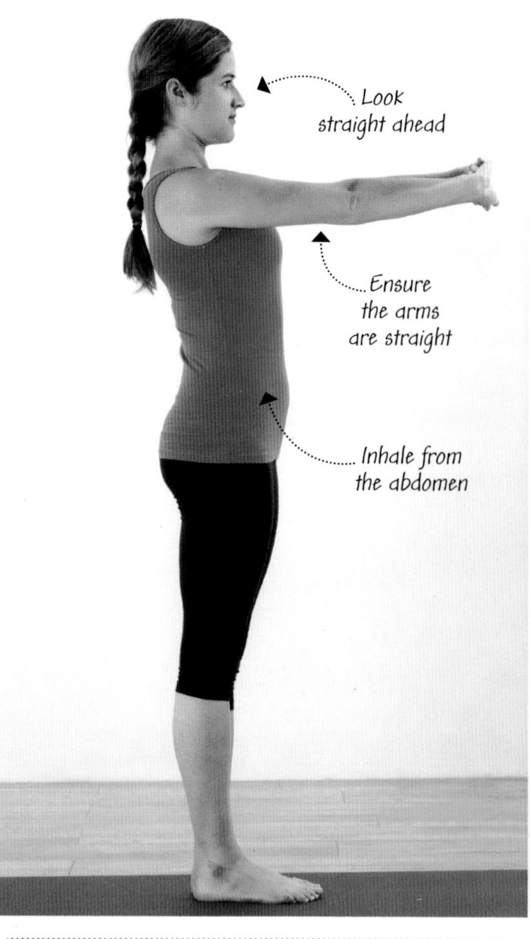

Look straight ahead
Ensure the arms are straight
Inhale from the abdomen

1 Adopt a standing position with your feet together. Clasping the hands together, bring them up to chest height and rest them lightly on the chest. Focus on your breath, feeling the rise and fall of your chest as you inhale and exhale.

2 As you inhale, stretch out your arms, with fingers interlocked and palms facing outward until your arms are straight. As you exhale, bring your arms back to their original position.

Take care...

A common mistake is to arch the lower part of your back (the lumbar region). Focus on retaining the natural curvature of your spine during this stretch.

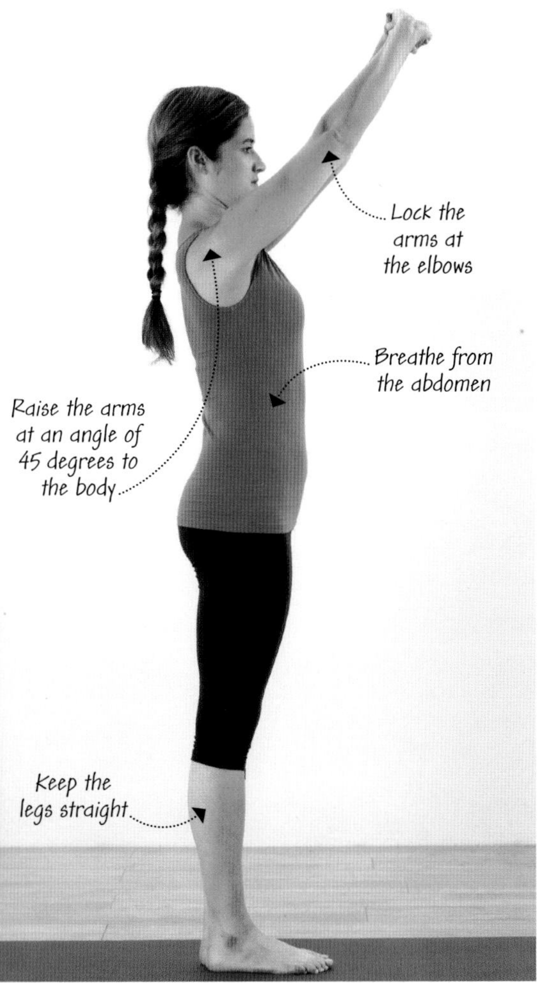
Lock the arms at the elbows
Breathe from the abdomen
Raise the arms at an angle of 45 degrees to the body
Keep the legs straight

Interlock the fingers and turn the palms upward

Keep the arms vertical, brushing the ears

Extend from the lower back

Breathe in as you reach upward

Pull your kneecaps up

3 Do the same movement as shown in step 2, except instead of extending your arms straight ahead, extend them at an angle of 45 degrees. Remember to inhale as you extend your arms and exhale as you return them to the start position.

4 Keeping the shoulders relaxed, repeat steps 1 and 2, but this time extend your arms upward, lengthening your spine. Be aware of coordinating movements with the breath. Exhaling, return to the start position. Repeat at least five times.

Leg Raise 1

Strengthen Abdominal and Leg Muscles • **Limber** Hips

Elevating the leg provides a strong stretch to the hamstring and calf muscles. This pose develops the flexibility and strength needed for forward-bend poses.

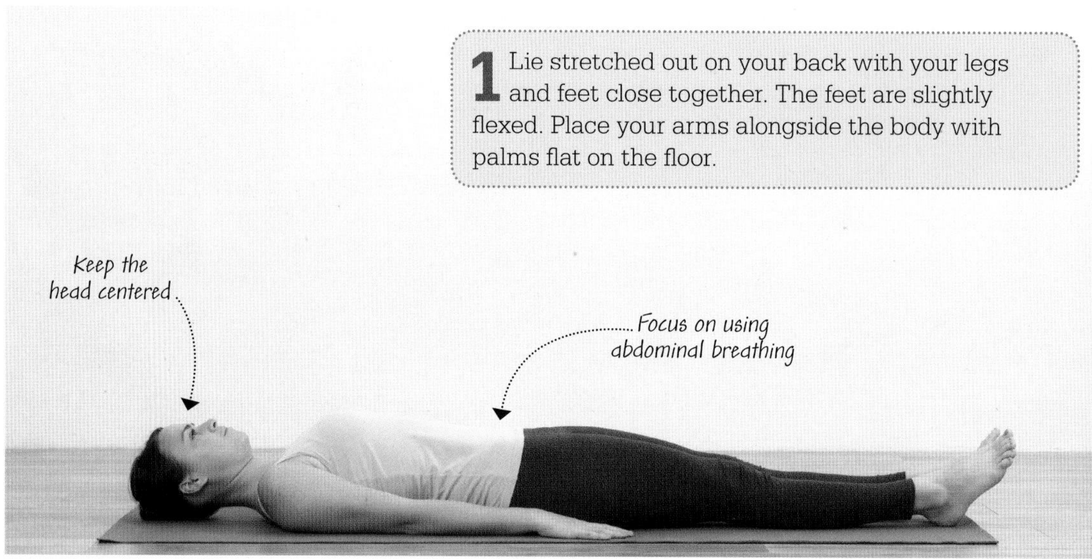
Keep the head centered
Focus on using abdominal breathing

1 Lie stretched out on your back with your legs and feet close together. The feet are slightly flexed. Place your arms alongside the body with palms flat on the floor.

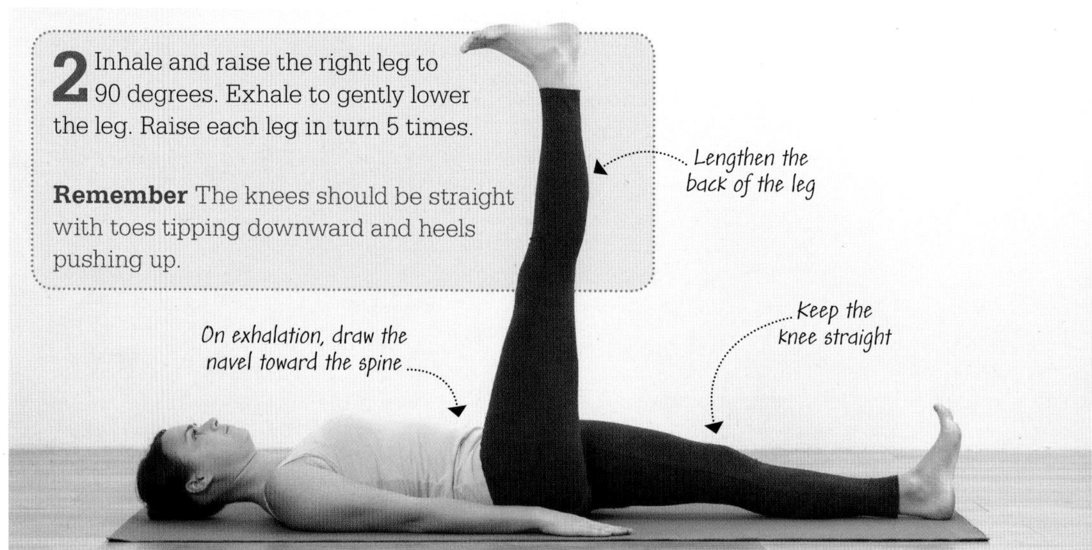
Lengthen the back of the leg
On exhalation, draw the navel toward the spine
Keep the knee straight

2 Inhale and raise the right leg to 90 degrees. Exhale to gently lower the leg. Raise each leg in turn 5 times.

Remember The knees should be straight with toes tipping downward and heels pushing up.

Leg Raise 2

Strengthen Neck • **Tone** Legs

In this exercise, the action of drawing the head to the knee compresses the abdomen, which means that the pose not only works the neck and legs, but also acts as an internal cleanser.

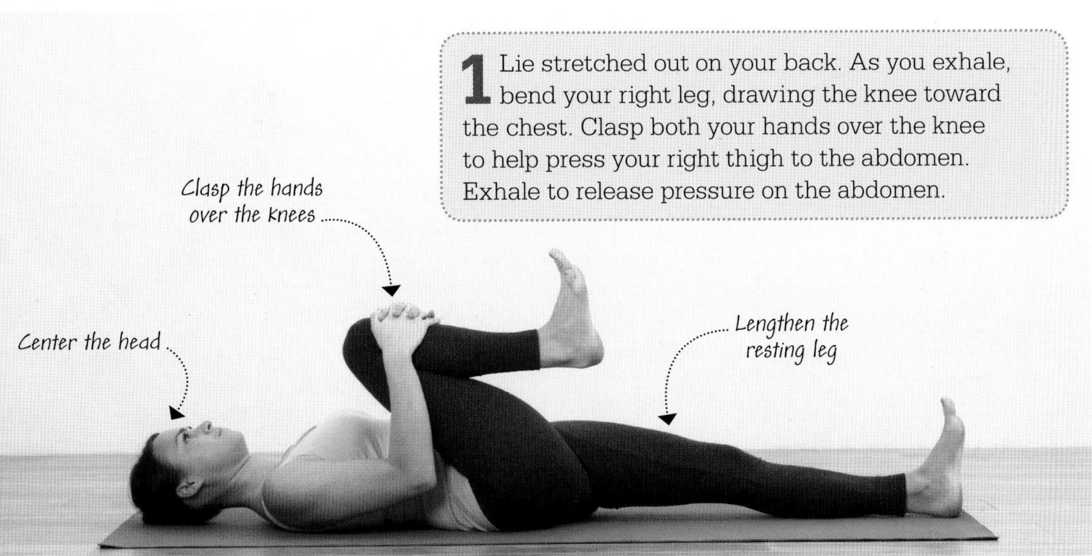
Clasp the hands over the knees
Center the head
Lengthen the resting leg

1 Lie stretched out on your back. As you exhale, bend your right leg, drawing the knee toward the chest. Clasp both your hands over the knee to help press your right thigh to the abdomen. Exhale to release pressure on the abdomen.

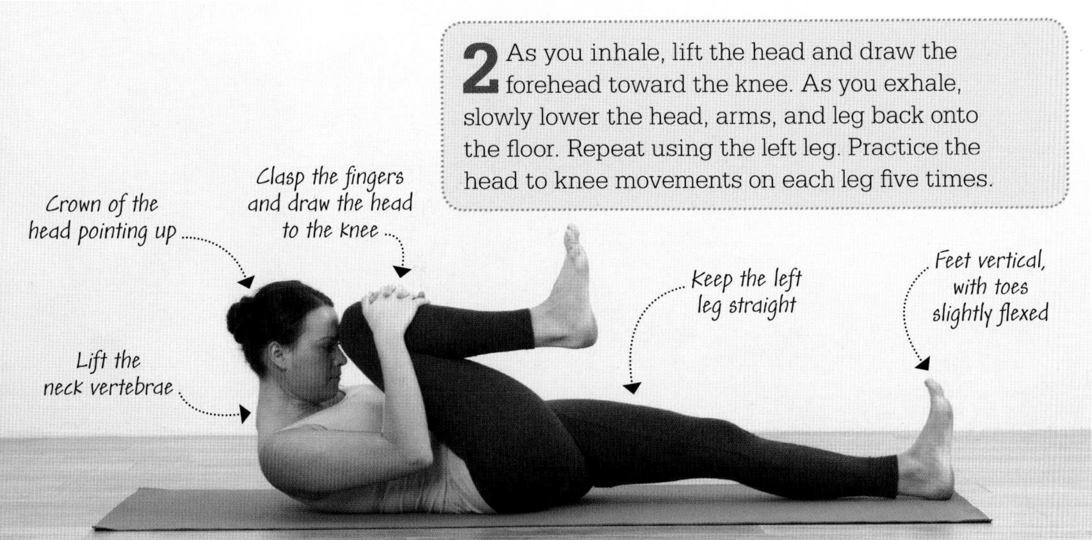
Crown of the head pointing up
Clasp the fingers and draw the head to the knee
Keep the left leg straight
Feet vertical, with toes slightly flexed
Lift the neck vertebrae

2 As you inhale, lift the head and draw the forehead toward the knee. As you exhale, slowly lower the head, arms, and leg back onto the floor. Repeat using the left leg. Practice the head to knee movements on each leg five times.

Triangle

Strengthen Body Length • **Tones** Hips

This side-bending posture is an excellent pose for strengthening the back and core muscles. It also improves the flexibility of the hip joints and opens up the chest.

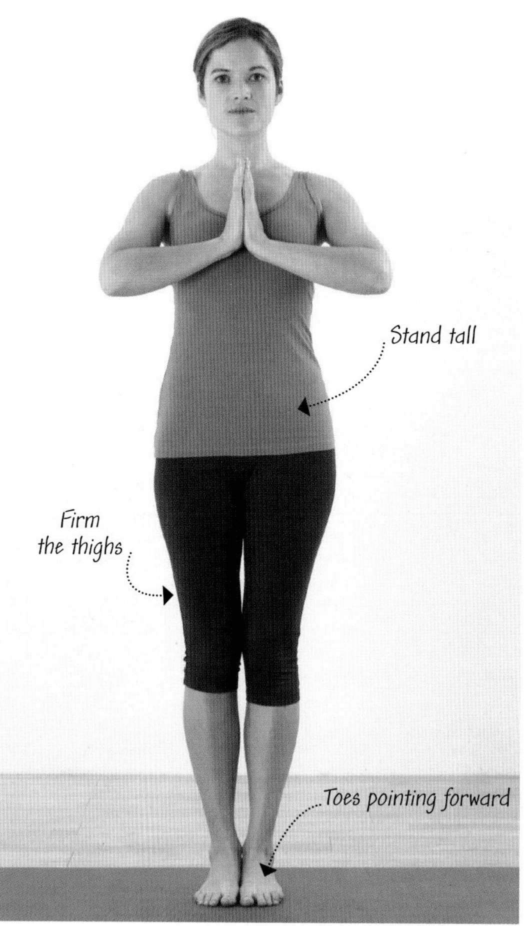
Stand tall
Firm the thighs
Toes pointing forward

1 Stand sideways on the mat with feet together and focus on your breathing. Feel the movements of the ribs and diaphragm as you breathe in and out.

Make it easier

If you are unable to touch the floor with your fingers, try using a foam block positioned behind your right foot. Press your palm onto the block. Keep the left palm open, aligned with the arm and work on extending the left hand upward.

Alternatively, begin by resting your hand on your lower right leg at a comfortable level (see below). Work on this sideways extension and move the hand a little farther down the leg as you exhale. Avoid tilting the torso forward as a way of moving your hand farther.

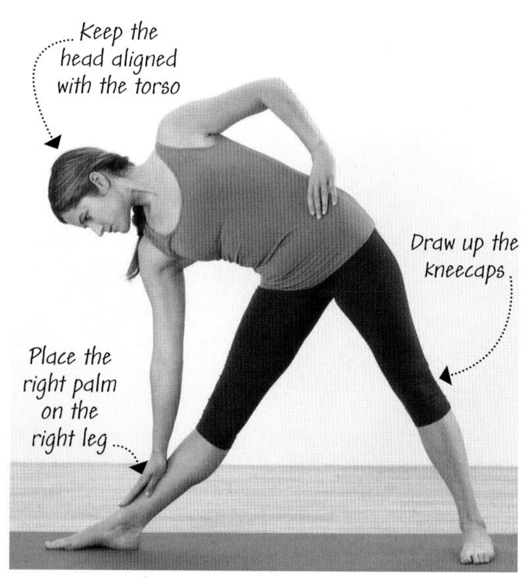
Keep the head aligned with the torso
Draw up the kneecaps
Place the right palm on the right leg

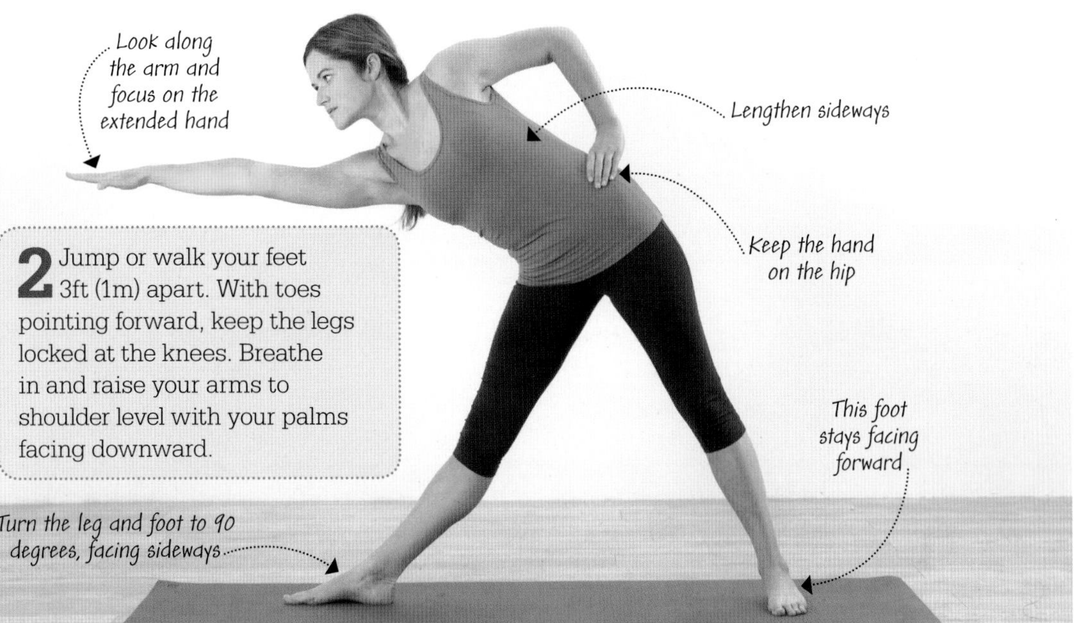
Look along the arm and focus on the extended hand
Lengthen sideways
Keep the hand on the hip
This foot stays facing forward
Turn the leg and foot to 90 degrees, facing sideways

2 Jump or walk your feet 3ft (1m) apart. With toes pointing forward, keep the legs locked at the knees. Breathe in and raise your arms to shoulder level with your palms facing downward.

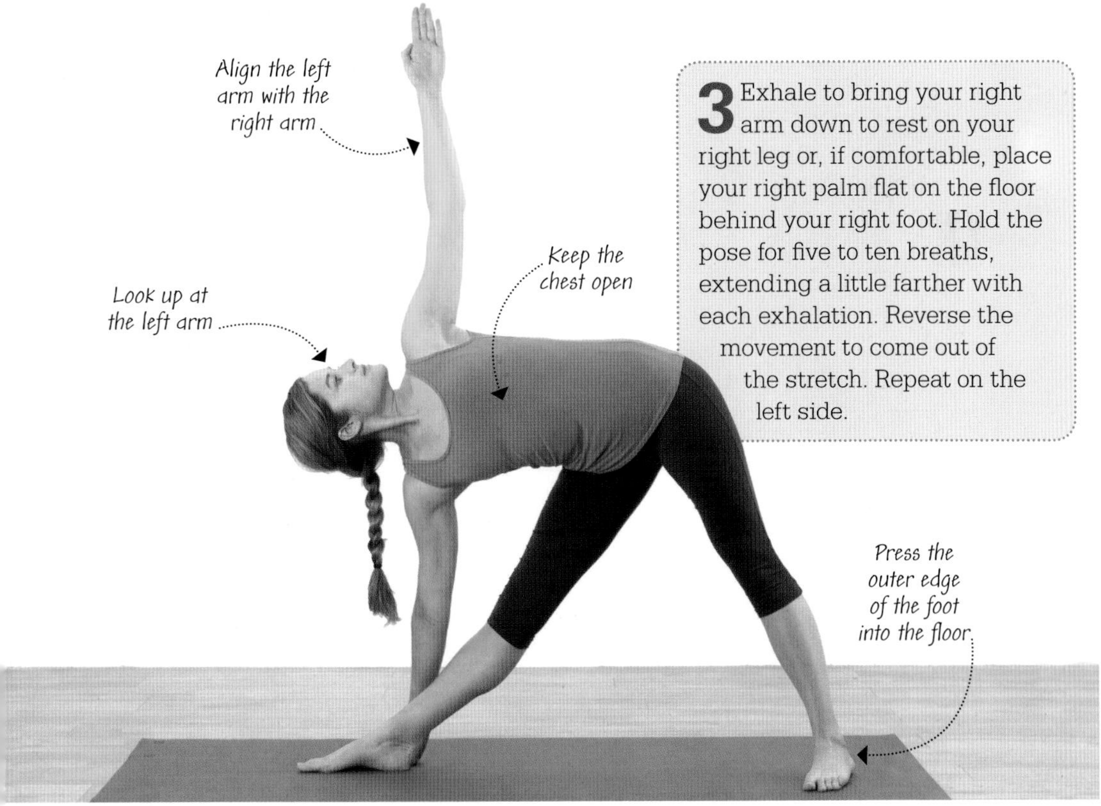

Align the left arm with the right arm

Look up at the left arm

Keep the chest open

Press the outer edge of the foot into the floor

3 Exhale to bring your right arm down to rest on your right leg or, if comfortable, place your right palm flat on the floor behind your right foot. Hold the pose for five to ten breaths, extending a little farther with each exhalation. Reverse the movement to come out of the stretch. Repeat on the left side.

Standing Forward Bend

Tone Legs • **Refresh** Mind

This posture gives the spine and legs, from the middle of your back to your heels, an intense stretch. It is also a useful counter-pose to the backward bends.

1 Stand in the mountain pose with your feet hip-width apart and your hands by your sides, fingers pointing down. Center yourself and be mindful of your breath as you root down.

2 Inhaling deeply, lock your arms at the elbow and slowly sweep them upward until they are shoulder-width apart. Tilt your head back to look up at the hands.

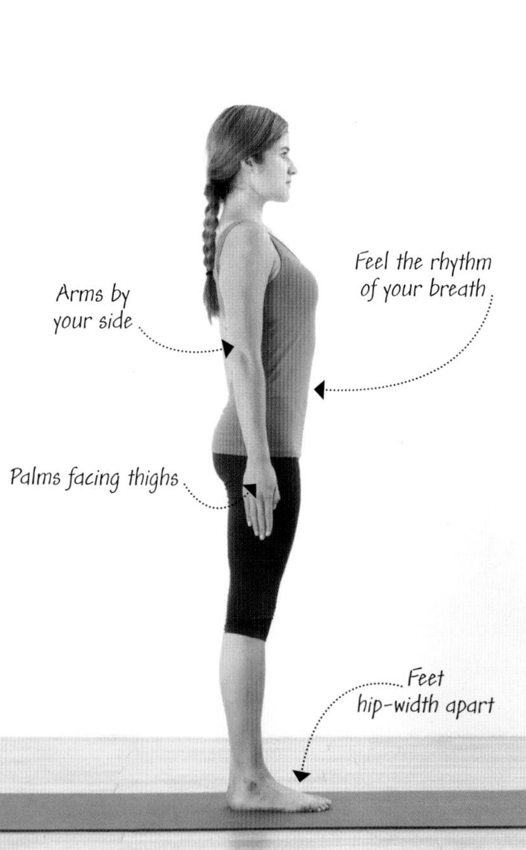
Arms by your side
Feel the rhythm of your breath
Palms facing thighs
Feet hip-width apart

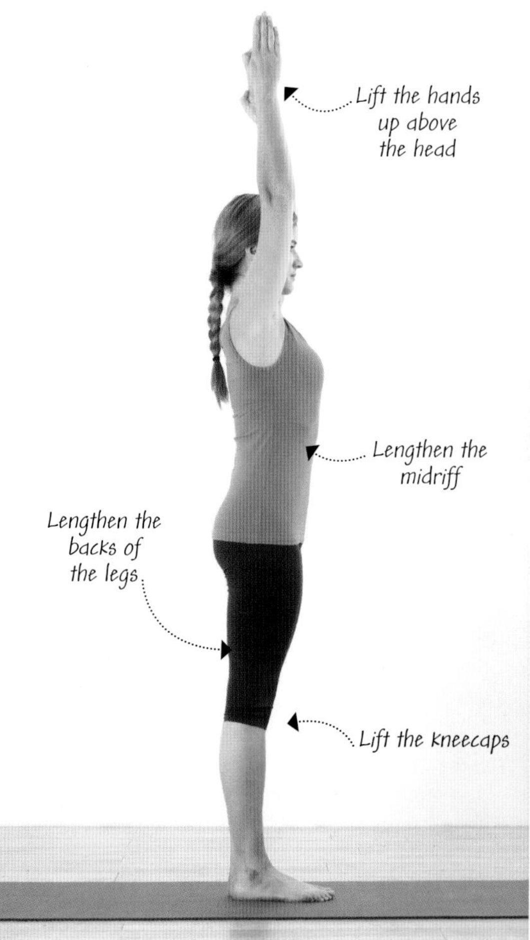
Lift the hands up above the head
Lengthen the midriff
Lengthen the backs of the legs
Lift the kneecaps

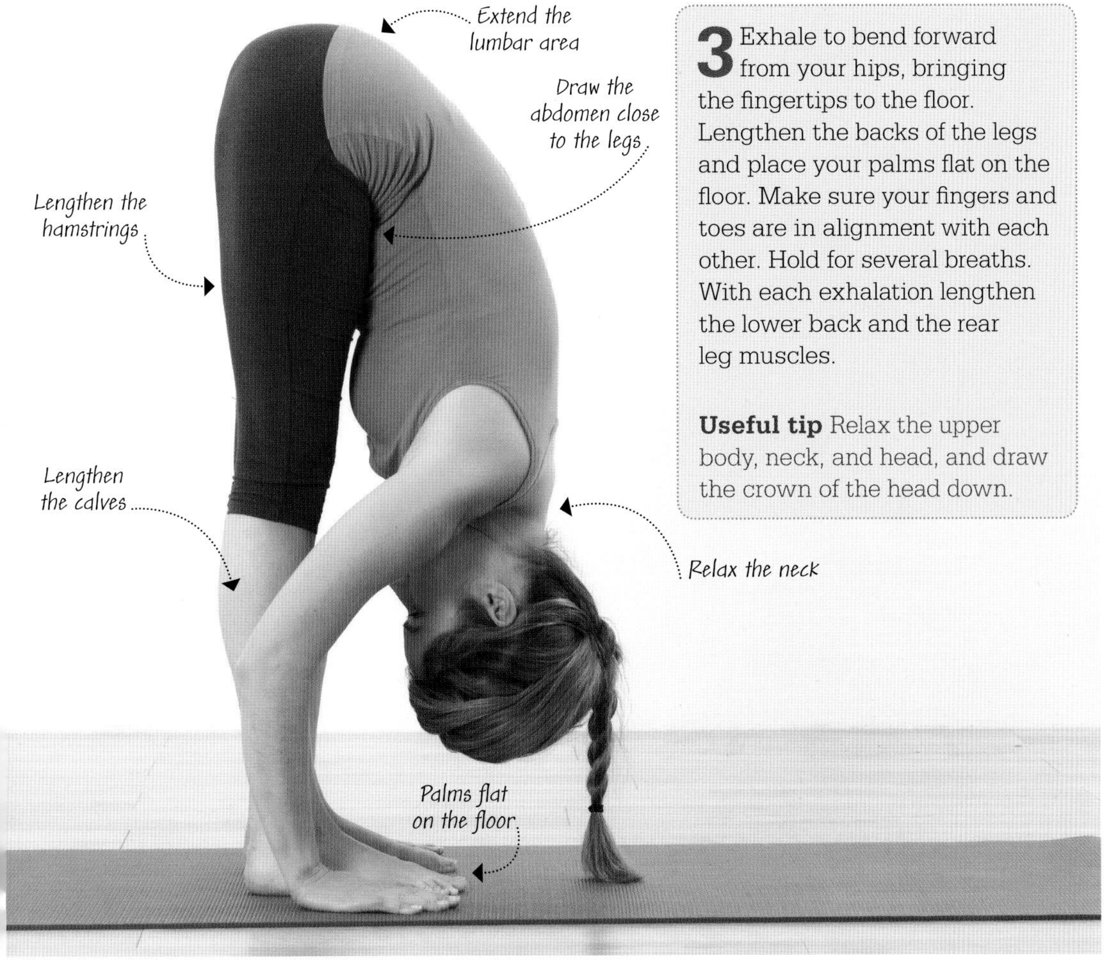

Extend the lumbar area

Draw the abdomen close to the legs

Lengthen the hamstrings

Lengthen the calves

Relax the neck

Palms flat on the floor

3 Exhale to bend forward from your hips, bringing the fingertips to the floor. Lengthen the backs of the legs and place your palms flat on the floor. Make sure your fingers and toes are in alignment with each other. Hold for several breaths. With each exhalation lengthen the lower back and the rear leg muscles.

Useful tip Relax the upper body, neck, and head, and draw the crown of the head down.

Make it easier

Bend your knees a little to allow your palms to sit flat on the floor.

Place your hands on a block with palms resting flat on it.

Practice Half Forward Bend, placing your hands on a chair, with your arms level with your shoulders and hips at 90 degrees (see page 40).

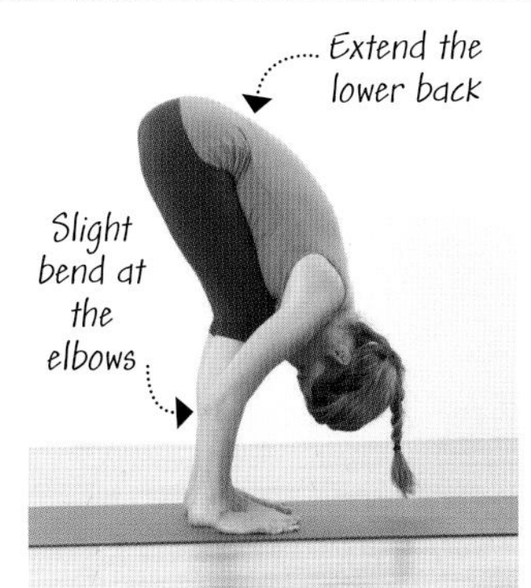
Extend the lower back
Slight bend at the elbows

Bend the knees

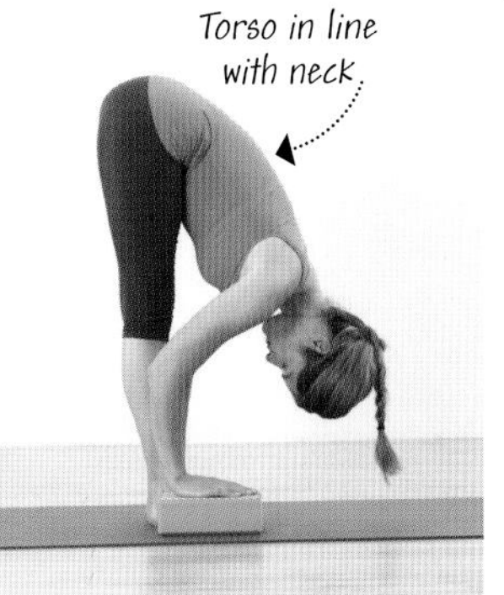
Torso in line with neck

Use a block

Plank Pose

Strengthen Arms and Upper Body
Develop Body Awareness

An all-around strengthening posture, the Plank Pose is also good for releasing stress in the neck and lengthening the spine.

1 Sit on the mat with your legs folded under, and the toes pointing away. Place your hands on the thighs with fingers pointing forward. Align the neck and back, with your chin parallel to floor. Let your breath flow in and out.

Useful tip Move your shoulders around in small circles, in both directions, to release tension.

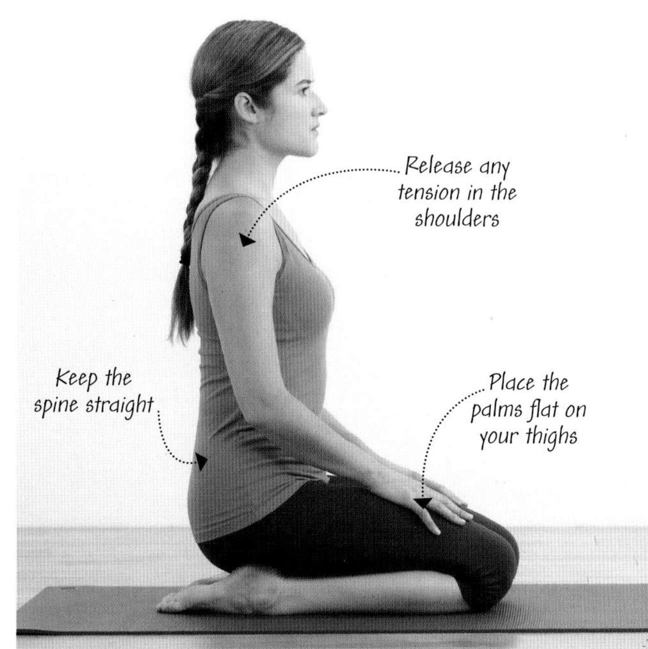
Release any tension in the shoulders
Keep the spine straight
Place the palms flat on your thighs

Take care...

A common mistake is for the middle part of the body to sag in the Plank Pose. Make sure you're maintaining a straight line by looking along the underside of your body.

Placing your palms incorrectly will strain the wrists. The arms should be at 90 degrees to the mat, so they can bear the weight of the upper body.

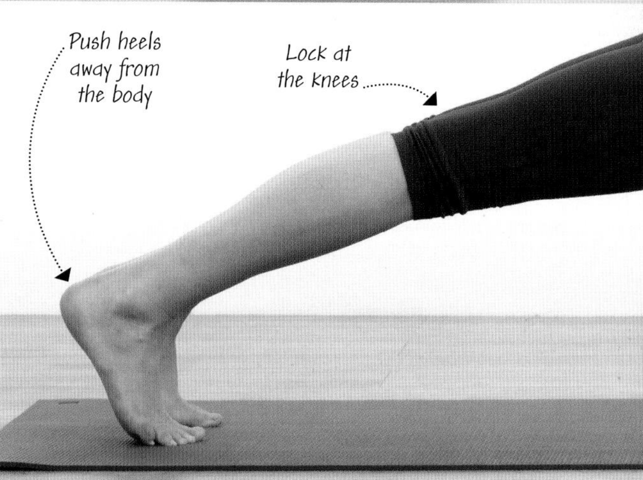
Push heels away from the body
Lock at the knees

2 Move onto all fours, keeping your shoulders and knees aligned with your hips. Pull the abdomen in toward the spine, flattening your back.

Useful tip Imagine a square box that can fit perfectly under your trunk, between your limbs.

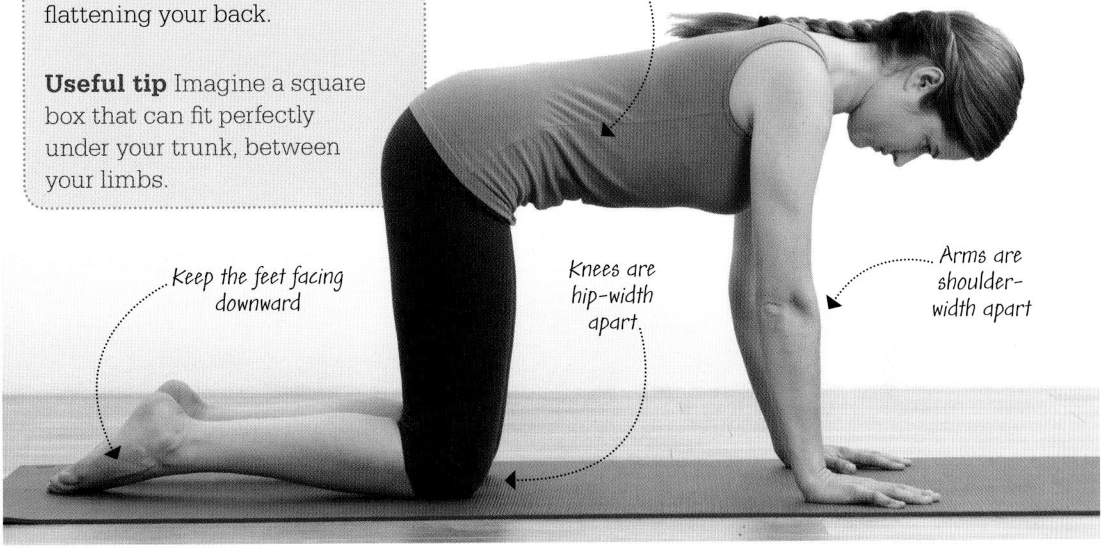

Pull in the abdomen toward the spine

Keep the feet facing downward

Knees are hip-width apart

Arms are shoulder-width apart

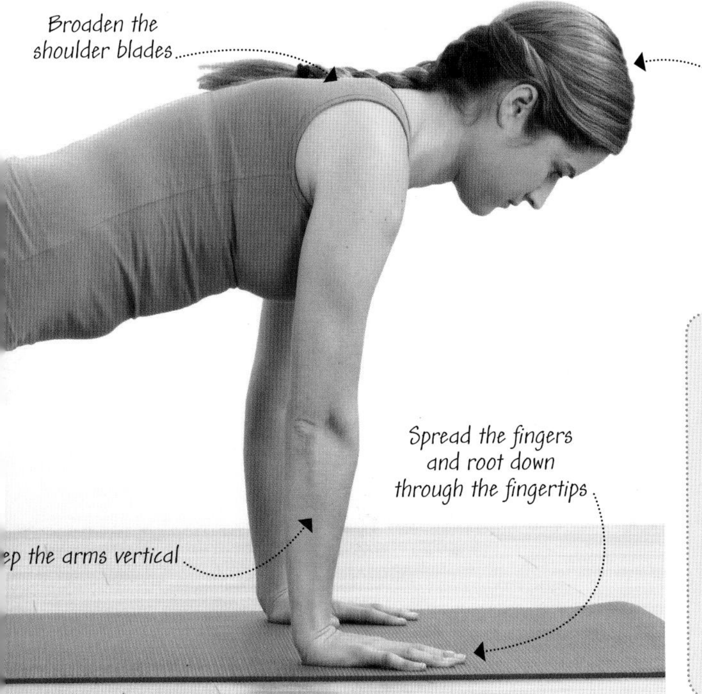
Broaden the shoulder blades
The head and neck follow the angle of the body
Spread the fingers and root down through the fingertips
ep the arms vertical

3 As you inhale, extend the legs, locking your knees and elbows and keeping your body as straight as possible. Using the toes to grip the mat, try to push your heels backward.

Useful tip Keep your belly and lower back from sagging by using inhalations to pull your stomach in and inflate your lower back.

Downward-facing Dog

Lengthen Back and Legs • **Energize** Body

This pose energizes the whole body while calming the mind and providing a strong stretch for the shoulders, hamstrings, and calves.

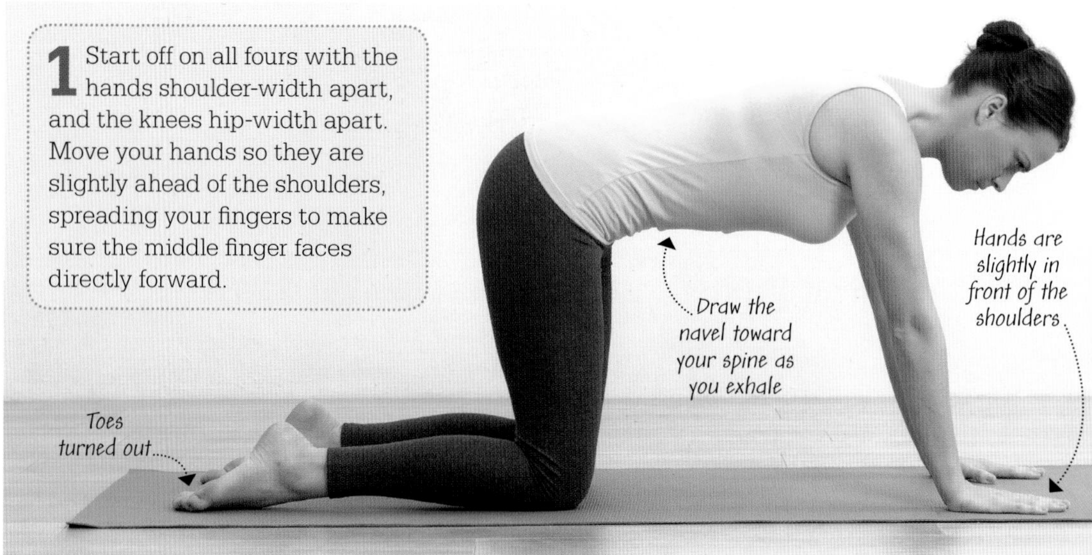
Draw the navel toward your spine as you exhale
Hands are slightly in front of the shoulders
Toes turned out

1 Start off on all fours with the hands shoulder-width apart, and the knees hip-width apart. Move your hands so they are slightly ahead of the shoulders, spreading your fingers to make sure the middle finger faces directly forward.

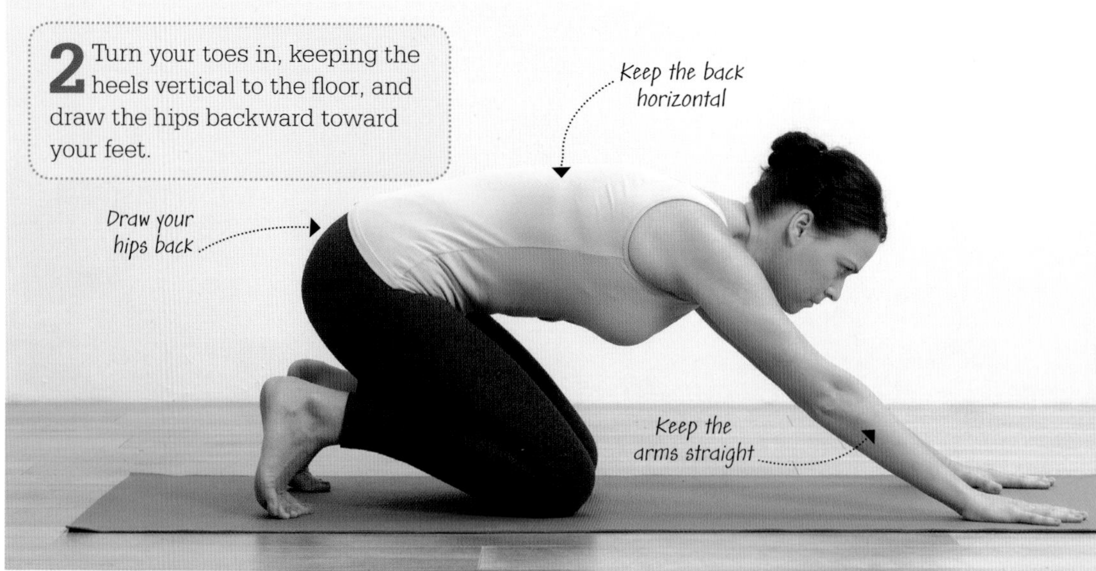
Keep the back horizontal
Draw your hips back
Keep the arms straight

2 Turn your toes in, keeping the heels vertical to the floor, and draw the hips backward toward your feet.

3 Exhale and lift your knees off the floor, drawing your tailbone upward. Keep your knees slightly bent and heels off the floor. Spread your toes, using them to root down.

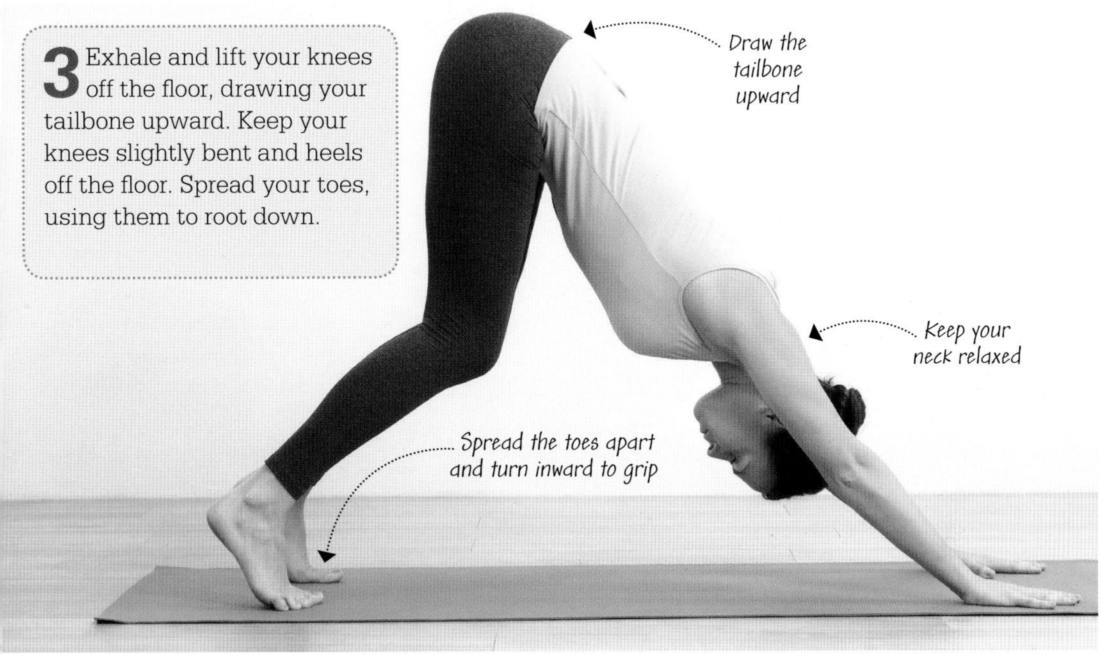

Draw the tailbone upward

Keep your neck relaxed

Spread the toes apart and turn inward to grip

4 Straighten your arms and legs as far as you can and push back into the heels. Relax your neck, keeping your breath steady and even. With each exhalation, lengthen your spine.

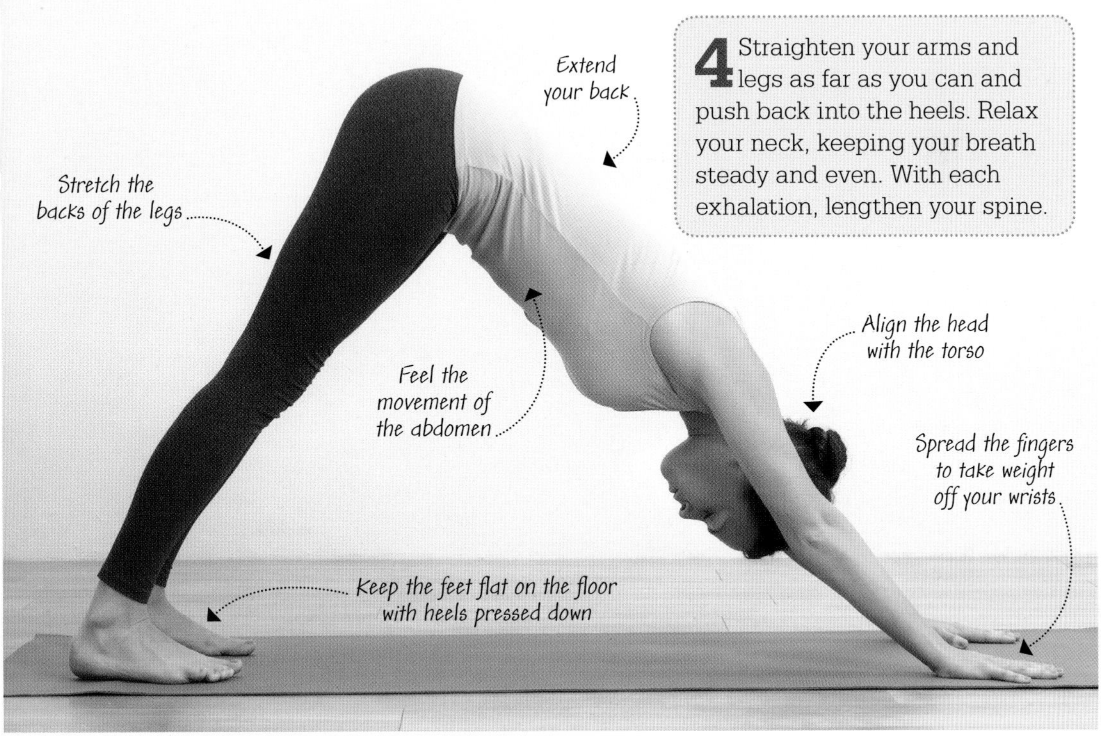

Extend your back

Stretch the backs of the legs

Align the head with the torso

Feel the movement of the abdomen

Spread the fingers to take weight off your wrists

Keep the feet flat on the floor with heels pressed down

Diagonal Stretch

Strengthen Core • **Release** Tension

This gentle, horizontal stretch will help to increase the flexibility of your spine and back muscles safely. Smoothing the flow of energy through the spine will also energize your body.

1 Lie on your stomach, arms alongside the body, head to one side, and feet relaxed with big toes touching. Relax and listen to your breathing.

Useful tip Tense then relax your limbs, starting from the feet, to feel proper relaxation.

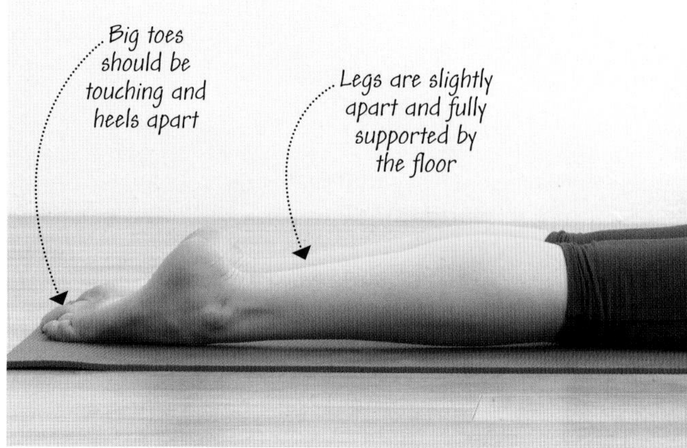
Big toes should be touching and heels apart
Legs are slightly apart and fully supported by the floor

2 Begin by extending both arms straight out in front. Inhale to raise your right arm and upper body off the mat. At the same time, lift your left leg up to a similar height and angle as your right arm. Hold for five to ten breaths. Exhale to release the limbs back to the floor. Repeat with the opposite limbs.

Useful tip Imagine a diagonal line from your right hand to your left foot. Focus on lengthening this line withn your limbs as you lift them up.

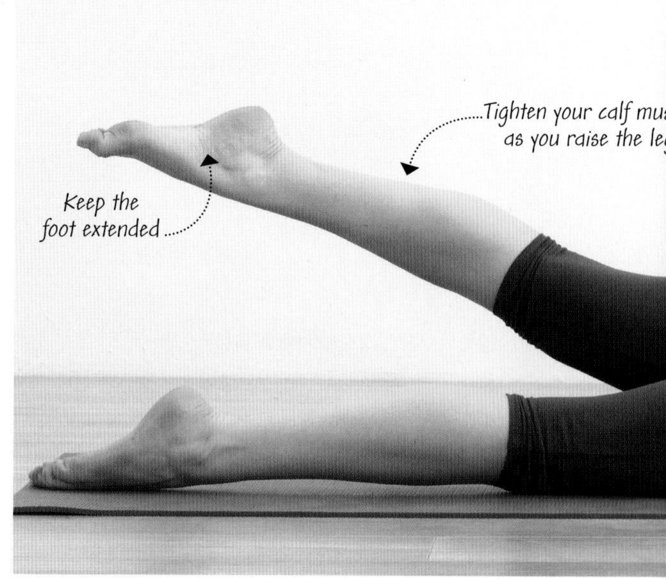
Keep the foot extended

Make it easier

From the step 1 position, extend both arms straight out in front. Keep the right arm straight. Bend the left arm at the elbow, placing the palm flat on the mat, and rest your forehead on the left hand. The arm left on the mat will help you to press down and stabilize as you raise each limb up diagonally.

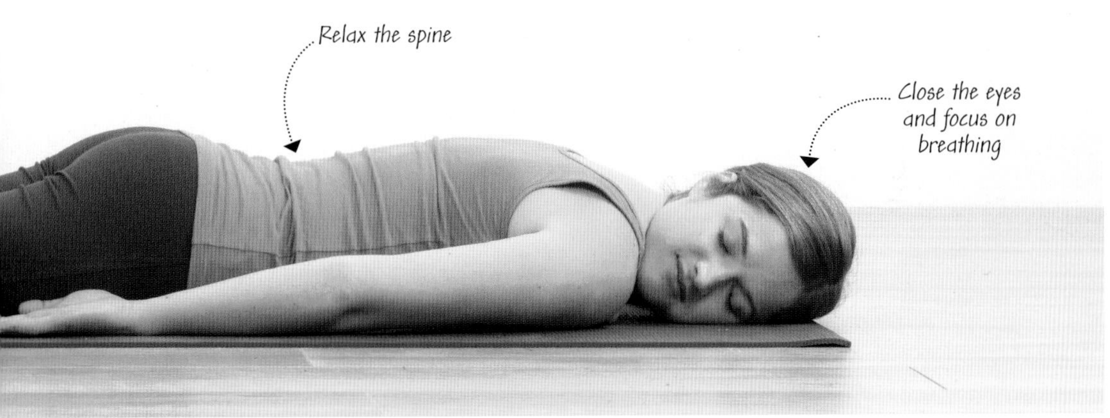
Relax the spine
Close the eyes and focus on breathing

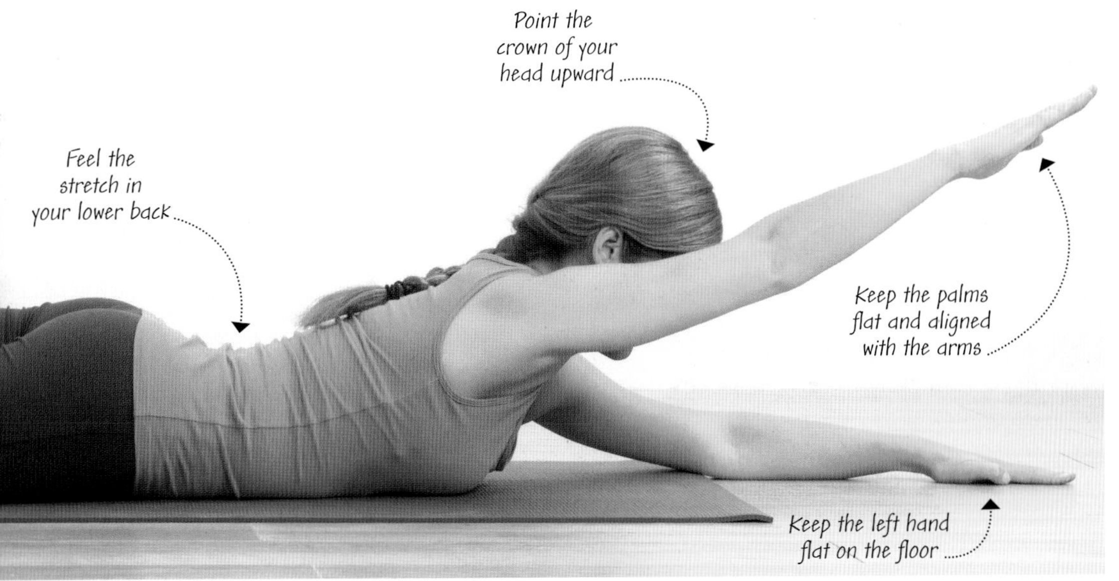
Point the crown of your head upward
Feel the stretch in your lower back
Keep the palms flat and aligned with the arms
Keep the left hand flat on the floor

Cobra

Strengthen Spine • **Energize** Body

This pose involves lifting the upper body using the arms, strengthening the arms and wrists, while the backward bend adds flexibility to the spine.

1 Start by lying stretched in a prone position on the mat, with your forehead resting on the mat and with the arms by your sides, palms turned upward. Stretch your legs and extend the toes away from the body.

Useful tip Engage the muscles of the legs and press the pubis, thighs, and the tops of the feet firmly into the mat.

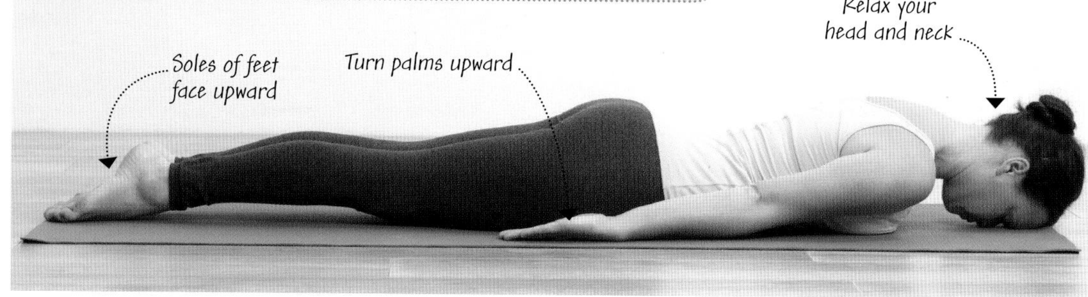
Relax your head and neck
Soles of feet face upward
Turn palms upward

2 Keeping your head tilted downward and your forehead on the floor, bend your arms and bring the palms of your hands flat on the floor, roughly in line with your chest.

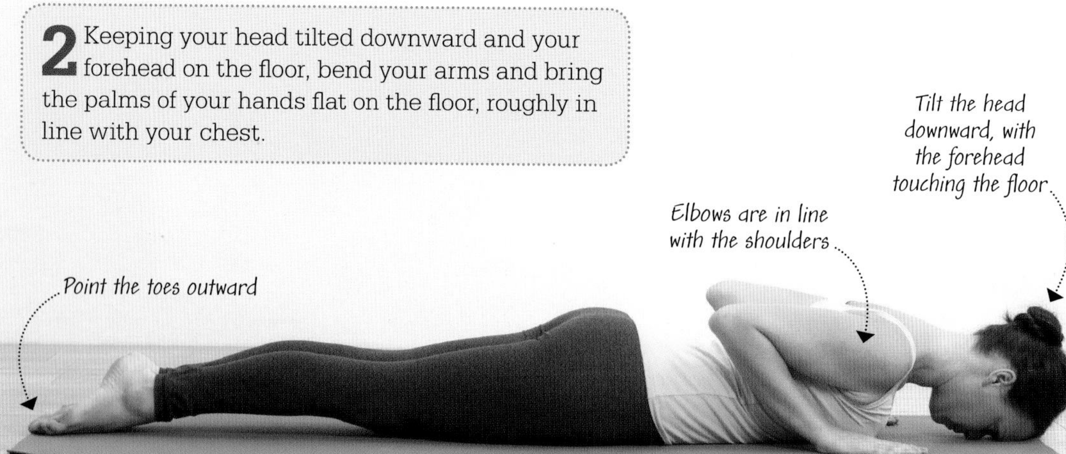
Tilt the head downward, with the forehead touching the floor
Elbows are in line with the shoulders
Point the toes outward

3 Inhale deeply and raise your head and chest, arching the spine and pulling your shoulder blades toward each other. Hold for five to ten breaths before gently returning to the start position.

Useful tip Focus on drawing your lower abdomen away from the mat to even out the spinal bend.

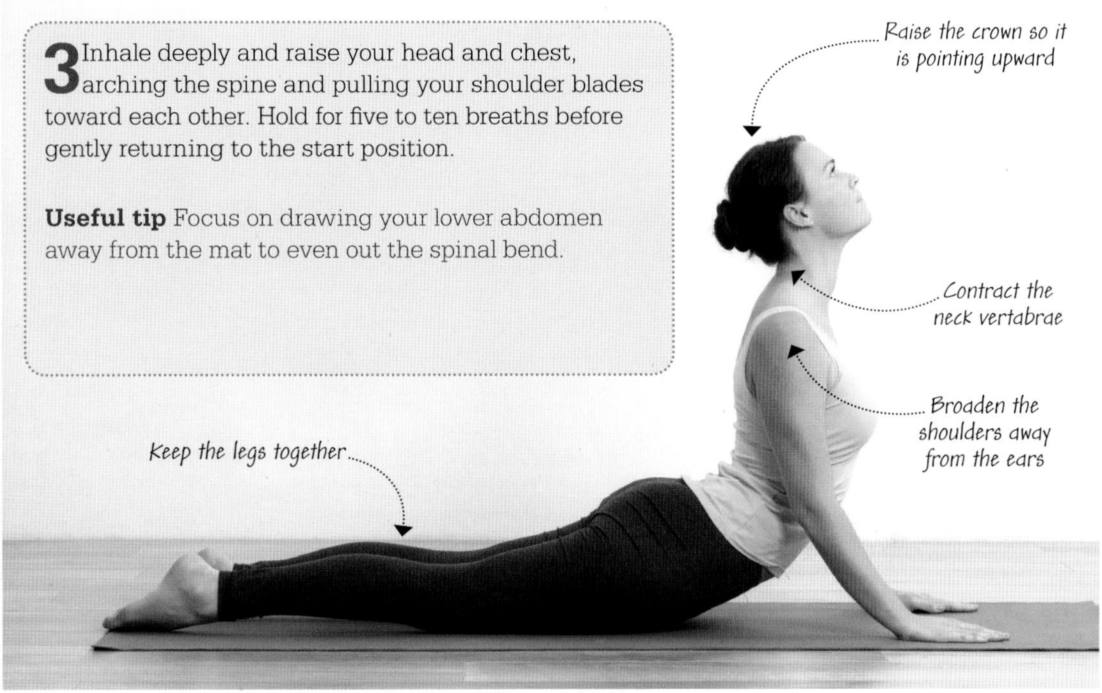

Raise the crown so it is pointing upward
Contract the neck vertabrae
Broaden the shoulders away from the ears
Keep the legs together

Take care...

A common mistake is to lock the arms to bring the head higher. Keep them bent and slowly work on lifting your head to a level that is comfortable for you.

Avoid hunching the shoulders up toward the ears as this will strain the neck vertebrae.

Do not overbend the spine. Raise your torso to a height that is comfortable for you.

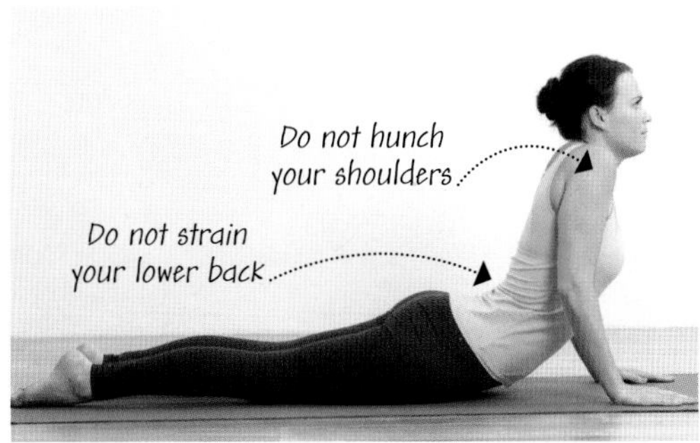

Do not hunch your shoulders
Do not strain your lower back

Make it easier

Practice the Baby Cobra pose—place your elbows parallel to your shoulders and the lower arms flat on the mat. Inhale to raise your chest, shoulders, and head into a "Sphinx" shape. Look forward and hold for five to ten breaths.

To release tension in the neck, inhale and rotate your head 90 degrees. Hold for one to two breaths and repeat on the other side.

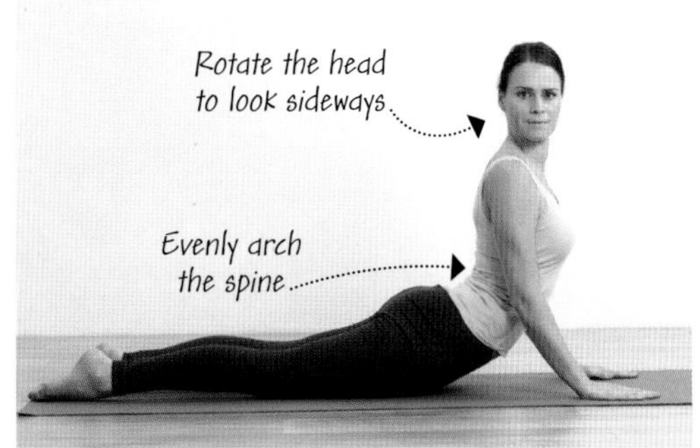

Rotate the head to look sideways
Evenly arch the spine

Child's Pose

Calm Mind • **Relax** Neck and Back Tension

This relaxing pose provides a counter-stretch to backward bends and recharges the muscles by normalizing circulation after inversions. The Child's Pose can be used either to prepare for, or recover from, any pose.

1 Kneel on the floor, with your big toes touching. Sit back on your heels, keeping your knees hip-width apart and your spine straight. Clasp one wrist with the other hand.

Useful tip Soften your facial muscles and release tension in your shoulders.

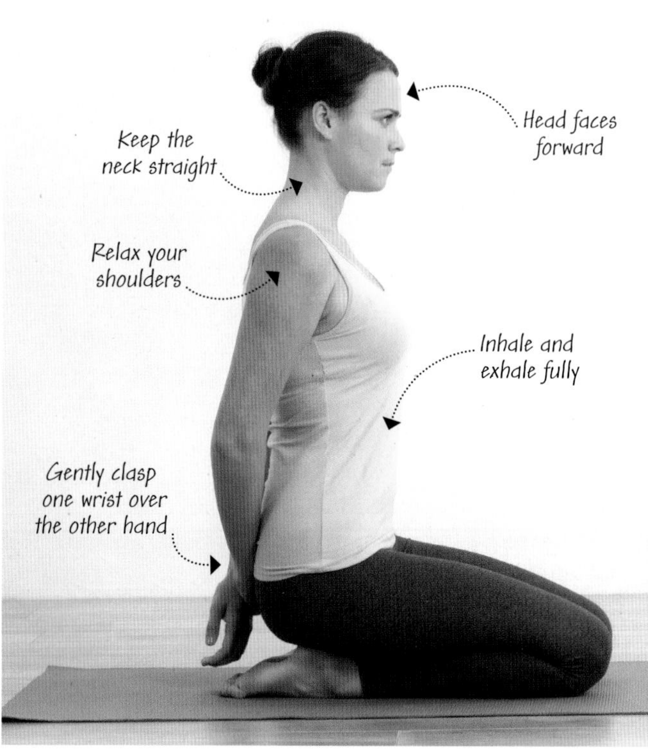
Head faces forward
Keep the neck straight
Relax your shoulders
Inhale and exhale fully
Gently clasp one wrist over the other hand

Make it easier

If you cannot get your forehead to rest on the mat, use a cushion instead (see right). Ensure that your nostrils are not pressed into the cushion as this will restrict your breathing.

If the compression in the belly is uncomfortable, then take your knees and feet about 2–4in (5–10cm) apart to reduce the pressure on your abdomen.

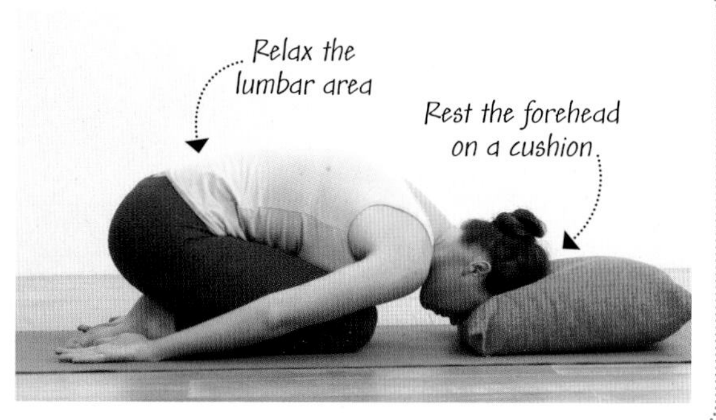
Relax the lumbar area
Rest the forehead on a cushion

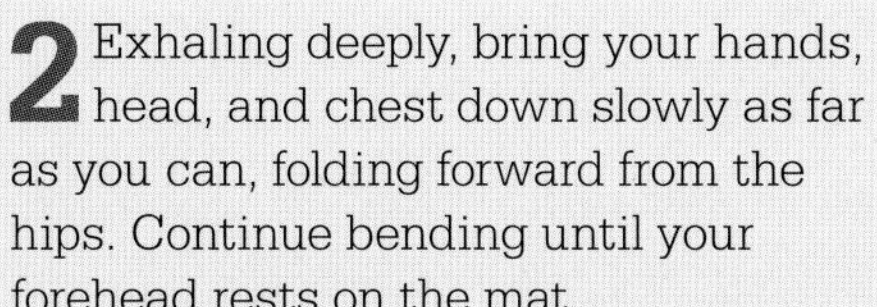

2 Exhaling deeply, bring your hands, head, and chest down slowly as far as you can, folding forward from the hips. Continue bending until your forehead rests on the mat.

Useful tip Broaden the sacrum and pull the shoulder blades wide to nestle the chest and belly on your thighs.

Feel the breath at the back of the ribcage

Touch your forehead onto the mat

Relax the lower legs and feet

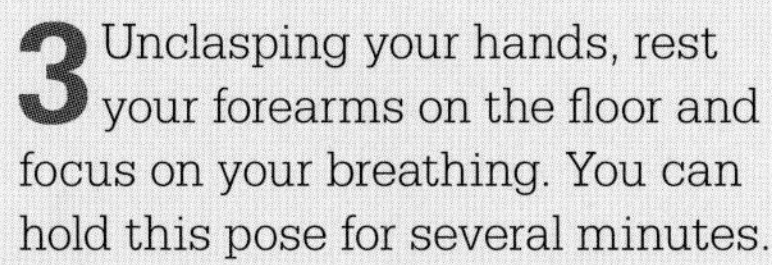

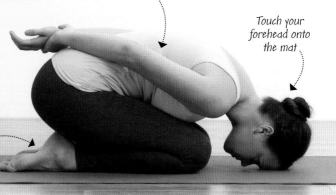

3 Unclasping your hands, rest your forearms on the floor and focus on your breathing. You can hold this pose for several minutes.

Useful tip Relax your back muscles to lengthen the spine into a dome shape.

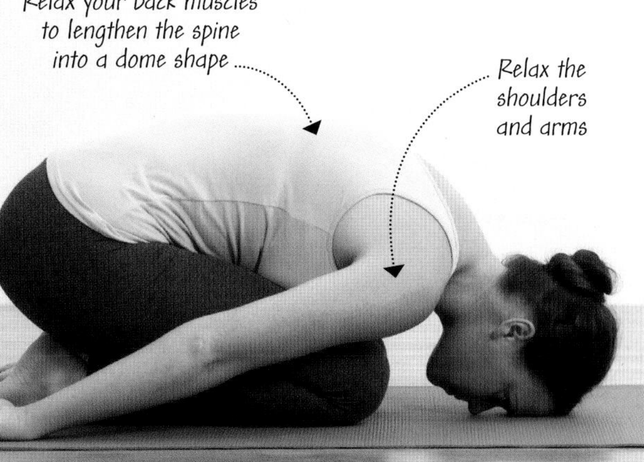
Relax your back muscles to lengthen the spine into a dome shape
Relax the shoulders and arms

Sun Salutation

Build Strength and Flexibility • **Increase** Harmony

Traditionally performed at dawn to greet the rising sun, this flowing cycle of postures warms the muscles, flexes the spine, and synchronizes the breath with body movements.

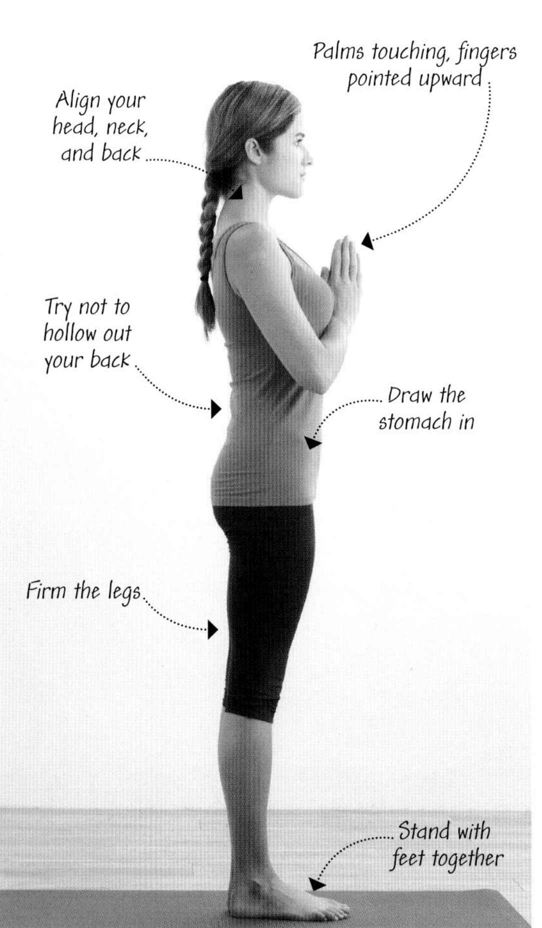
Palms touching, fingers pointed upward
Align your head, neck, and back
Try not to hollow out your back
Draw the stomach in
Firm the legs
Stand with feet together

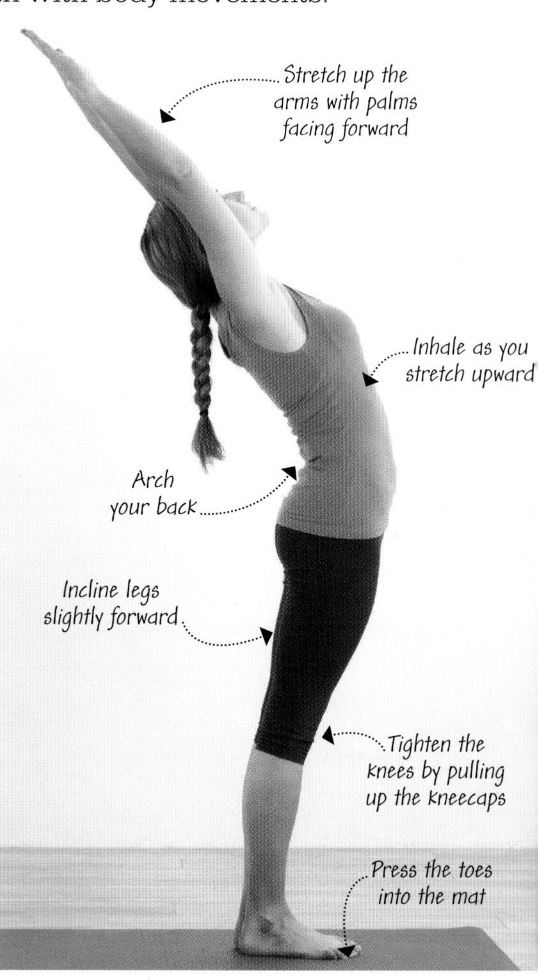
Stretch up the arms with palms facing forward
Inhale as you stretch upward
Arch your back
Incline legs slightly forward
Tighten the knees by pulling up the kneecaps
Press the toes into the mat

1 Start in Mountain Pose (see pp.44–45). Look straight ahead and focus on your alignment and breathing. As you exhale, bring your hands up into the prayer position in front of your chest. Firm your legs and root down through the feet.

2 Inhaling deeply, draw the arms up, palms forward, and bend backward from the waist, pushing out your hips and keeping the legs straight. Try to keep your shoulders relaxed and arms apart as you raise your hands.

3 Exhaling, bend forward from the hips, bringing the palms to rest beside the feet. Position the hands correctly as they stay in this position for the next seven steps. Keep the leg muscles fully engaged to support the downward movement of the torso.

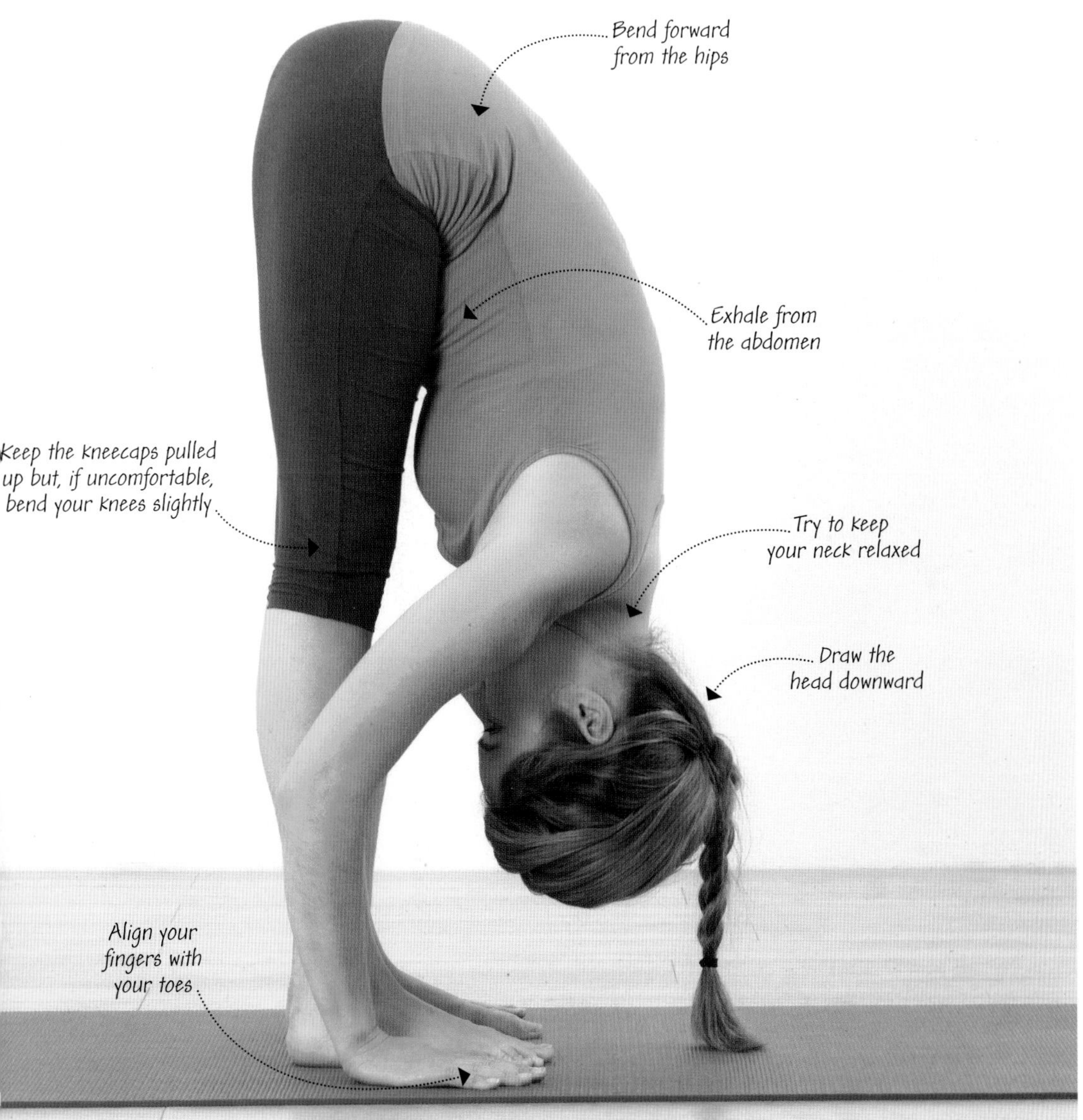
Bend forward from the hips
Exhale from the abdomen
Keep the kneecaps pulled up but, if uncomfortable, bend your knees slightly
Try to keep your neck relaxed
Draw the head downward
Align your fingers with your toes

4 As you inhale, bend your left leg and extend your right leg backward, resting your knee on the floor. Draw the shoulder blades closer together and steady the arms by pressing your fingertips on the mat. Arch your back farther by tilting your face upward to make a crescent shape with your body.

Useful tip Before stepping back, bend the knee of the right leg slightly.

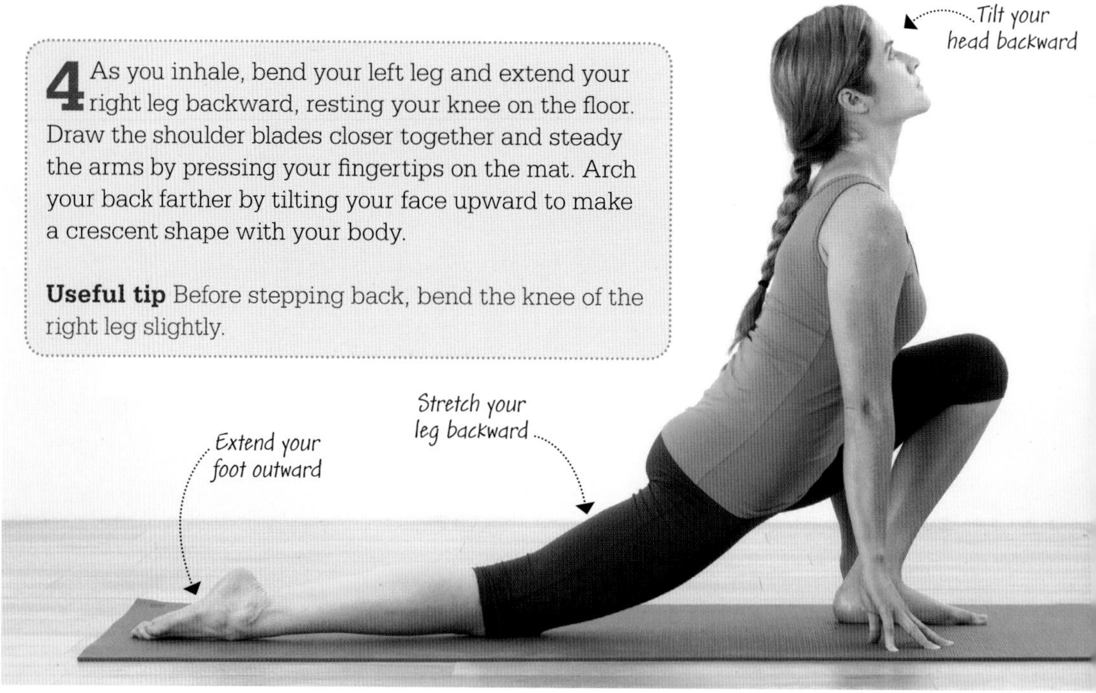

Tilt your head backward

Stretch your leg backward

Extend your foot outward

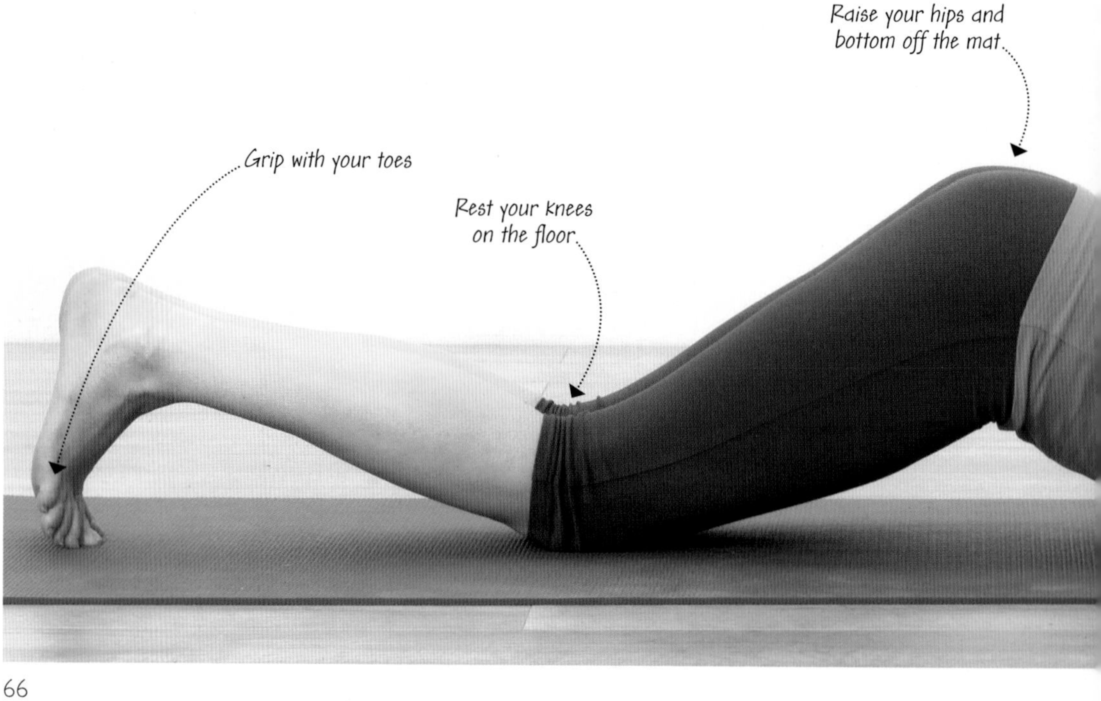

Raise your hips and bottom off the mat

Grip with your toes

Rest your knees on the floor

5 Retain your breath as you bring your other foot back so that your head, neck, legs, and back are in an inclined plane.

Useful tip Check that the palms are shoulder-width apart and the feet are hip-width apart.

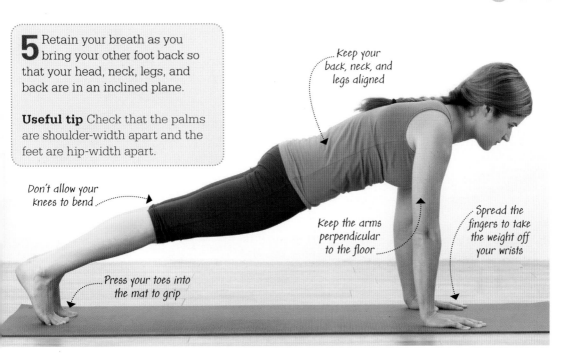

Keep your back, neck, and legs aligned

Don't allow your knees to bend

Keep the arms perpendicular to the floor

Spread the fingers to take the weight off your wrists

Press your toes into the mat to grip

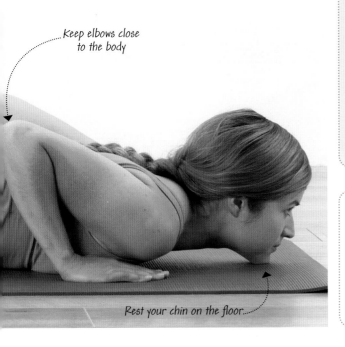
Keep elbows close to the body
Rest your chin on the floor

6 Exhaling, lower your knees to the floor. Aligning your shoulders with your fingertips, and with your toes turned inward, bring your head and chest down until they are also touching the mat, while keeping your hips raised.

Useful tip Keep your elbows close by your sides.

Make it easier

It may be difficult when learning the sequence to synchronize your breath with the movements. If you cannot execute a movement with the required inhalation or exhalation, then hold the position for a breath before moving to the next stage.

1 2 3

7 Inhale as you lower your hips and extend your feet backward. Raise your torso using your arms, and arch your upper spine to look upward. Try to keep your abdomen and legs relaxed.

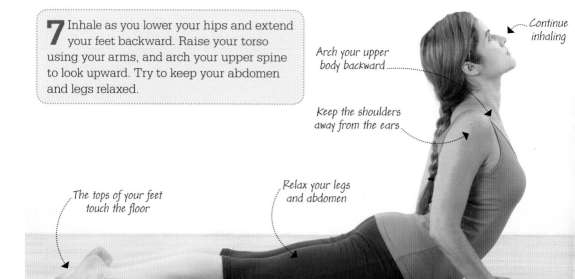

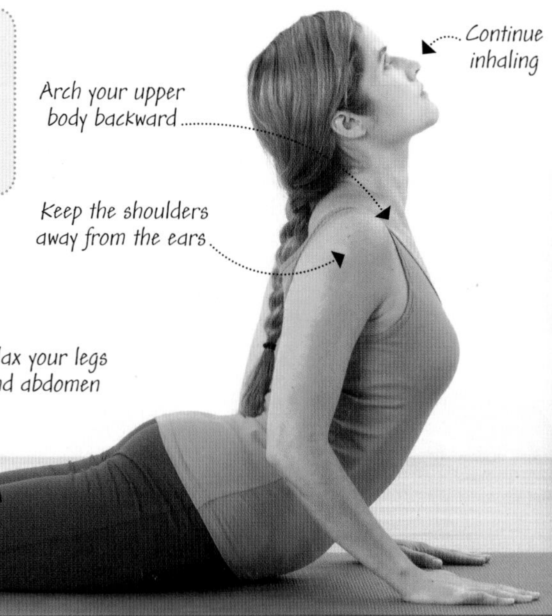
Continue inhaling
Arch your upper body backward
Keep the shoulders away from the ears
Relax your legs and abdomen
The tops of your feet touch the floor

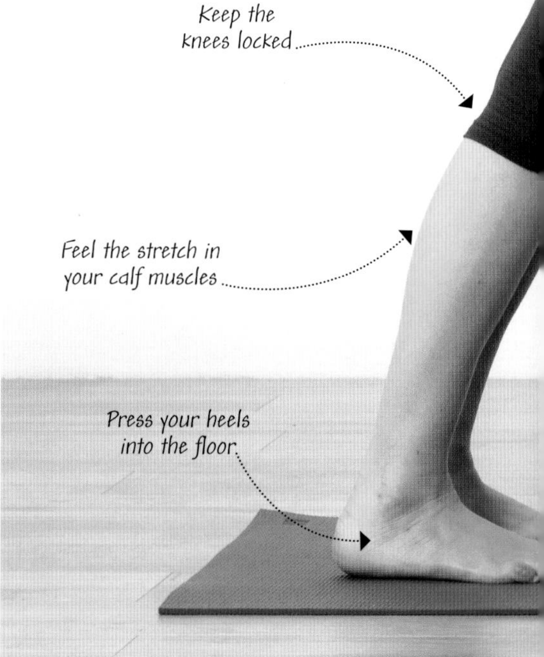
Keep the knees locked
Feel the stretch in your calf muscles
Press your heels into the floor

8 On exhalation, turn your toes in as you raise your hips high to create an inverted V-shape. Push your hips back as far as you can. Keep your back as straight as possible and the heels pressed downward.

Useful tip If your heels are high off the mat, move your feet forward to bring the heels down farther or onto the floor.

Take care...

There is a tendency in step 7 to tense the shoulders toward the ears and overcompress the cervical vertebrae by arching the head too far back. Flex at the elbows a little more to help draw your shoulders downward. Try to be aware of the position of your neck and head, and lengthen through the neck to tilt the head back gently.

A common mistake is to position your limbs incorrectly as you perform the sequence, which results in poor execution of the poses and misalignment. Try to practice each pose in turn. When you combine them all, start with your toes at the front end of the mat. In the final pose (see p.71), the feet should return to their original position.

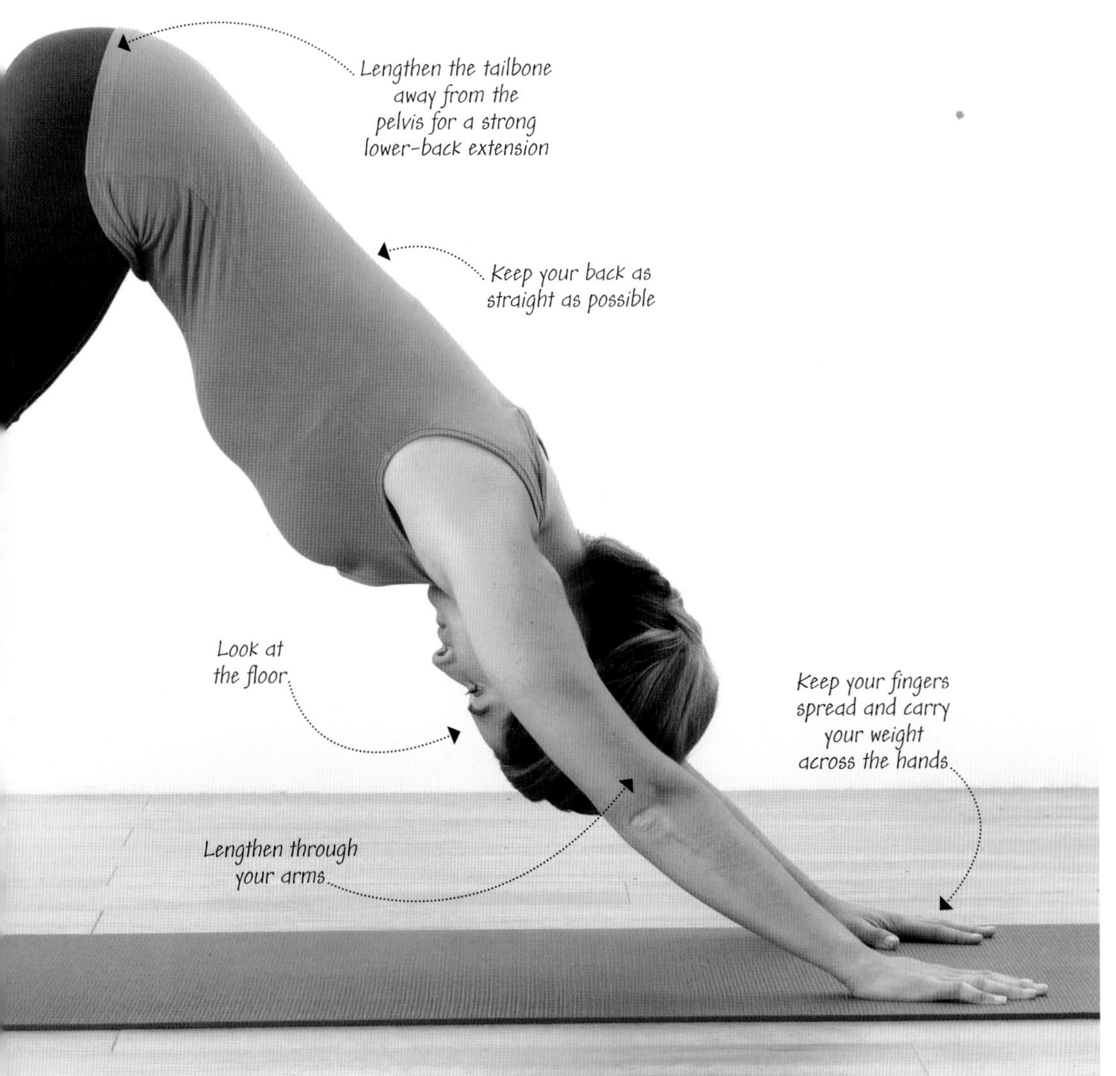
Lengthen the tailbone away from the pelvis for a strong lower-back extension
Keep your back as straight as possible
Look at the floor
Keep your fingers spread and carry your weight across the hands
Lengthen through your arms

9 Inhaling deeply, move your right leg forward, bringing the toes and fingers into alignment. Resting your left knee on the floor, arch your back and look upward. Press down on your fingers and right foot to anchor yourself.

Useful tip Relax the hips and draw them forward, leaning toward the folded leg. This gives a crescent shape to the body.

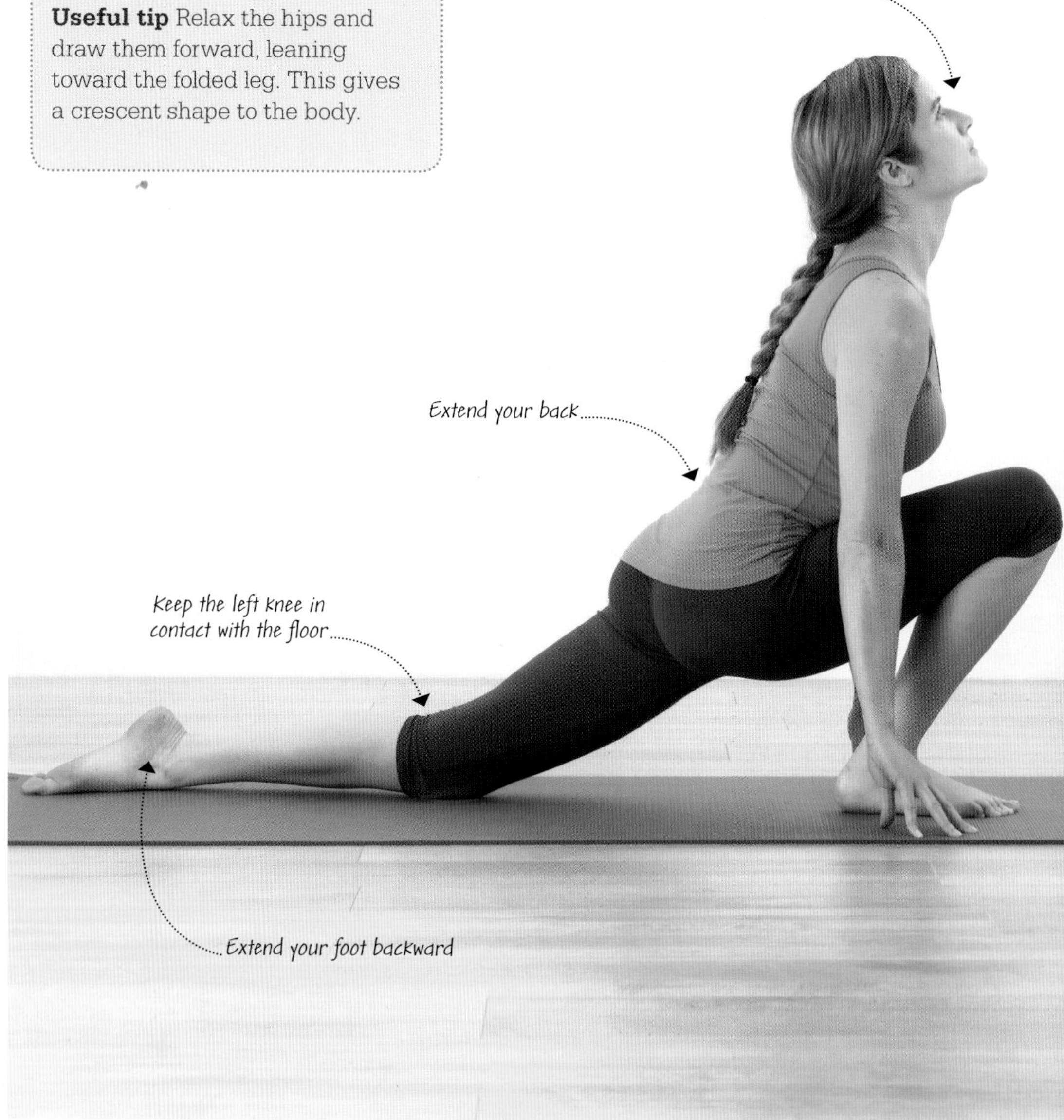
Turn your face upward
Extend your back
Keep the left knee in contact with the floor
Extend your foot backward

10 On exhalation, bring your left foot forward until it meets your right foot and straighten your legs. Bend forward as far as possible with your head touching your legs.

11 Inhaling deeply, straighten to a standing position. Draw your arms upward, then bend backward from the waist, pushing the hips out while keeping the legs straight.

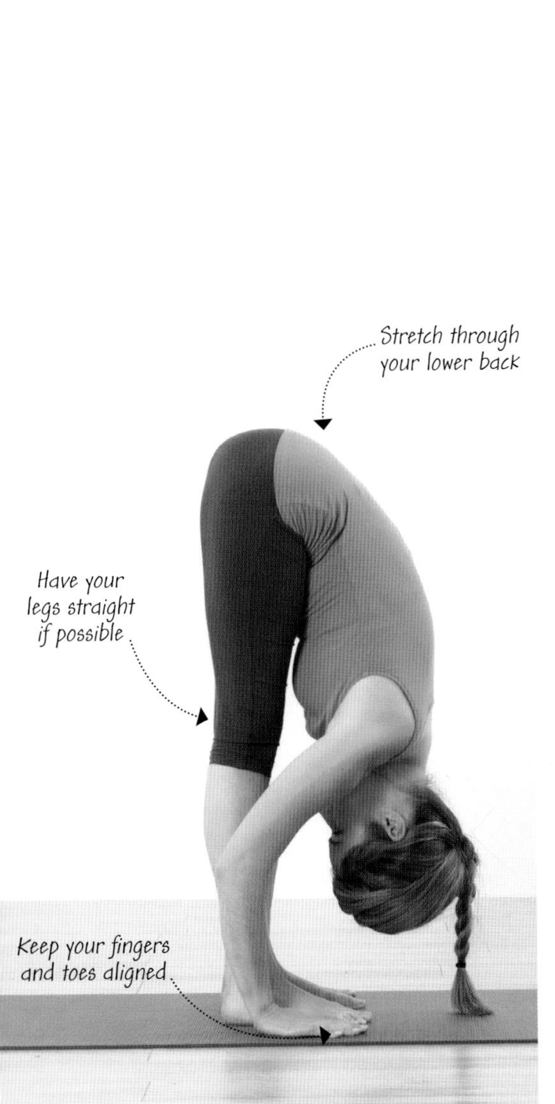
Stretch through your lower back
Have your legs straight if possible
Keep your fingers and toes aligned

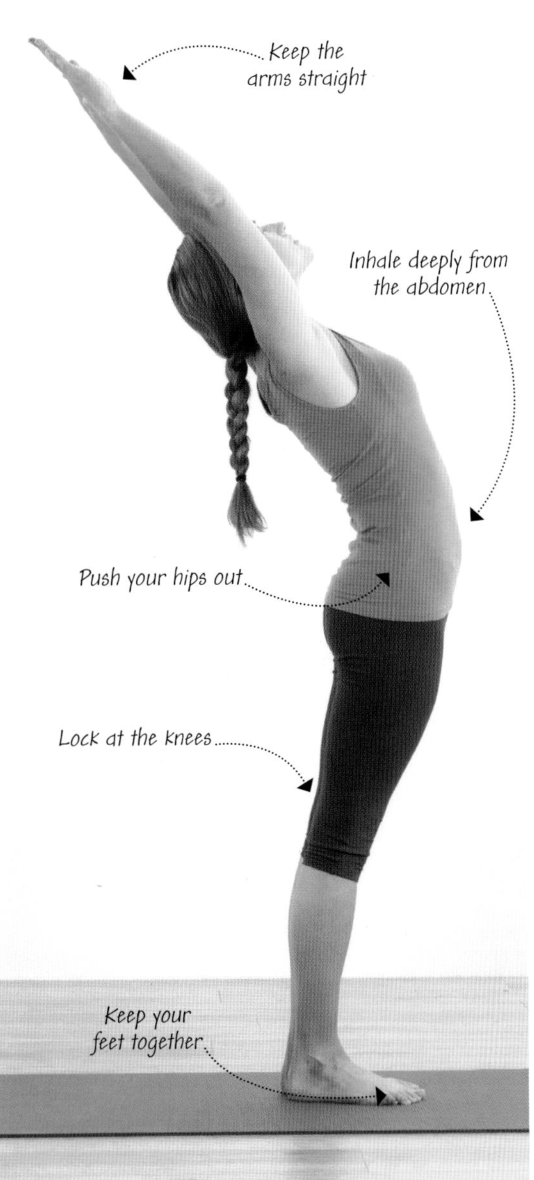
Keep the arms straight
Inhale deeply from the abdomen
Push your hips out
Lock at the knees
Keep your feet together

Easy Floor Twist

Relieve Back Tension • **Practice** Cleansing

This energizing posture stretches and relaxes the spine and legs to relieve built-up tension. Twisting the torso helps to reinvigorate and detoxify organs in the abdominal region.

1 To start, lie on your back with shoulders relaxed, arms away from the body, and palms facing upward.

Useful tip To prepare your spine for the twist, breath out any tension that you can feel in the back.

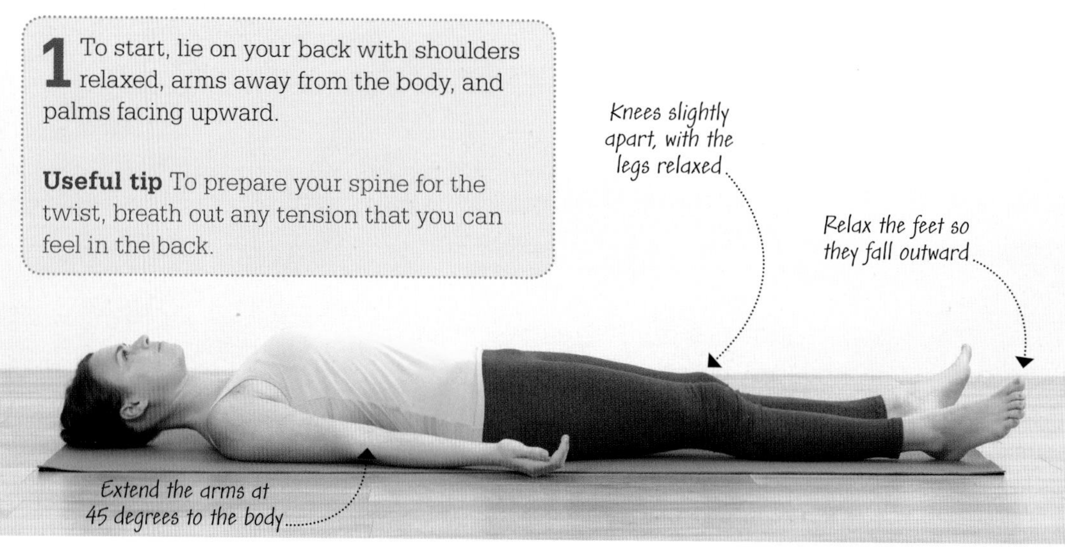
Knees slightly apart, with the legs relaxed
Relax the feet so they fall outward
Extend the arms at 45 degrees to the body

2 Bend the right knee so the toes are by your left knee. As you exhale, use your left hand to guide the folded leg over the left leg with the toes pressing into the left leg. Start to move your right arm away from the body.

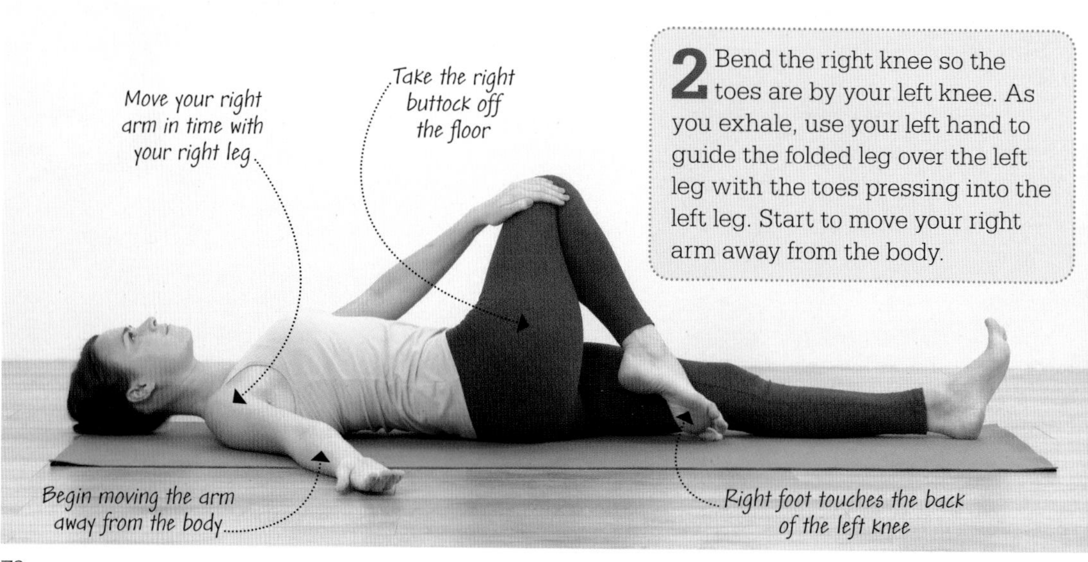
Move your right arm in time with your right leg
Take the right buttock off the floor
Begin moving the arm away from the body
Right foot touches the back of the left knee

3 Exhale again to rotate farther, bringing your right knee to rest on the floor. At the same time, stretch the right arm out at 90 degrees and turn your head in the same direction. Hold for five to ten breaths. Inhale to release and return to the Step 1 position.

Useful tip Gently press the folded right leg with the left hand to twist the lower vertebrae and encourage the right shoulder to root down, so continuing the twist through the upper vertebrae.

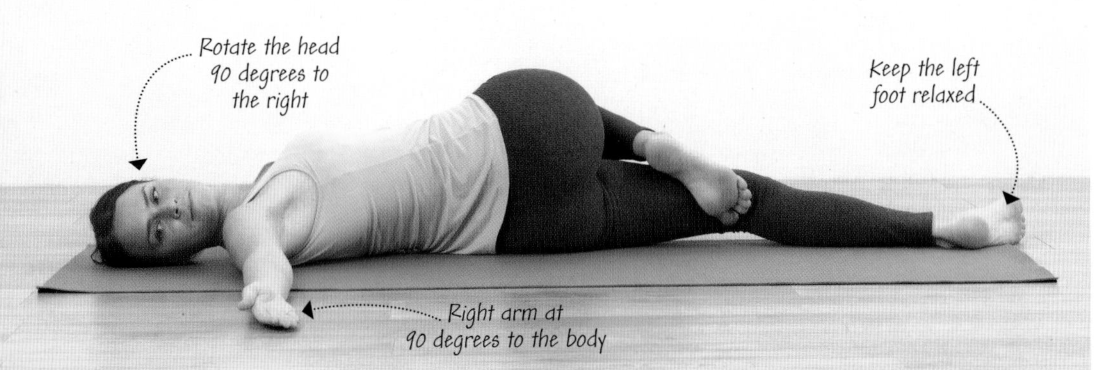
Rotate the head 90 degrees to the right
Keep the left foot relaxed
Right arm at 90 degrees to the body

4 Now twist in the opposite direction with the left leg rolling over to the right side and the left arm extending out from the side at 90 degrees. Hold for five to ten breaths. Inhale to slowly reverse the movements back to the start position.

Make it easier

Rest the knee of your folded leg on a cushion if you cannot comfortably place your knee on the mat.

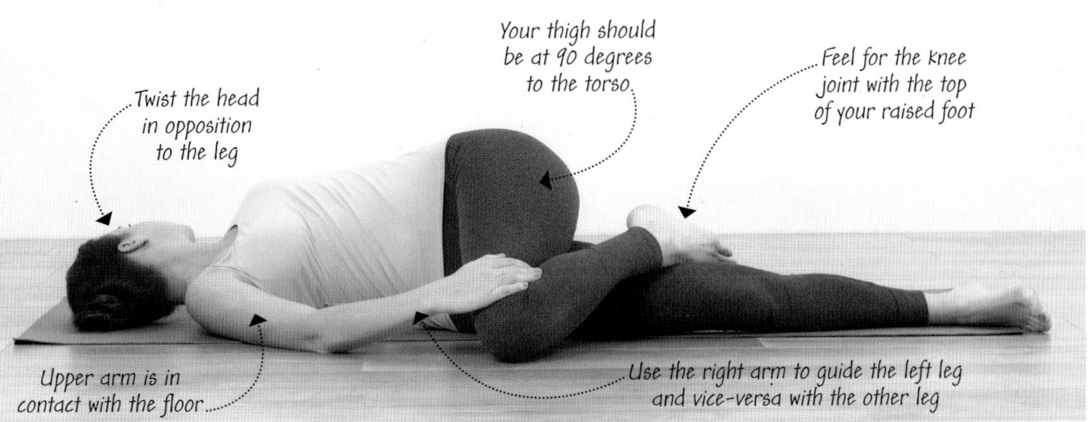
Your thigh should be at 90 degrees to the torso
Feel for the knee joint with the top of your raised foot
Twist the head in opposition to the leg
Upper arm is in contact with the floor
Use the right arm to guide the left leg and vice-versa with the other leg

Cobbler

Strengthen Hips • **Improve** Circulation

Aside from the benefits, such as opening up the hips and improving circulation, this pose helps to release tension in the hips, legs, and lower back, making it a great stress reliever.

1 Start from a sitting position with your legs extended in front of you. Bend your knees and draw your feet together until the soles are pressed together. Keep your back straight.

Useful tip Press your fingers or the palms of your hands down behind the thighs and lengthen the back. Inhale to draw the shoulders slightly back and open the chest.

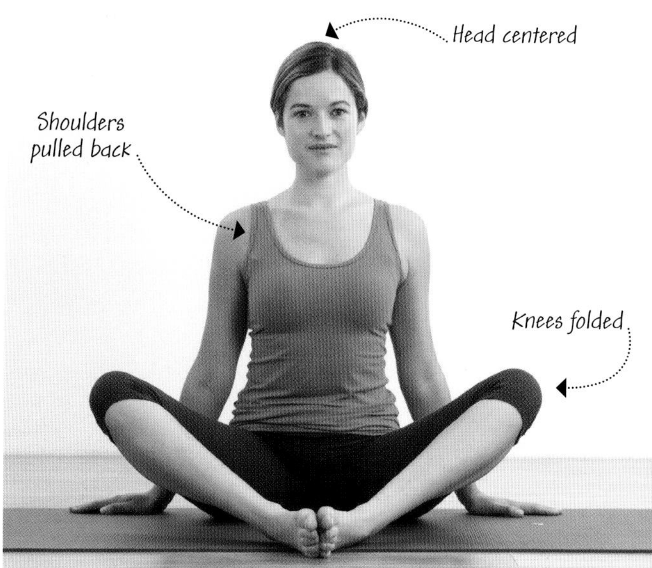
Head centered
Shoulders pulled back
Knees folded

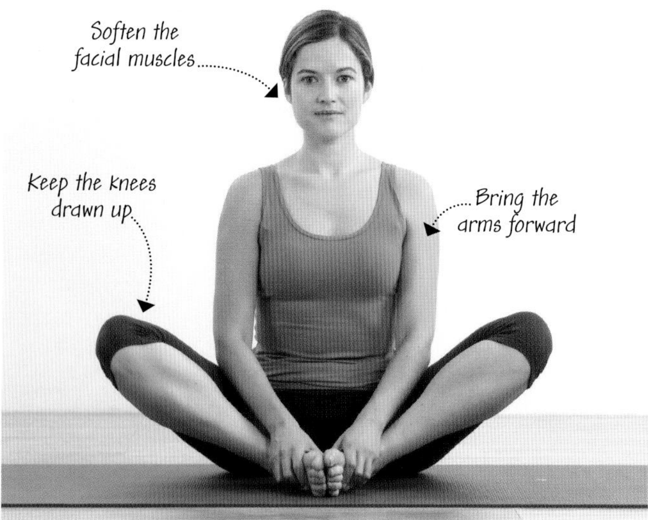
Soften the facial muscles
Keep the knees drawn up
Bring the arms forward

2 With your feet pressed firmly together, bring your hands around to the front of your body in order to clasp your feet. Keep your spine elongated and the head centered.

Useful tip To get a firm hold of your feet, tuck the thumbs into the arches of the feet and curl the fingers over the tops of the feet.

3 As you breathe out, gently draw your knees a fraction farther toward the floor, allowing the hips to open. At the same time, lengthen the spine.

Useful tip Hold your feet firmly with your hands to provide a central anchor to enable you to lengthen your back.

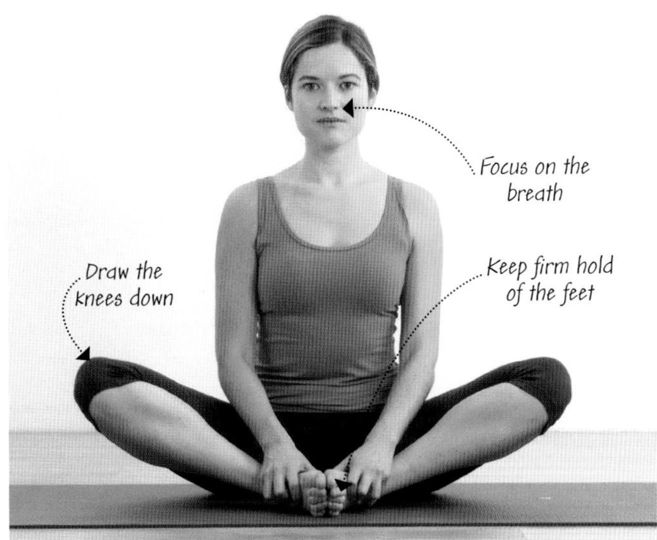
Focus on the breath
Draw the knees down
Keep firm hold of the feet

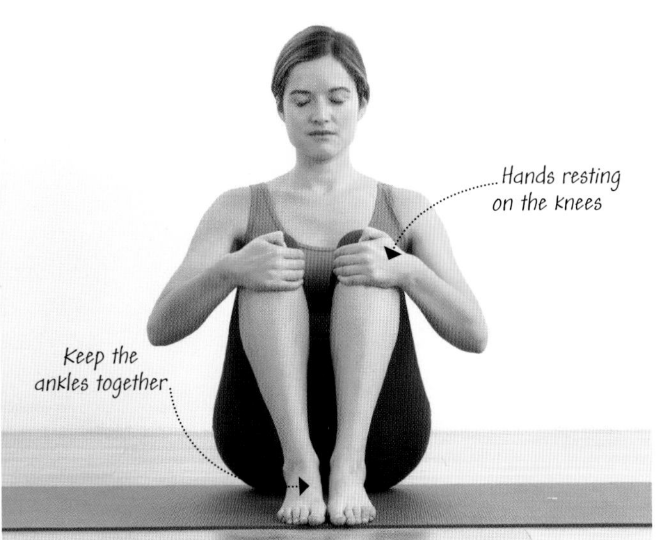
Hands resting on the knees
Keep the ankles together

4 To release the pose, raise your knees up to your chest while sliding your hands up to your knees. Rock yourself from side to side, feeling the stretch in your hip area.

Useful tip Use the palms of the hands to gently bring the knees close together.

Make it easier

Use a strap to provide extra pressure to keep the feet together. Loop the strap under the feet and hold one end in each hand, close to the feet.

If your knees experience pain, support them by placing a bolster under each knee.

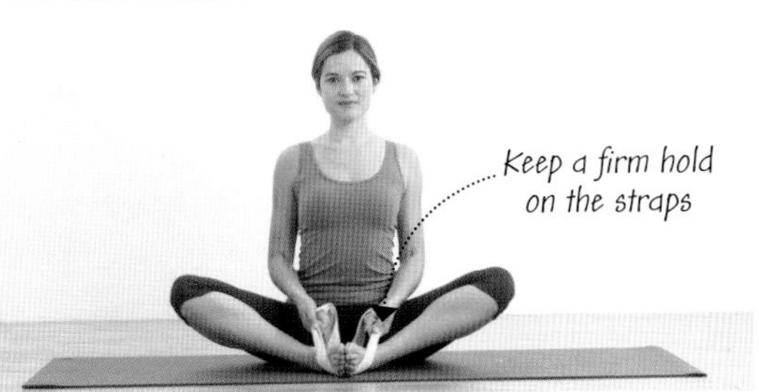
Keep a firm hold on the straps

Legs up the Wall

Tone Legs • **Improve** Circulation

In this pose, the upper body is fully supported and the legs partially so as they are extended upward. This pose is ideal as preparation for the more advanced inverted poses.

1 With hips and legs at an angle of 90 degrees, sit with your left hip and shoulder pressed against the wall. Rest your palms on your thighs.

Remember Keep a straight back and avoid leaning against the wall.

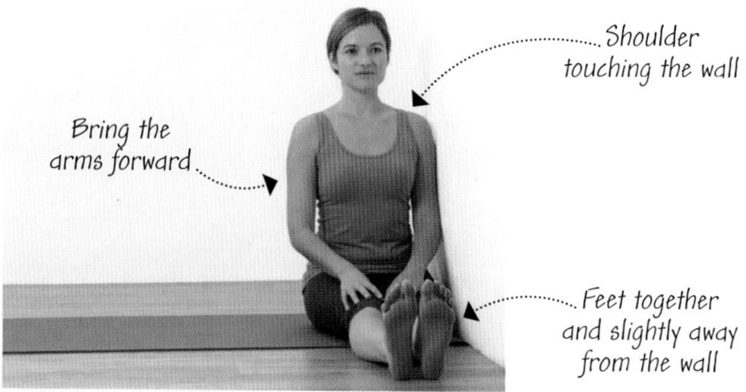
Shoulder touching the wall
Bring the arms forward
Feet together and slightly away from the wall

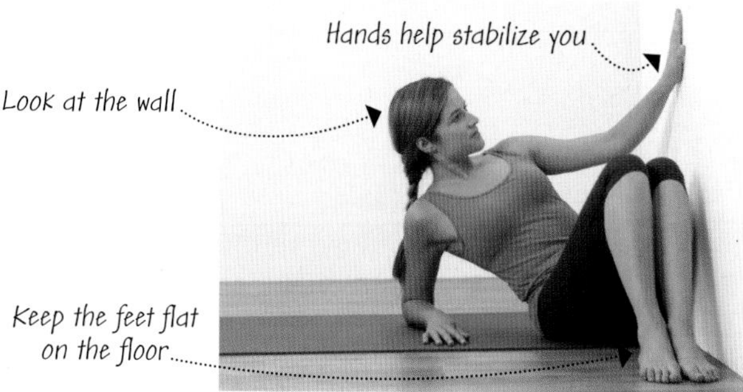
Hands help stabilize you
Look at the wall
Keep the feet flat on the floor

2 Place your left hand against the wall. Lean back, putting your weight on the right elbow, and draw up your knees.

Useful tip As you lean sideways, keep the feet and knees together.

3 Swivel your hips as you extend your legs up the wall and rest your back flat on the ground, hands on your stomach.

Useful tip Align the head with your feet so that the legs are at 90 degrees to the floor.

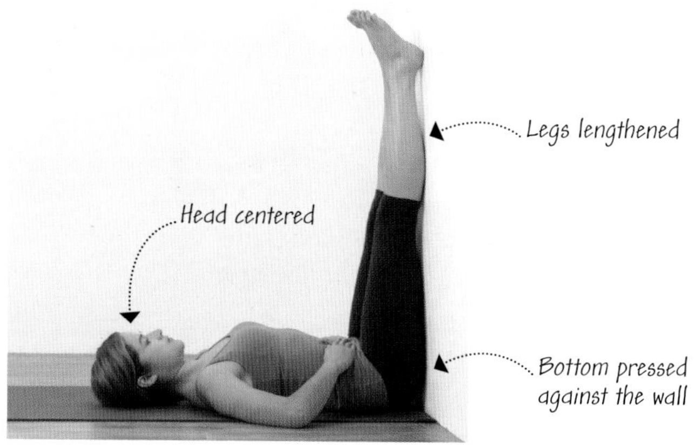
Legs lengthened
Head centered
Bottom pressed against the wall

4 Spread your legs in a V-shape while allowing your arms to rest by your sides, palms upward and fingers lightly curled. Keep your legs and heels against the wall. Hold for several breaths.

Useful tip Relax the arms, shoulders, and back. Soften the muscles of the face and inhale and exhale slowly.

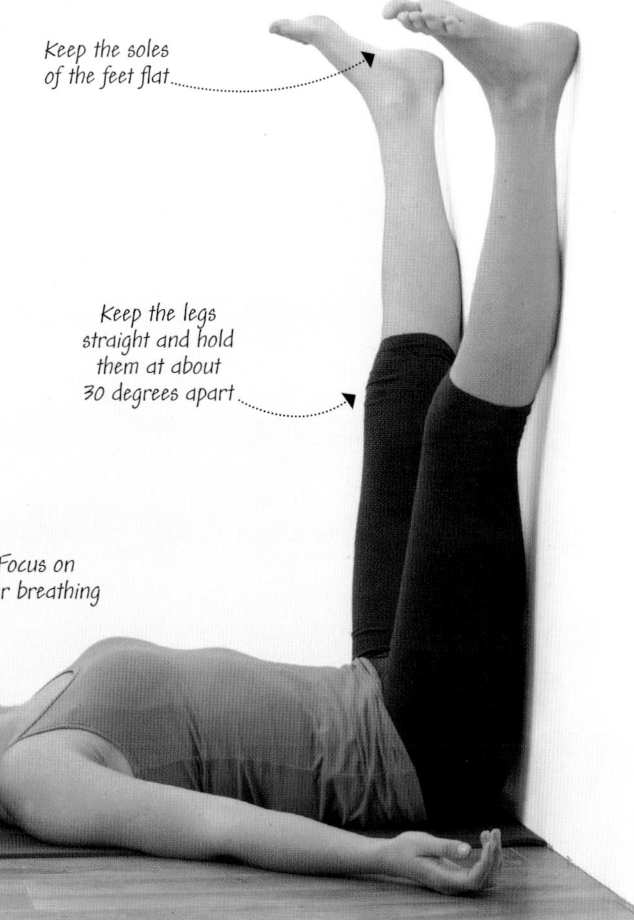
Keep the soles of the feet flat
Keep the legs straight and hold them at about 30 degrees apart
Focus on your breathing

Increase the stretch

Stretch the arms past the head, so that they are resting on the mat with your upper arms next to the ears.

The hips can be slightly elevated by placing a rolled towel under the lower back.

Take the legs farther apart, at about 45 degrees to stretch the inner thighs more fully.

Bend at the knees, sliding the heels down. Keep the feet hip-width apart and draw them down a little farther.

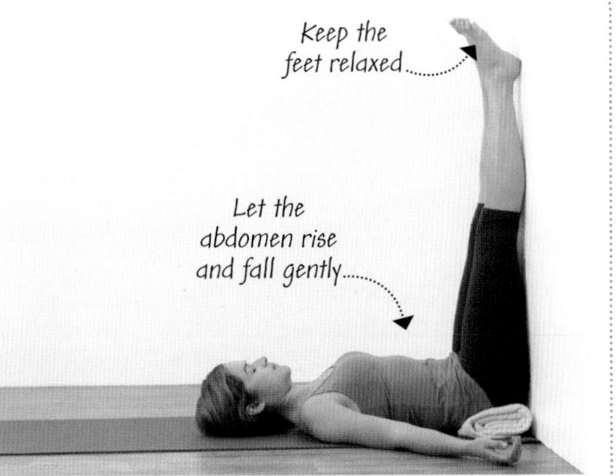
Keep the feet relaxed
Let the abdomen rise and fall gently

Corpse: Final Relaxation

Relax Muscles • **Energize** Mind and Body

In this pose the entire length of the body is aligned and fully supported by the floor, enabling all the muscles of the body to relax deeply.

1 Lie stretched out on the floor with your knees bent and feet flat on the floor. Interlock your fingers and place behind the head. Using the hands to assist, lift the head up to look at the knees.

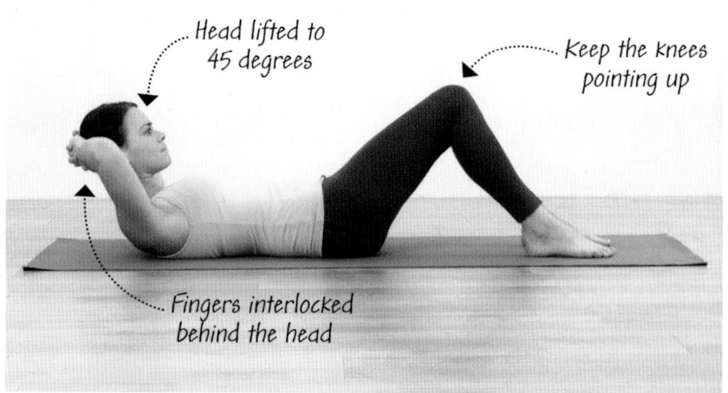
Head lifted to 45 degrees
Keep the knees pointing up
Fingers interlocked behind the head

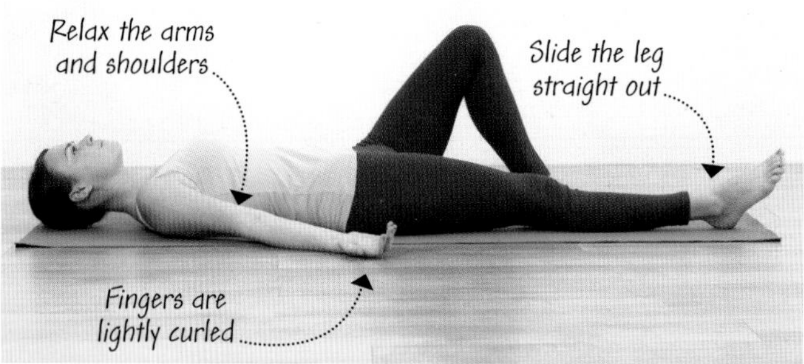
Relax the arms and shoulders
Slide the leg straight out
Fingers are lightly curled

2 Gently lay your head back on the floor and bring the arms to rest by the sides of the body. The arms are slightly angled away from the body and the palms turned up. Stretch each leg out in turn.

3 Lie fully extended and let your feet fall naturally outward. The limbs should feel fully supported, allowing all the muscles to relax. Close your eyes. Now, working from your feet to your head, ease away any tightness in your muscles.

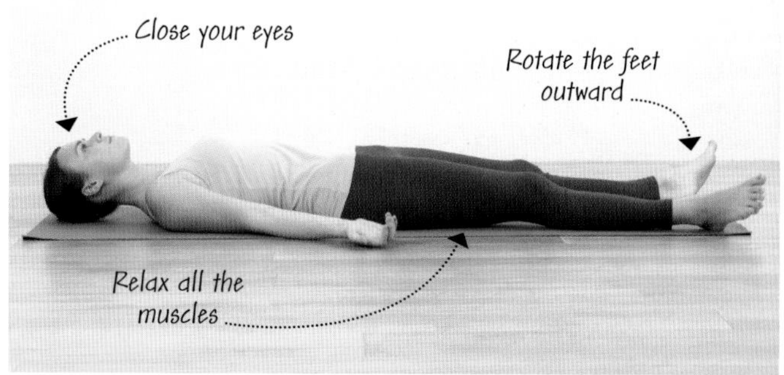
Close your eyes
Rotate the feet outward
Relax all the muscles

4 Inhale and lift your right leg about 1ft (30cm) off the floor. Tense all the muscles of your right leg only, keeping the torso and arms relaxed. As you hold for one breath, be aware of the tension. Exhale to lower the leg back onto the floor, relaxing all the muscles again. Repeat with your left leg.

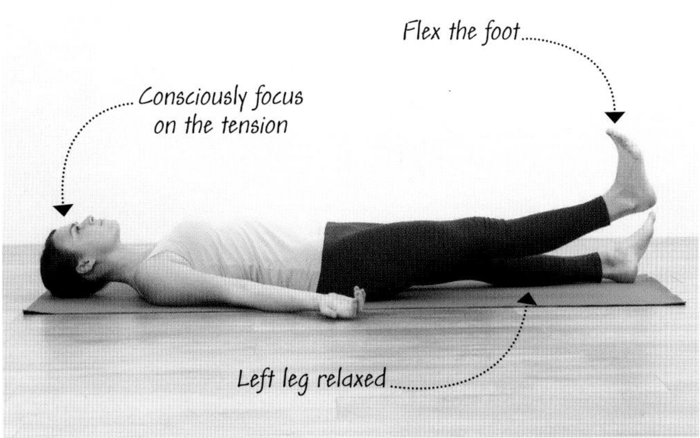
Flex the foot
Consciously focus on the tension
Left leg relaxed

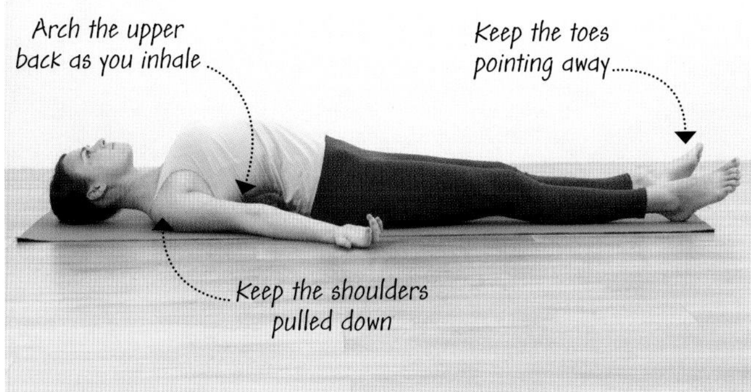
Arch the upper back as you inhale
Keep the toes pointing away
Keep the shoulders pulled down

5 Inhale and arch the upper back, pulling the shoulder blades closer to lift the chest and back slightly off the floor. Keep the head and bottom on the floor. Hold for a breath, observing the tightness in the muscles that have been activated. Exhale and relax back down to the floor.

6 Inhale to lift both your arms about 1ft (30cm) off the floor. Tense all the muscles in your arms, making fists with both the hands. Hold for one breath. Exhale to lower the arms onto the floor.

Useful tip Gaze upward and keep the muscles of the face soft and relaxed.

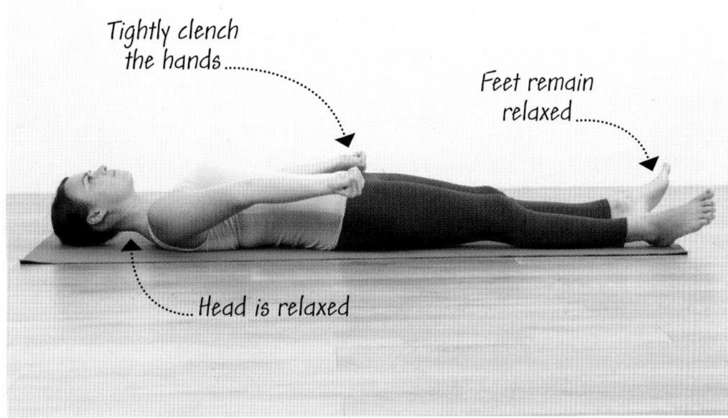
Tightly clench the hands
Feet remain relaxed
Head is relaxed

7 Inhale to lift both arms off the floor again. Tense your arm muscles, with palms open and fingers stretched apart. Hold for one breath. Exhale to lower the arms onto the floor.

Useful tip Extend the raised arms by pulling the arms and fingers away from the body.

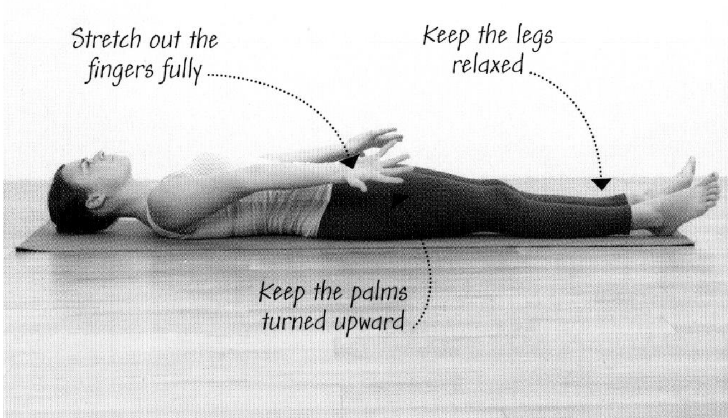
Stretch out the fingers fully
Keep the legs relaxed
Keep the palms turned upward

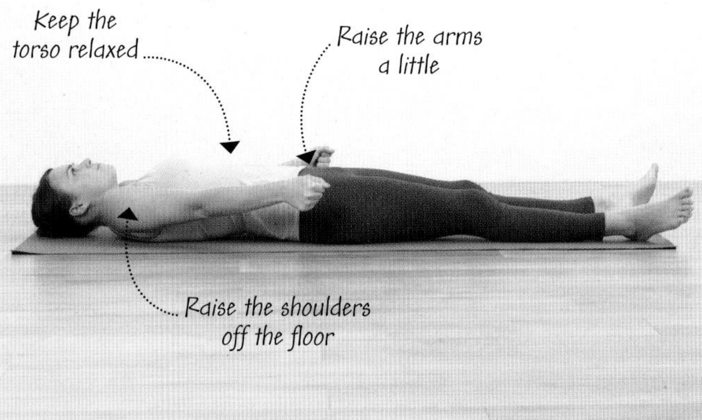
Keep the torso relaxed
Raise the arms a little
Raise the shoulders off the floor

8 Inhale to lift both your shoulders, hunching them toward the ears. Hold for one breath. Exhale to lower the arms onto the floor.

Useful tip Keep the head still and relaxed while the shoulders are consciously tensed.

9 Lie with every muscle in the body completely relaxed. Let go of all concerns and worries. With each exhalation, focus on the tension floating out of your body. Rest for a few minutes.

Useful tip Cover your eyes with a folded cloth or eye mask to help you deepen the relaxation.

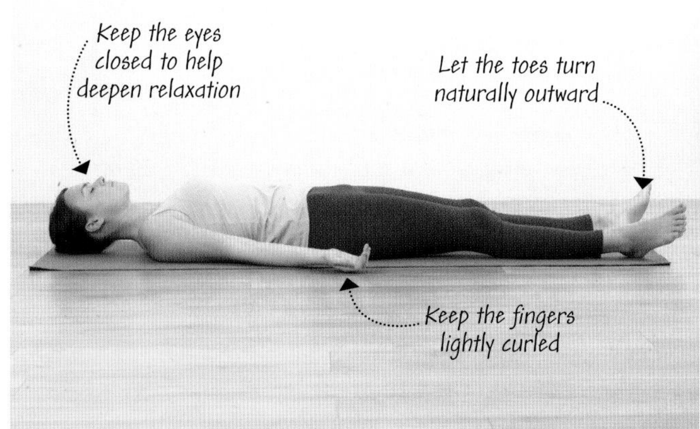
Keep the eyes closed to help deepen relaxation
Let the toes turn naturally outward
Keep the fingers lightly curled

10 When you are ready to come out of the relaxation pose, bend the knees and roll to rest on the side of your body. Stay here for a few moments and observe the effects of relaxing.

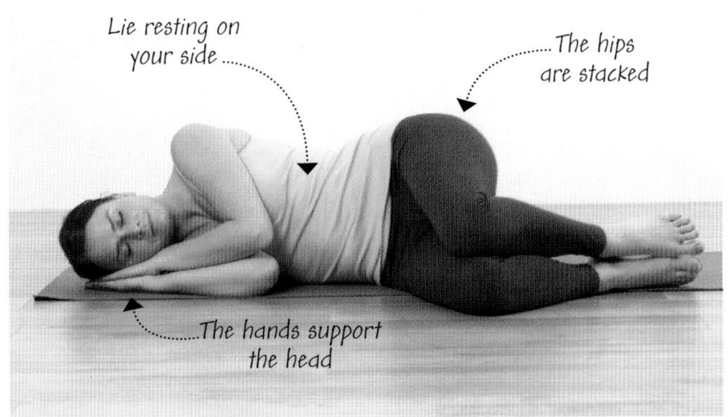
Lie resting on your side
The hips are stacked
The hands support the head

11 From lying on your side, use the hands to push the upper body off the floor and come into a kneeling position. Lower your bottom onto the folded legs. Bring your hands together in the prayer position. Focus on the internal calmness of the mind.

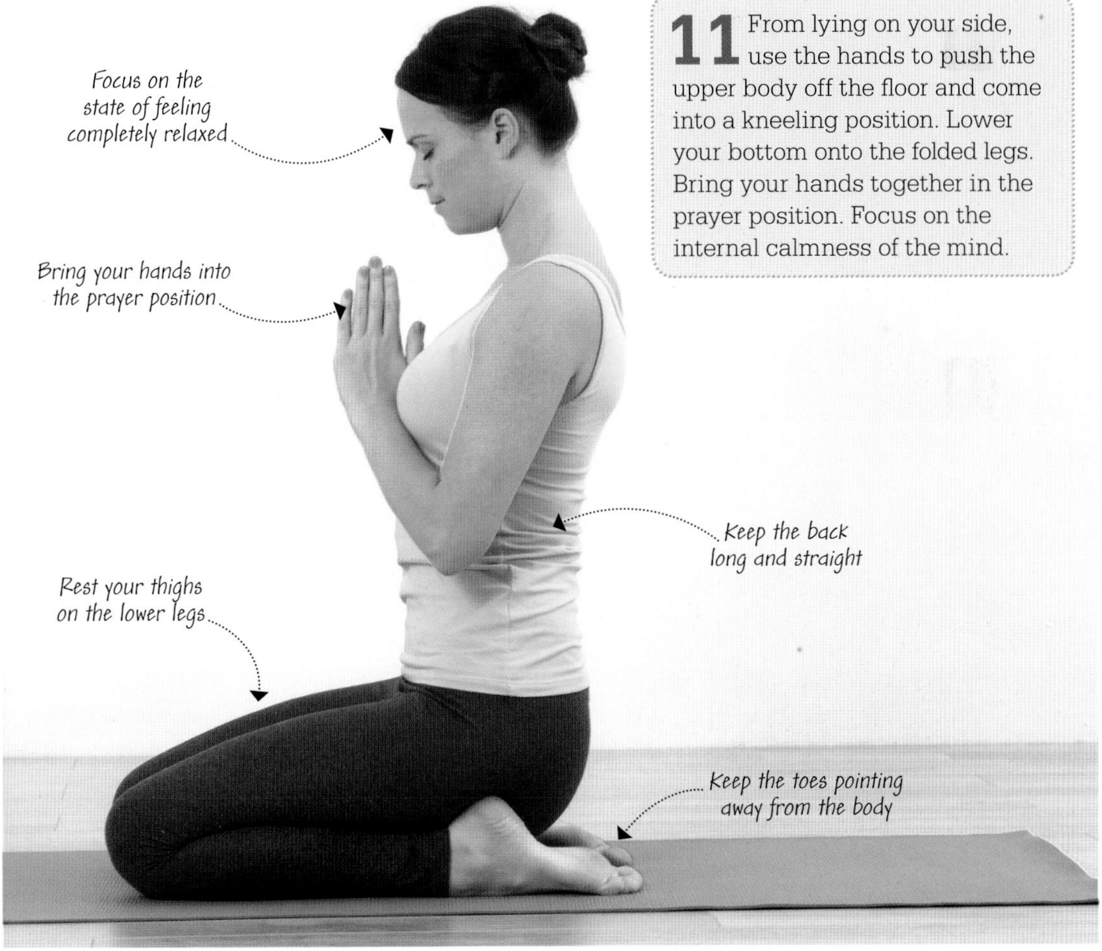

Focus on the state of feeling completely relaxed

Bring your hands into the prayer position

Keep the back long and straight

Rest your thighs on the lower legs

Keep the toes pointing away from the body

15-Minute Sequence

1 Mountain Pose
pp.44–45

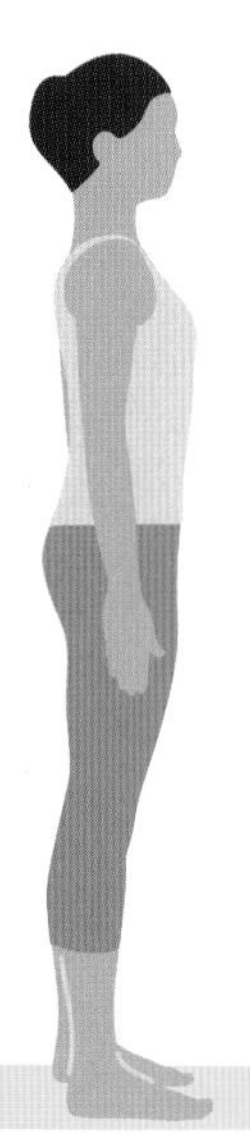

2 Standing Arm Stretches
pp.46–47

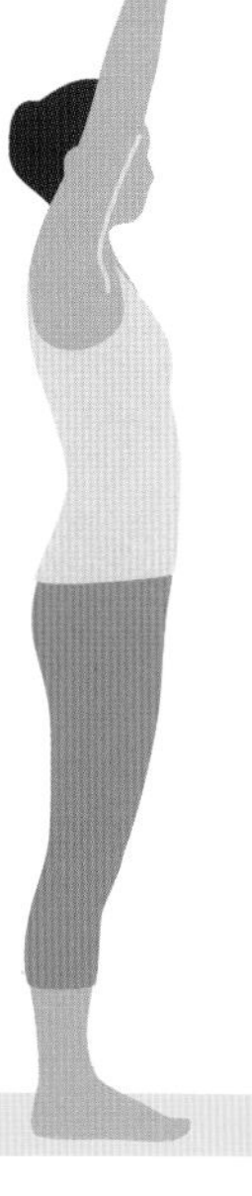

5 Downward-facing Dog pp.56–57

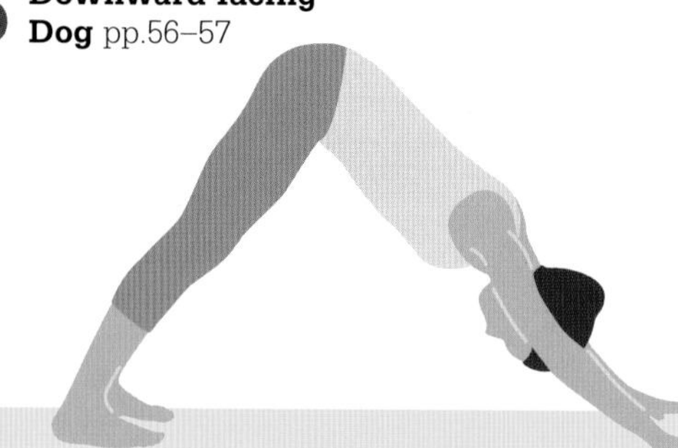

6 Child's Pose
pp.62–63

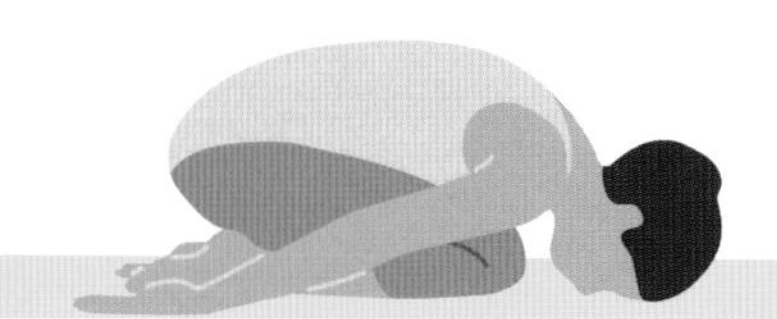

8 Easy Floor Twist
pp.72–73

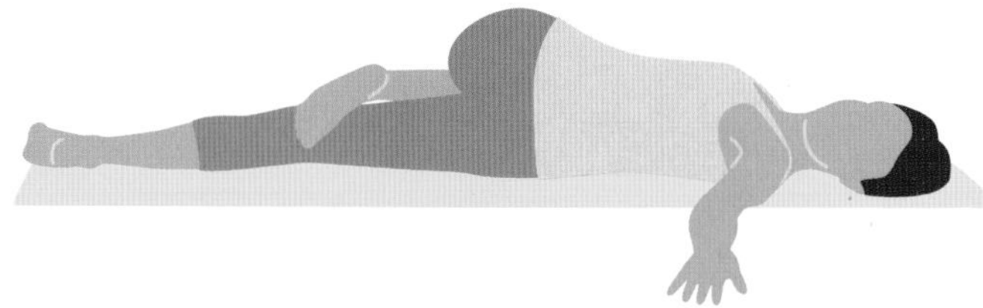

3 Triangle
pp.50–51

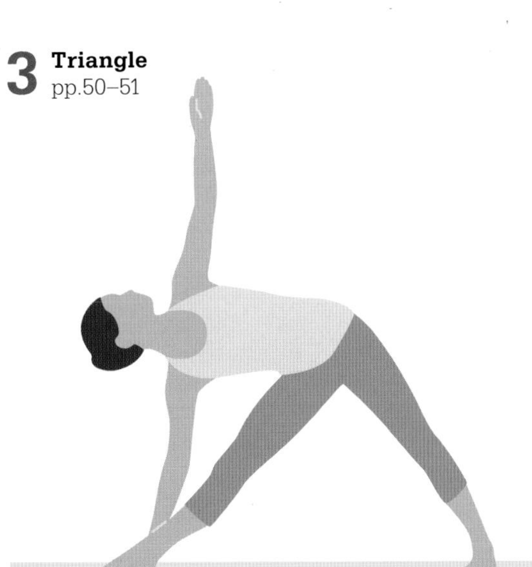

4 Standing Forward Bend
pp.52–53

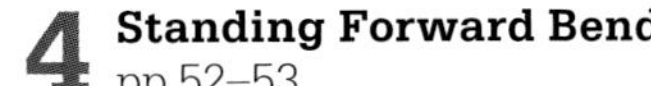

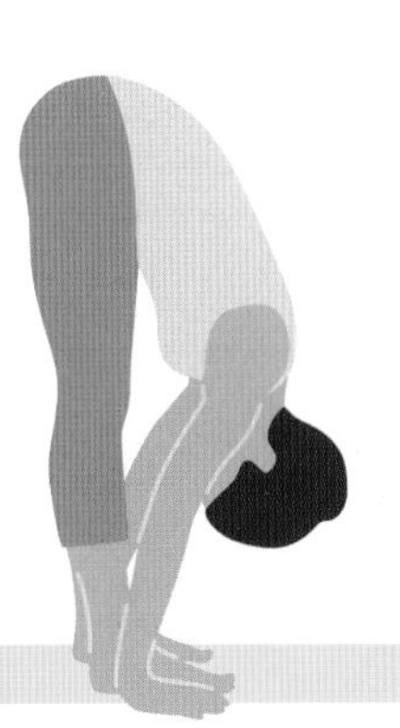

7 Cobra
pp.60–61

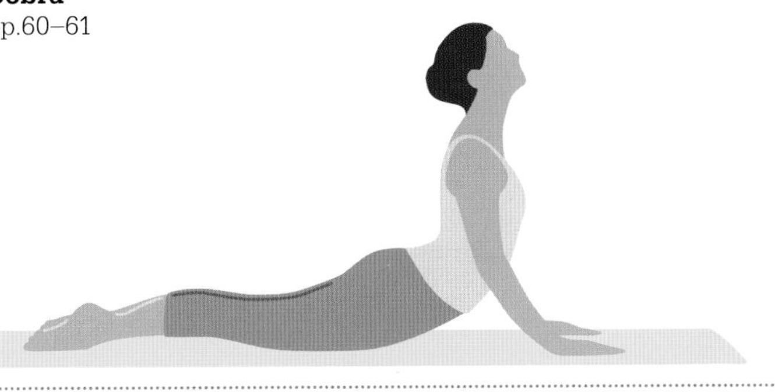

9 Corpse and Final Relaxation
pp.78–81

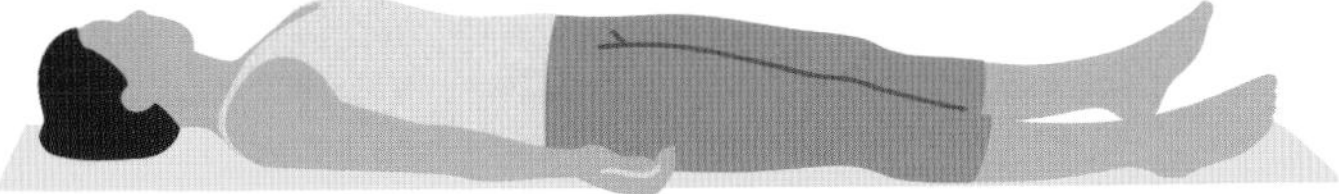

30-Minute Sequence

1 Sun Salutation
pp.64–71

2 Standing Arm Stretches
pp.46–47

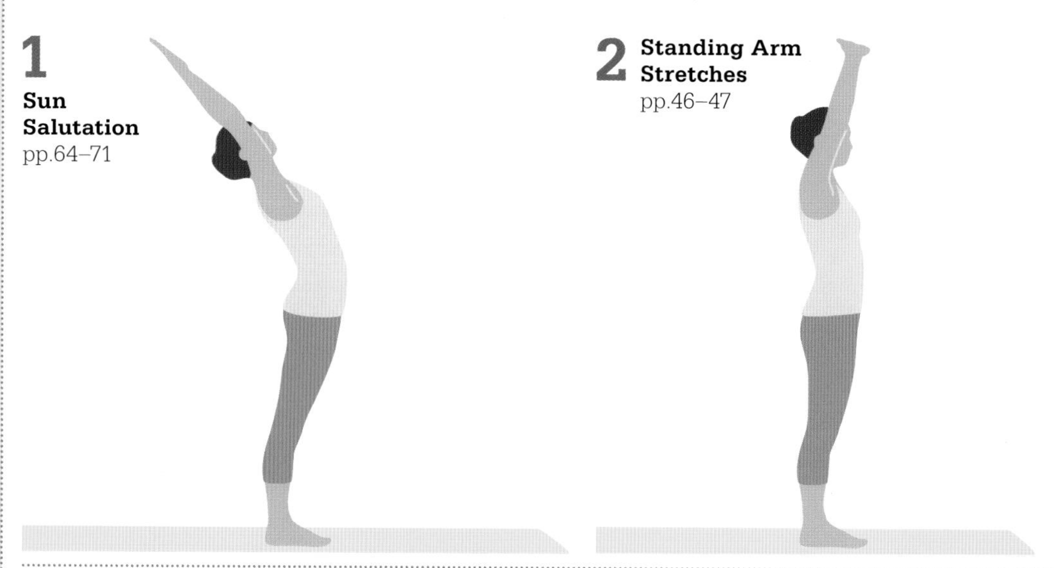

5 Diagonal Stretch
pp.58–59

8 Leg Raise
p.48

9 Easy Floor Twist
pp.72–73

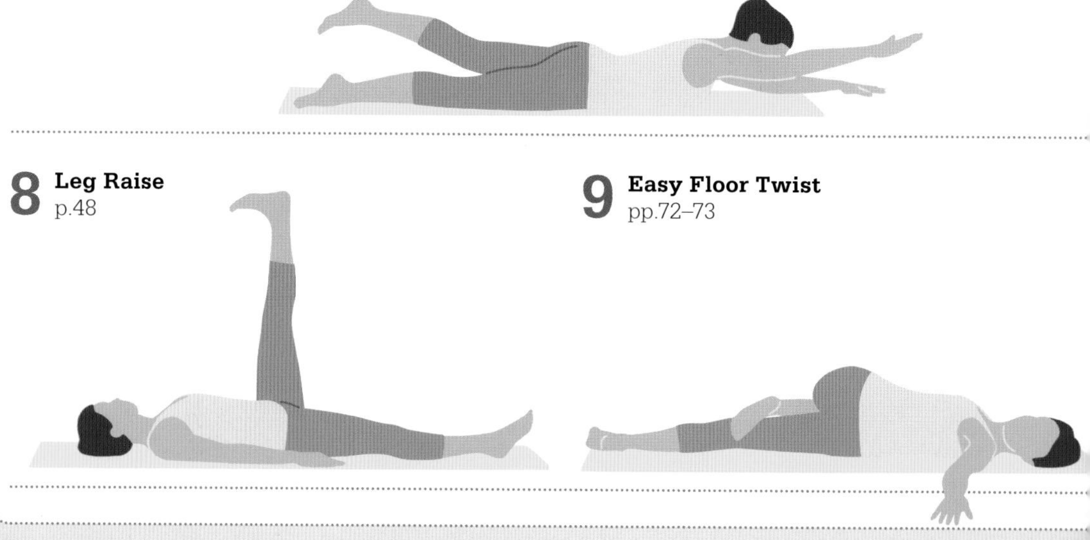

3 Triangle pp.50–51

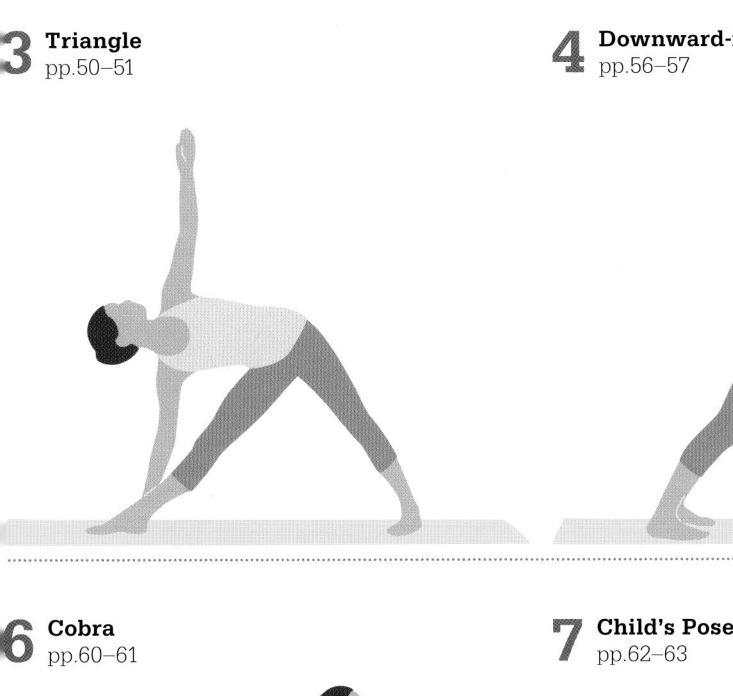

4 Downward-facing Dog pp.56–57

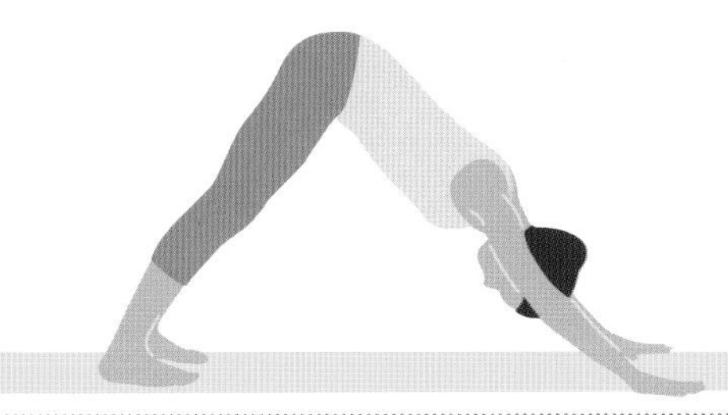

6 Cobra pp.60–61

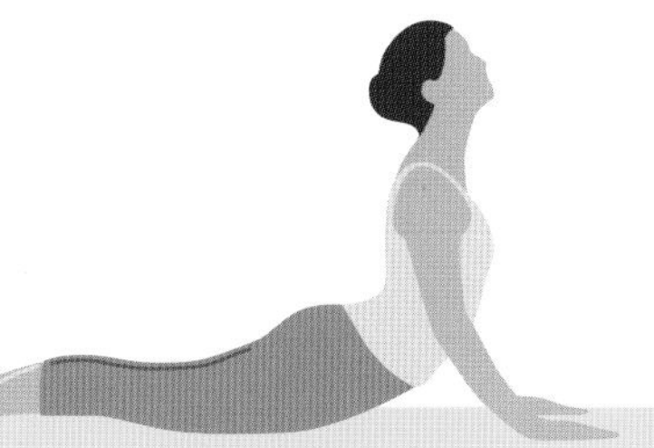

7 Child's Pose pp.62–63

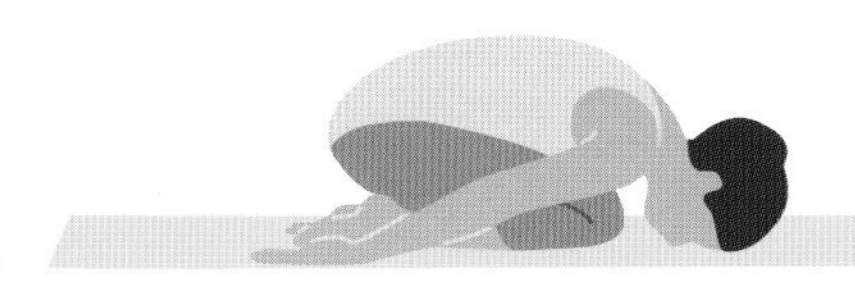

10 Corpse: Final Relaxation pp.78–81

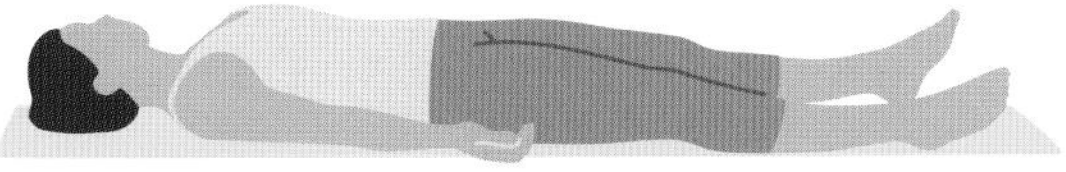

45-Minute Sequence

1 Sun Salutation × 2
pp.64–71

2 Standing Arm Stretch
pp.46–47

3 Triangle
pp.50–51

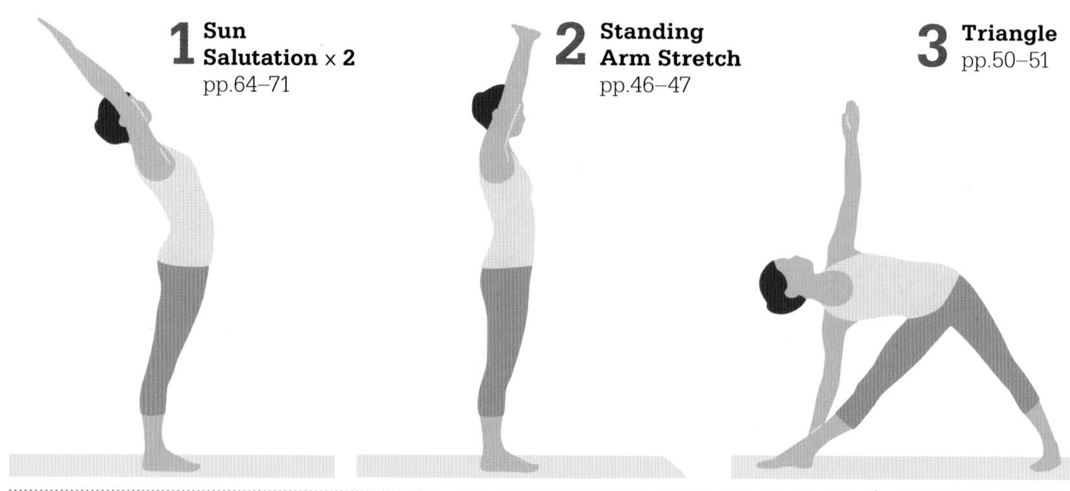

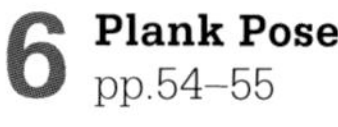

6 Plank Pose
pp.54–55

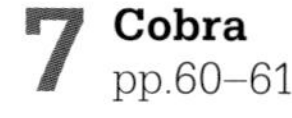

7 Cobra
pp.60–61

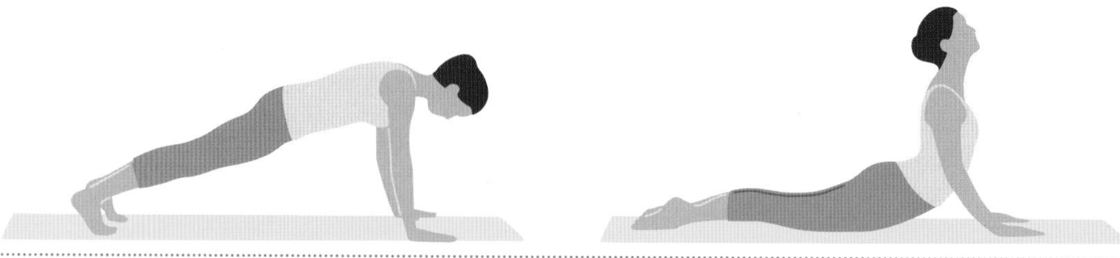

10 Cobbler
pp.74–75

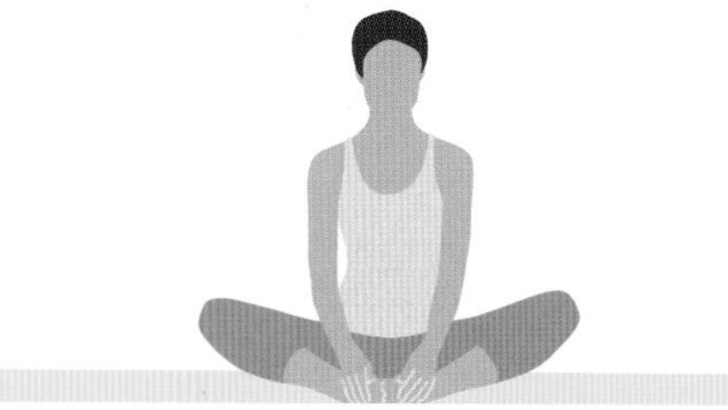

11 Legs up the Wall
pp.76–77

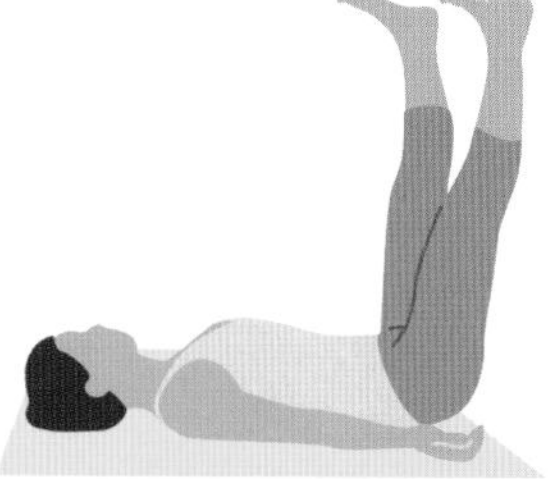

4 **Diagonal Stretch**
pp.58–59

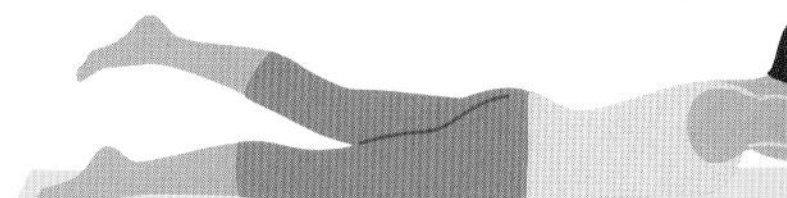
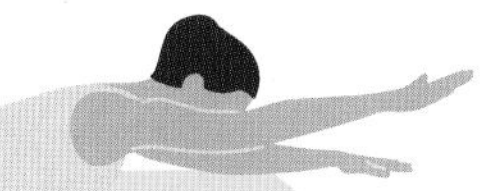

5 **Child's Pose**
pp.62–63

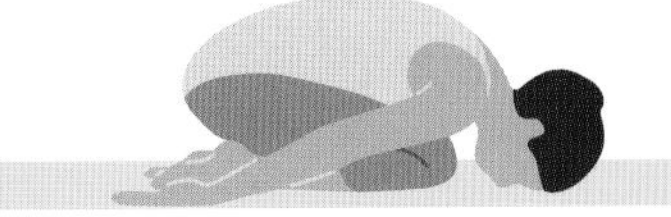

8 **Child's Pose**
pp.62–63

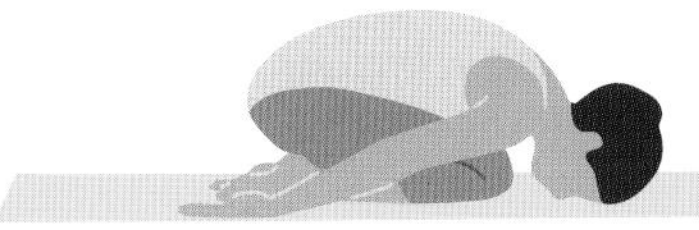

9 **Easy Floor Twist**
pp.72–73

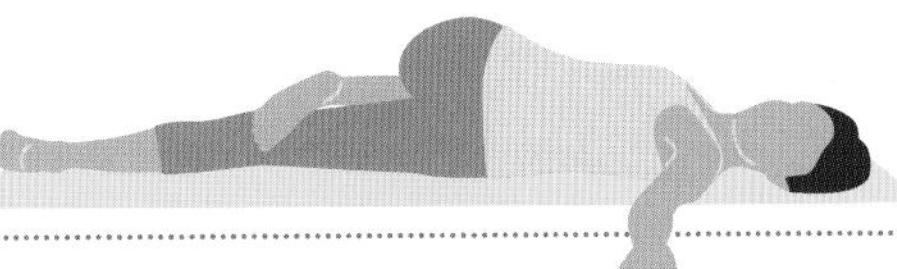

12 **Easy Floor Twist**
pp.72–73

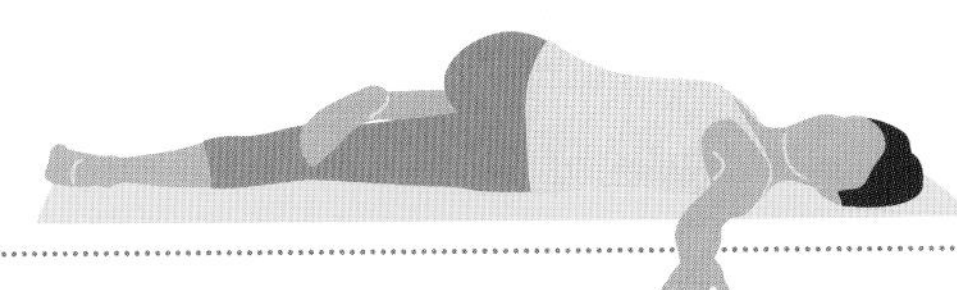

13 **Corpse and Final Relaxation** pp.78–81

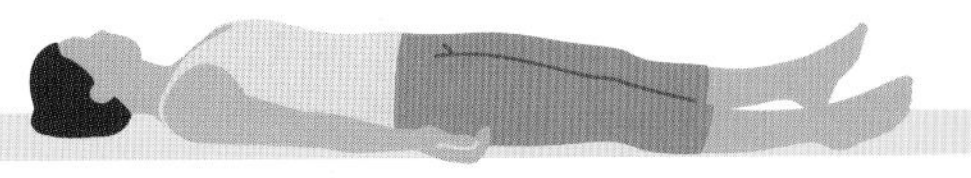

Assess your progress

Having explored the postures in the first section, it's worth taking some time out to reflect on the progress made so far. Yoga is a continual and open-ended process of self-improvement. By taking time to absorb and reflect on what you've achieved, you can build a firm foundation for future practice.

Reviewing your goals

The desirability and usefulness of goal-setting for establishing a benchmark of progress has already been mentioned. If you have done this, now is the time to look at your progress in a goal-orientated context. Have you achieved the targets you set for yourself? If so, you should be experiencing the satisfaction of a job well done. On the other hand, you may be experiencing the opposite—a sense of failure due to being unable to fulfill the goals you have set for yourself. It's most likely that you will experience elements of both success and failure as it becomes clear that some goals are easier to achieve than others.

Failure to achieve goals should not reduce your feelings of self-worth. Take time to review all your goals and think about why you were unable to achieve them. Then formulate a new set of goals that are more likely to be achievable. It is not uncommon to initially set goals that prove to be unrealistic because of the gulf between what was considered possible in theory and what is actually manageable in practice. It is important to modify goals before they induce a negative mindset. Remember, you are the one in control. Any goals you set for yourself are simply a means to an end rather than an end in themselves. There is no shame in starting over if you feel that would be best for you. Above all, do not feel under pressure to achieve your goals. Don't push yourself too hard, and pursue your practice as a way of reducing tension rather than causing it.

Perfecting the poses

As a student starting yoga, it is likely your practice will cause some stiffness and soreness in the joint areas—particularly around the spinal vertebrae and hips. This is actually a positive thing as it shows you are working on areas that have probably been neglected for a long time. Therefore building flexibility in these regions will be a very gradual process. For this, patience and commitment is needed.

It may help to list the postures that you are finding difficult and make sure that you are positioning your feet, hands, and limbs correctly. You may need to practice a modified version before attempting the full pose. Consider using supplementary equipment. The correct use of cushions, straps, and chairs may enable you to bridge the gap between where you are now and what you are trying to achieve. Even if you are already using supplementary equipment, it is worth considering whether it is being used in the most effective way.

Positive thinking

Always aim to review your progress in positive, rather than negative, terms, following the principle of positive thinking. Focus on what went right and what can be improved upon, rather than what went wrong. Yoga is a process of continual improvement. Through repeated practice, postures should begin to feel more natural as your positional awareness and flexibility begin to develop.

Keeping a yoga journal

If you have been keeping a journal of your progress, now is a good time to read it over. Notes on your physical and emotional responses to different postures will help you to produce a map of the self, leading to greater self-awareness and understanding of who you really are and what you want to be. This reflective practice will really help you to develop your practice. If you haven't kept a journal so far, then you should consider starting one. It is when facing challenges in your practice that the value of keeping a yoga journal becomes apparent. Your journal is a means of identifying, solidifying, and reinforcing your practice, thus making it fit for your own unique requirements.

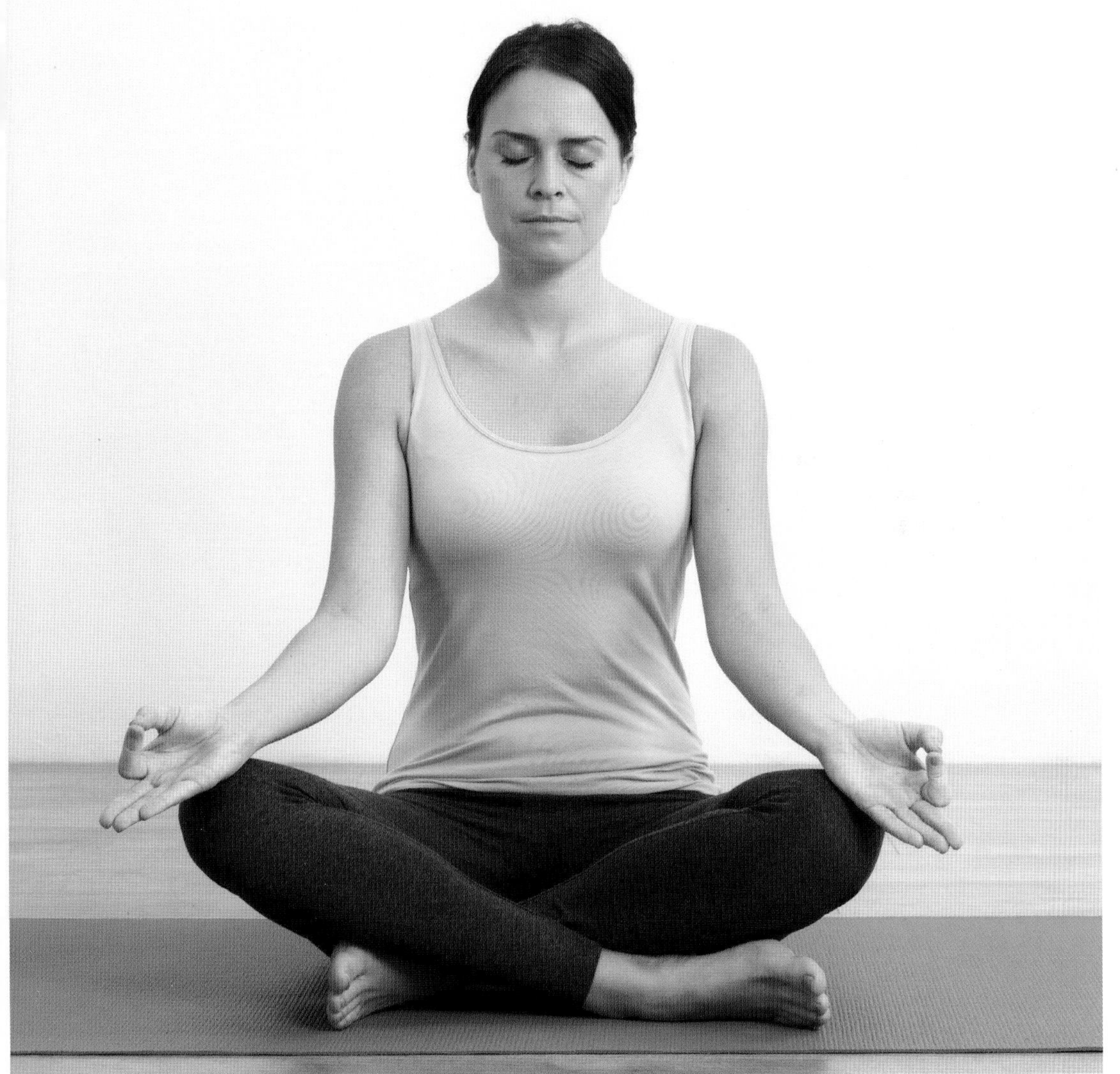

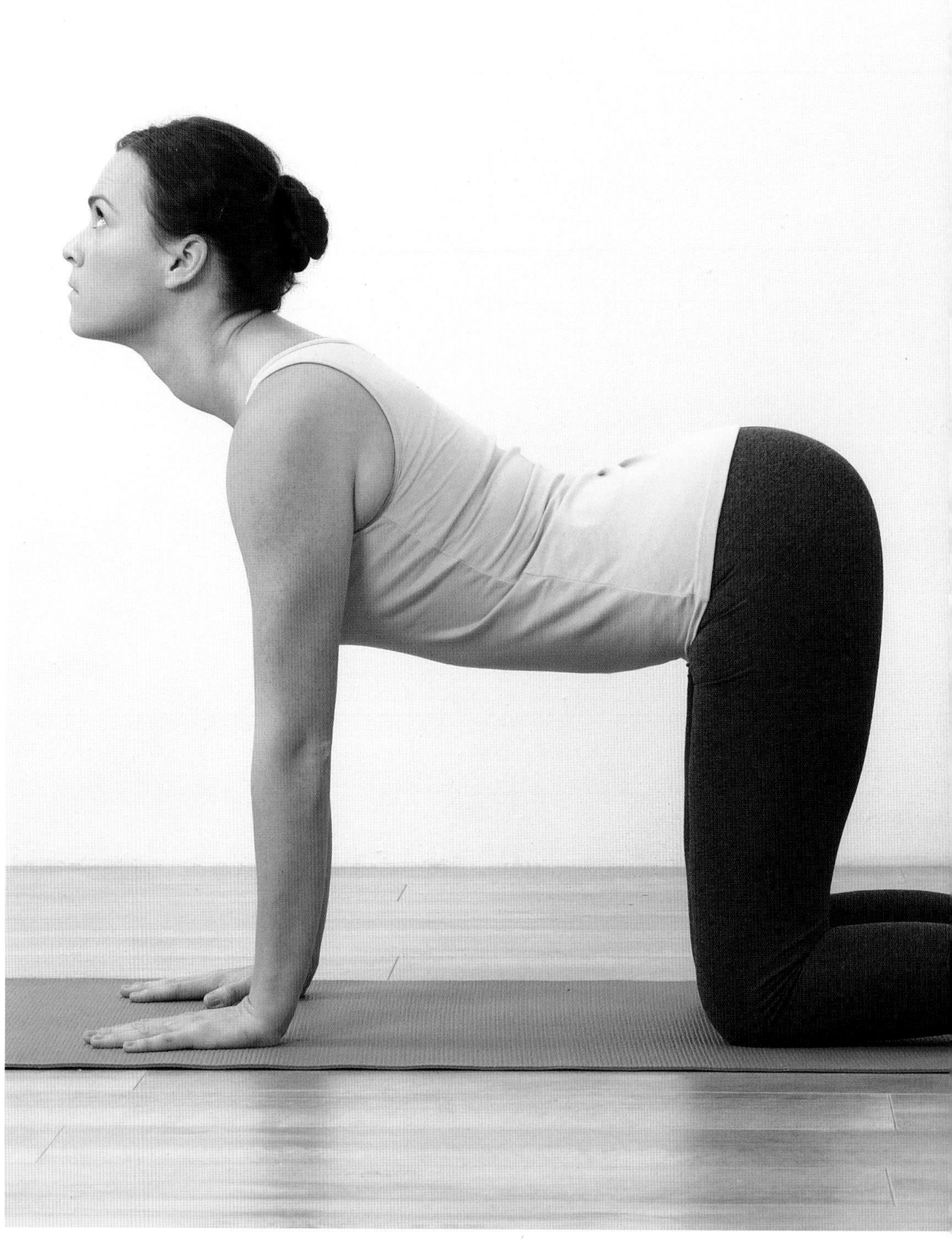

2

Build On It

Build on your achievements by taking the time to review and consolidate what you have learned so far. Read around the subject to increase your knowledge, thinking about positive ways in which you could improve the way you practice. This will help to ensure that your future practice is based on firm foundations and correct principles.

Sequences

One of the advantages of home practice is the freedom you have to experiment, improvise, and modify. Knowing the theory behind the practice will help you to perform the postures in a safe and progressive fashion. Postures can be grouped into eight different types, and it is useful to learn what these groups are and their optimum position in a sequence.

1. Standing postures

The Mountain Pose is one standing pose with which you'll be familiar as it is the first pose in the basic sequence (see pp.44–45). Other standing poses, such as the Tree Pose (see pp.94–95), help you establish correct alignment at the beginning of the practice.

2. Arm balance postures

These postures focus on building upper-body strength and stability through the use of the arms. This group includes postures such as the Plank Pose, which develops the upper body, and the Tree Pose, which relies on correct alignment to achieve balance.

3. Forward bends

Although some forward bends are executed from a standing position, this category includes only seated forward bends, the former being included in the standing poses described above. The effect on the organs of these poses is similar to that described for the twists (see right). In addition to aiding digestion, they are particularly effective poses for working on the hamstrings.

4. Twists

These postures involve twisting the torso, and are often performed while sitting on the floor. Organs and glands in the torso are gently compressed by these postures, allowing the release of built-up toxins.
As the pose is released, freshly oxygenated blood is absorbed, which has a rejuvenating effect. Another benefit of twists is their action on the spine, where they serve to improve strength and flexibility.

5. Back bends

This group of poses concentrates on the spine, which, as we have seen, is both the hub of the body's nervous communication system and the fulcrum of the musculo-skeletal system. Poses such as the Cobra (see pp.60–61) and the Locust (see pp.152–153) involve stretching the spine. These are great stress-busters as trapped tensions are often located in the spinal region.

6. Inversions

The group of poses known as inversions require vertical alignment and upper-body strength. The definition of an inverted posture is one where the head is below the heart. Inverted poses include the Half Shoulder Stand with Wall (see pp. 128–131). They are considered to have tremendous health benefits due to the unique cardiac workouts they provide.

7. Restorative postures

These postures play a vital, relaxing, and restorative role in your practice. It is in these poses that you have the chance to reflect on your practice and focus on the various sensations you are feeling. It is only by being able to truly relax that you will be able to take your practice to a higher level.

Key principles of sequences

- **Yoga sequences order** The order of poses broadly follows the list on the opposite page. Some poses in groups are interchangeable. For example, forward bends can be performed before the twist poses—as they prepare the spine and hips—and after back bends, as they provide a counter-stretch.
- **Balancing a pose with a counter-pose** A counter-pose moves in the opposite direction from the previous pose, thus helping to realign the body. So you might, for example, follow a back bend with a forward bend.
- **Ordering the poses in a hierarchy** Some poses are much more demanding than others. Knowing the hierarchy of postures prevents you from going too far, too fast, which can result in injury.
- **Holding ending poses for longer** Toward the end of the practice, poses are held for longer, allowing for greater inward focus.
- **Use the restorative and resting poses** Poses such as the Child's Pose (see pp.62–63) are a welcome interlude after a difficult pose. All sequences should finish with a relaxation pose, such as the Corpse.

Tree Pose

Strengthen Balance • **Improve** Memory

This elegant pose teaches balance through concentration, bringing strength and flexibility to the leg muscles.

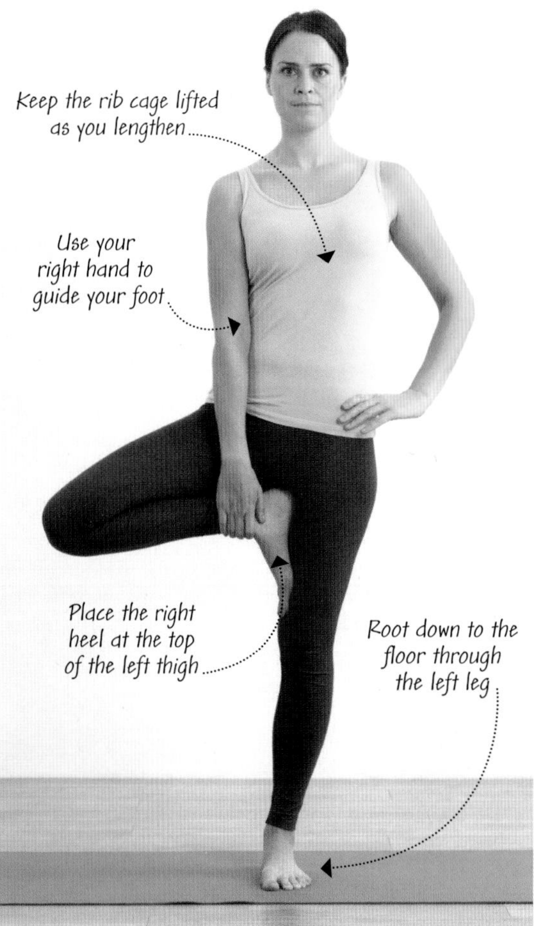
Keep the rib cage lifted as you lengthen
Use your right hand to guide your foot
Place the right heel at the top of the left thigh
Root down to the floor through the left leg

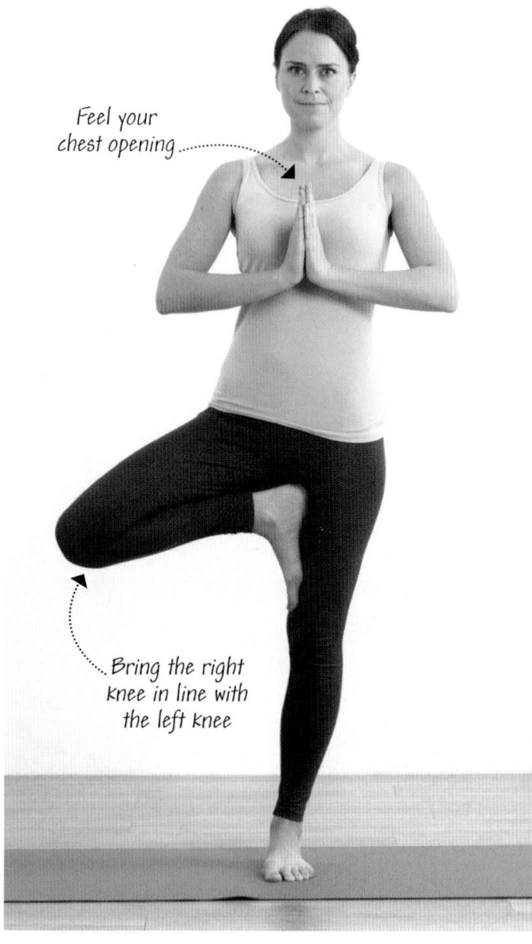
Feel your chest opening
Bring the right knee in line with the left knee

1 Stand with the feet together. Breathe in as you begin to transfer your body weight to the left foot. Then bend the right knee and raise up the right foot, placing it on the inside of the left leg. Use your right hand to draw your foot higher up the left leg.

2 Find your point of balance as you activate the standing leg further, pressing the foot down, and take even breaths to stabilize. Inhale to raise your hands up slowly into the prayer position. Take two or three breaths in this transition.

1 2 3

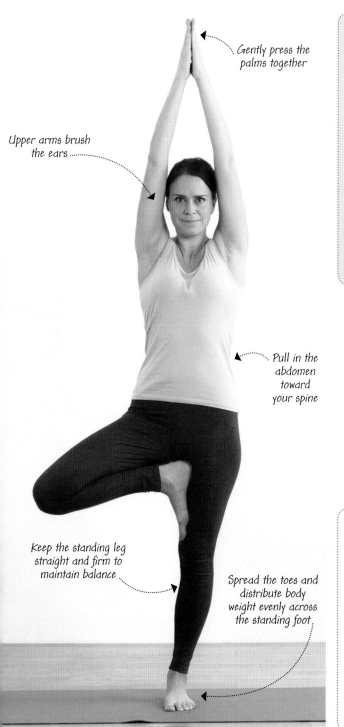

Gently press the palms together

Upper arms brush the ears

Pull in the abdomen toward your spine

Keep the standing leg straight and firm to maintain balance

Spread the toes and distribute body weight evenly across the standing foot

3 As you breathe in, fix your gaze on a point straight ahead and extend your arms upward, touching your palms together to make a steeple shape. Take a complete breath, then lower your arms and raised leg before repeating the pose on the other side.

Useful tip If you find maintaining concentration difficult, practice the pose against a wall to help you balance. Start by positioning both heels close to the wall.

Take care...

Position your raised foot lower down on the standing leg if you find it difficult to balance.

Use your hand to continue to hold the raised foot in position if you find that it keeps slipping down toward the knee. You can raise the arm that is not providing support up straight.

Check your clothing, as you may need to roll up your leg wear and rest the raised foot on the bare flesh.

Half Lotus Tree

Tone Arms and Legs • **Develop** Focus

This pose is a standing, hip-opening posture requiring balance and concentration rather than strength to perform.

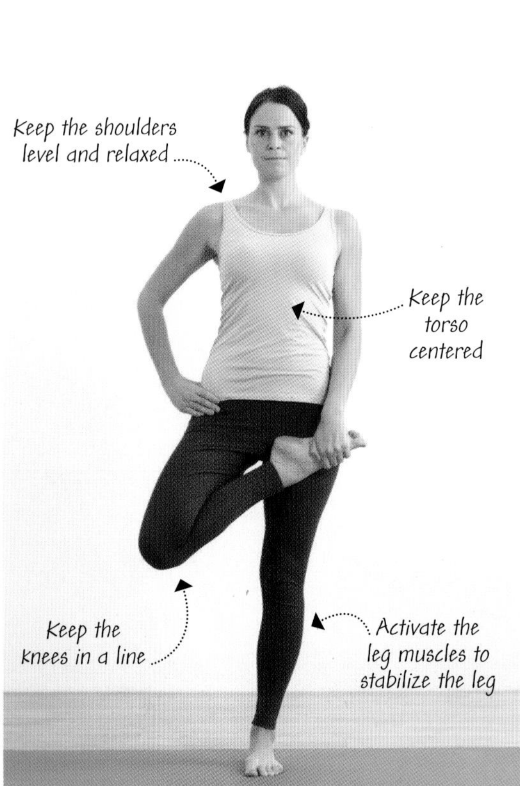
Keep the shoulders level and relaxed
Keep the torso centered
Keep the knees in a line
Activate the leg muscles to stabilize the leg

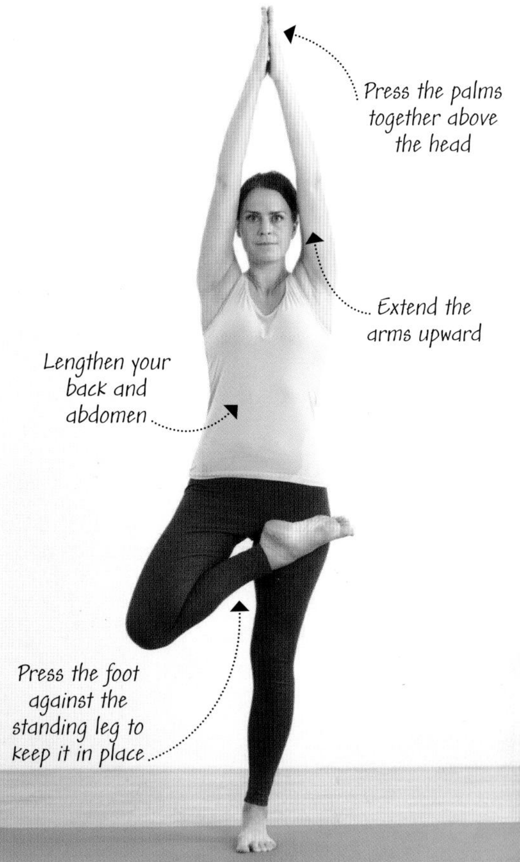
Press the palms together above the head
Extend the arms upward
Lengthen your back and abdomen
Press the foot against the standing leg to keep it in place

1 Stand with feet together and breathe in to transfer your body weight to the left foot. Bend the right knee and raise the right foot. Use your left hand to draw the foot as high on the left thigh as you can.

2 Find your point of balance and raise your arms slowly until your palms are pressed together above your head. Straighten your arms, extending upward. Breathing steadily, hold for five to ten breaths before gently lowering the arms and releasing the foot. Repeat with the left leg.

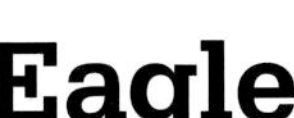

Eagle

Strengthen Wrists and Ankles
Develop Concentration

This pose works on centering and alignment by strengthening your core. The increased blood flow nourishes the joints.

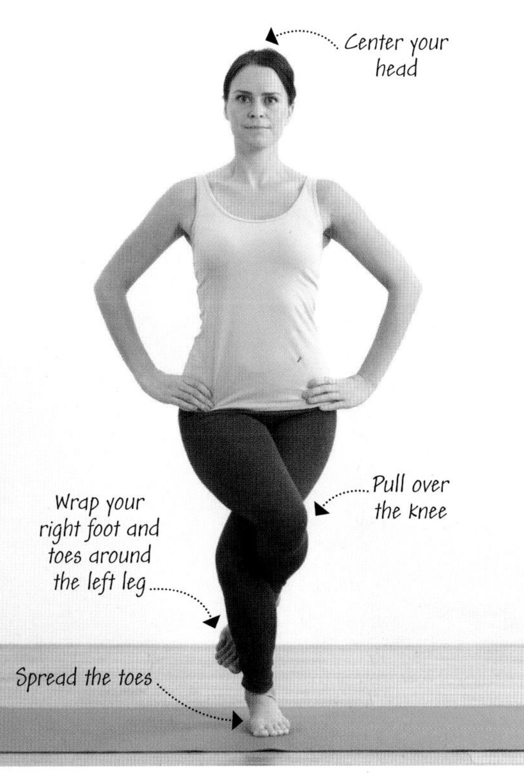
Center your head
Pull over the knee
Wrap your right foot and toes around the left leg
Spread the toes

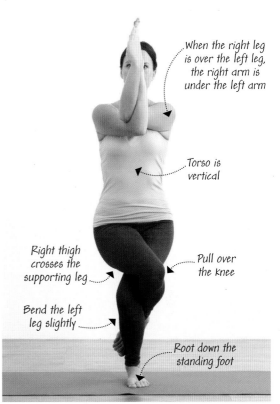

When the right leg is over the left leg, the right arm is under the left arm
Torso is vertical
Right thigh crosses the supporting leg
Pull over the knee
Bend the left leg slightly
Root down the standing foot

1 From a standing position, bend the knees slightly and, balancing on the left foot, cross your right thigh over your left and hook your right foot behind your standing leg.

2 Holding firm with your standing leg, raise your arms with the elbows bent. Wrap your right arm and hand around the left arm, and press the palms together. Repeat, swapping limbs.

Useful tip To hold balance poses, fix your gaze on one spot on the floor or wall to stabilize the head, and breathe evenly.

Warrior 2

Tone Hips • **Prepare** For Life Challenges

Practicing the Warrior 2 pose helps tone the abdomen as well as strengthen the limbs and open the chest and shoulders.

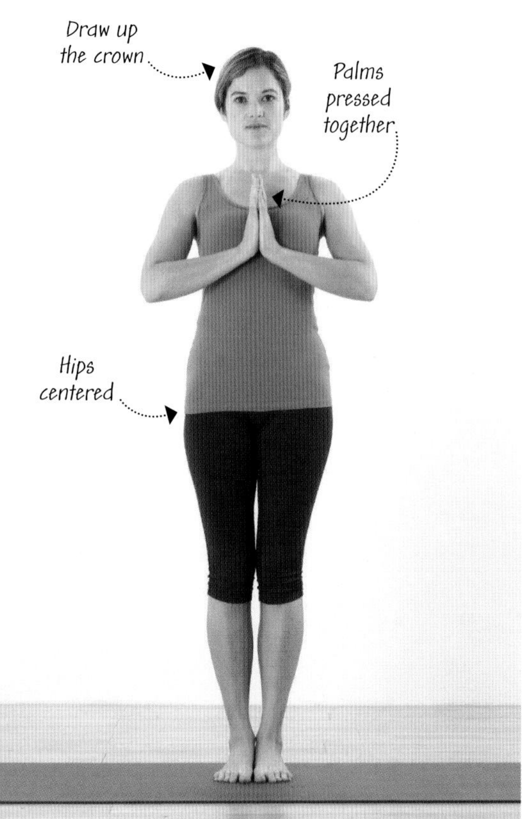
Draw up the crown
Palms pressed together
Hips centered

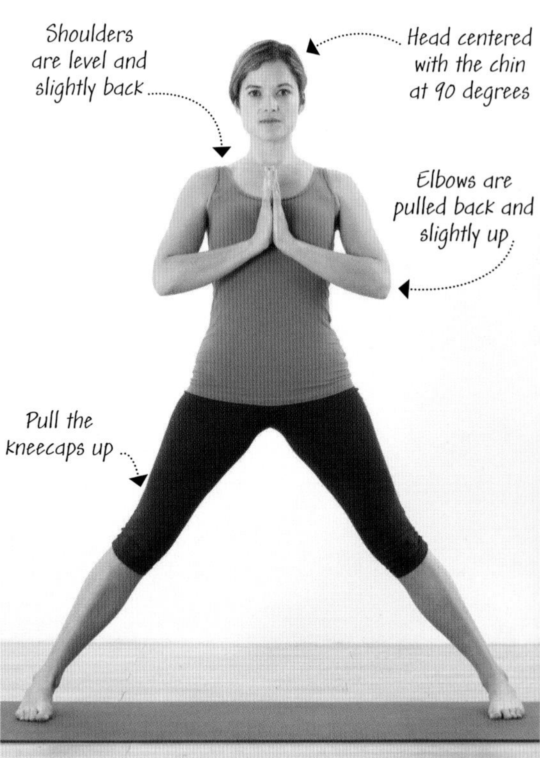
Shoulders are level and slightly back
Head centered with the chin at 90 degrees
Elbows are pulled back and slightly up
Pull the kneecaps up

1 Stand sideways on the mat with your feet together and hands in front of your chest in the prayer position. Focus on your breath, and look straight ahead as you center yourself.

2 Step sideways so your feet are 3ft (1m) apart, pressing the outer edges of the feet downward to provide stability. Keep your back straight and your breathing regular.

Useful tip Point the toes forward and root down through the feet to anchor your position.

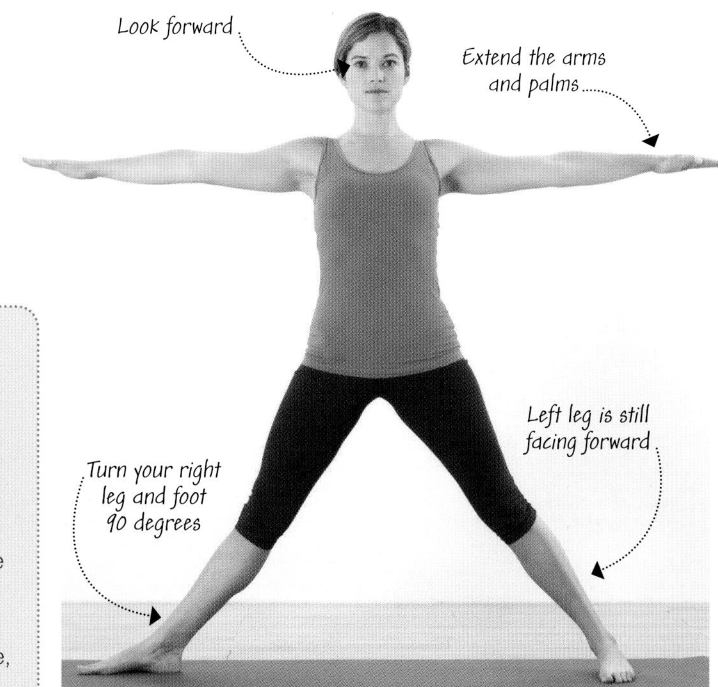

Look forward
Extend the arms and palms
Left leg is still facing forward
Turn your right leg and foot 90 degrees

3 On inhalation, sweep the arms up level with your shoulders, rotating the right foot until it is pointing in the same direction as your right hand. The left foot remains facing forward.

Useful tip Focus on opening the chest by pushing the fingertips away from you. The oppositional force is worked through your core, shoulders, and arms.

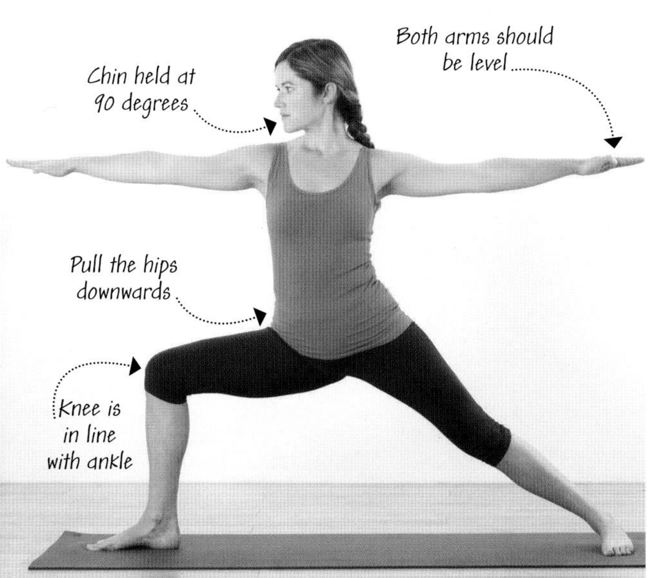

Both arms should be level
Chin held at 90 degrees
Pull the hips downwards
Knee is in line with ankle

4 Rooting down through both feet, bend your right knee, pushing forward until it aligns with the ankle. Move your head in the same direction, and look along your right arm. Hold for five breaths and release on inhalation. Repeat on the other side.

Useful tip Imagine there is a downward pull through the center of your body, pulling the torso down.

Extended Side Stretch

Strengthen Core • **Develop** Body Awareness

This pose tones and strengthens the legs, improves lung capacity, and stimulates the organs in the abdomen.

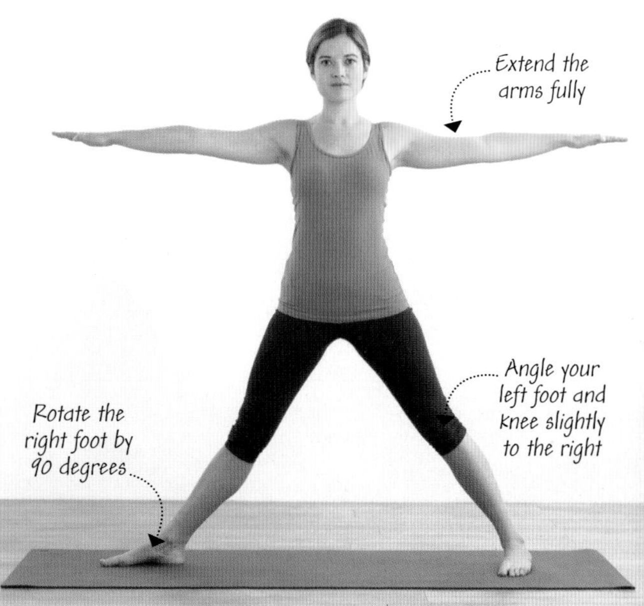
Extend the arms fully
Angle your left foot and knee slightly to the right
Rotate the right foot by 90 degrees

1 Stand sideways on the mat, feet about 3ft (1m) apart. Inhale, raising your arms parallel to the floor, with palms pointing downward. Turn your left foot slightly to the right and your right foot to the right by 90 degrees.

Useful tip Ground yourself by pressing the outer edge of your left foot into the mat.

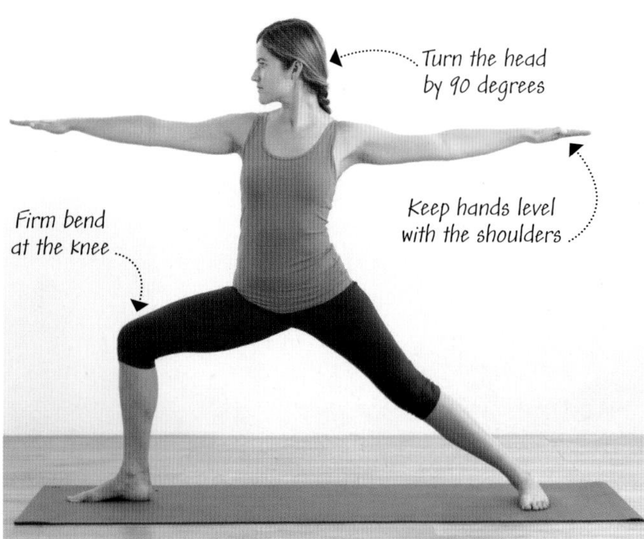
Turn the head by 90 degrees
Keep hands level with the shoulders
Firm bend at the knee

2 Inhale deeply, then exhale, bending your right knee so that it is vertically aligned above your right ankle. Stretch the arms out wide, locked at the elbows and with your hands level with the shoulders. Try to bring the right thigh parallel to the floor.

Useful tip If your left foot lifts off the floor, try supporting your heel against a wall.

3 Exhale to lean your upper body forward, supporting the right forearm on your thigh. Fold your left arm and place this hand on the small of your back.

Useful tip Before moving into the pose, make adjustments to ensure you are in alignment.

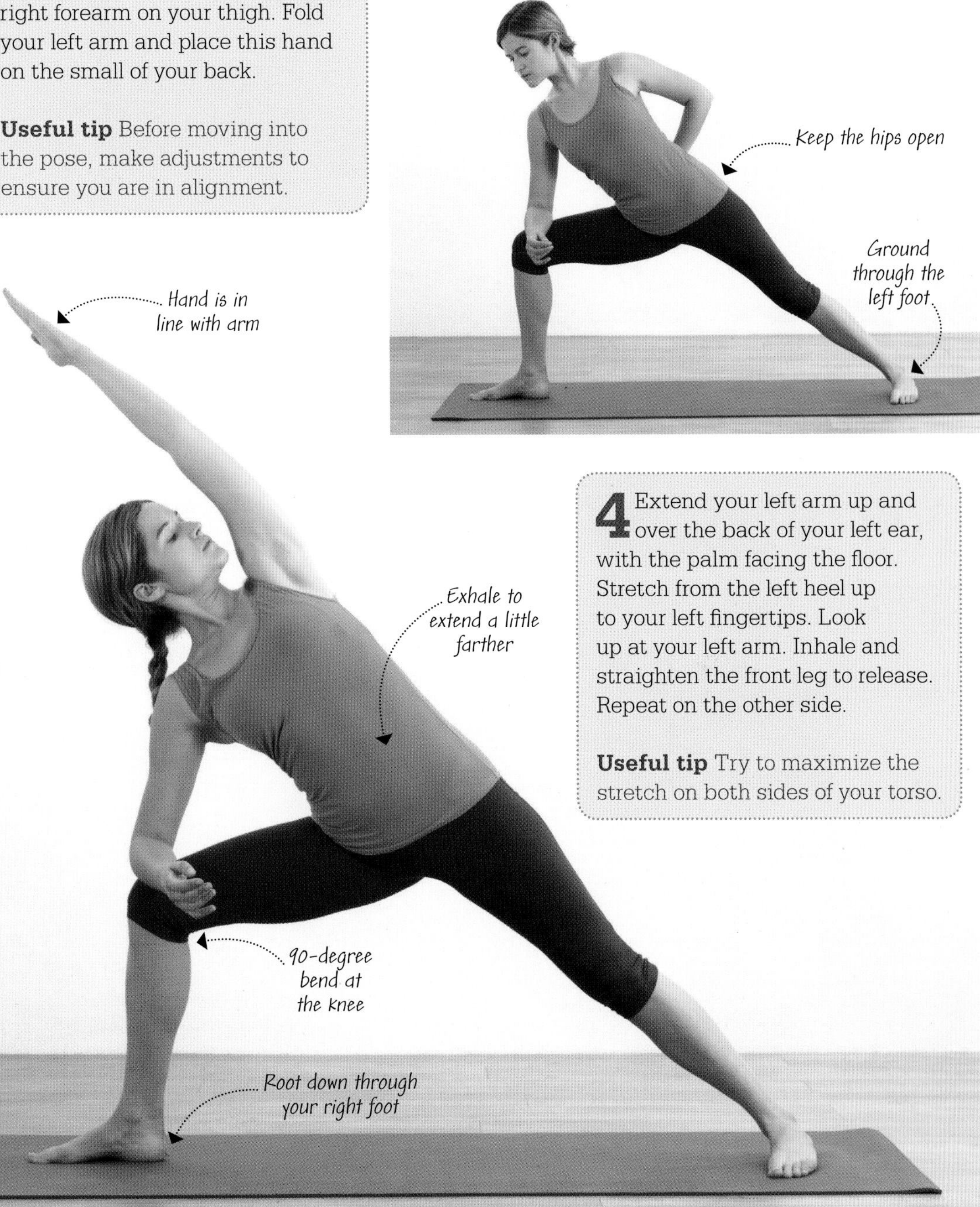
Keep the hips open
Ground through the left foot
Hand is in line with arm
Exhale to extend a little farther
90-degree bend at the knee
Root down through your right foot

4 Extend your left arm up and over the back of your left ear, with the palm facing the floor. Stretch from the left heel up to your left fingertips. Look up at your left arm. Inhale and straighten the front leg to release. Repeat on the other side.

Useful tip Try to maximize the stretch on both sides of your torso.

Horse

Strengthen Hamstrings • **Assist** Digestion

This pose strengthens your core and stretches the leg muscles. It counteracts the adverse effects of prolonged sitting by elongating the spine and opening up the hips.

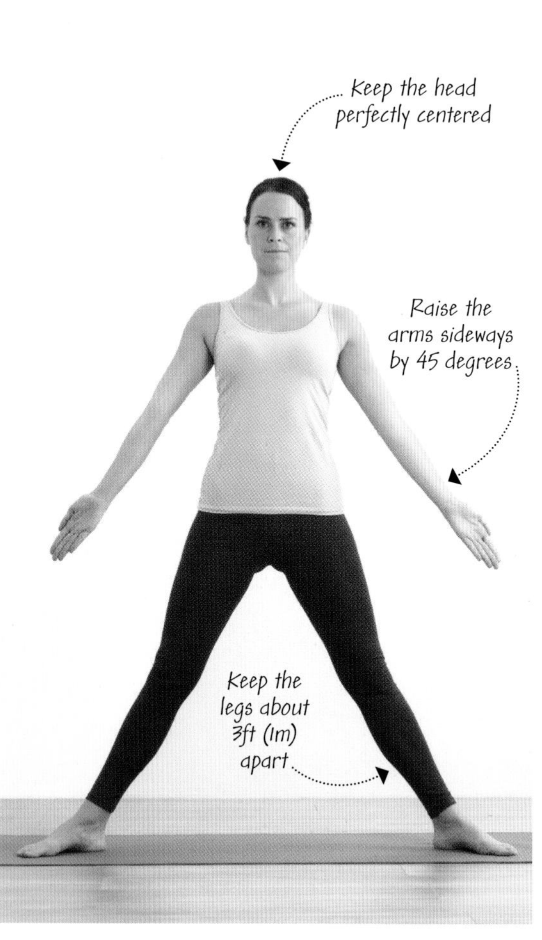
Keep the head
perfectly centered
Raise the
arms sideways
by 45 degrees
Keep the
legs about
3ft (1m)
apart

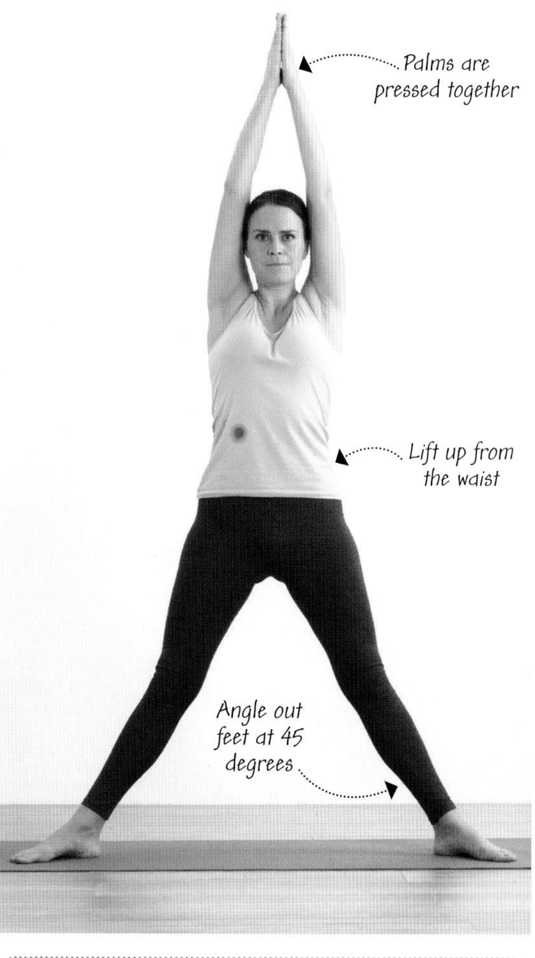
Palms are
pressed together
Lift up from
the waist
Angle out
feet at 45
degrees

1 Start with the feet together and jump or step sideways so the feet are about 3ft (1m) apart and turned outward at an angle of 45 degrees. Inhale and raise the arms 45 degrees, palms facing forward.

2 Firm your leg muscles and press your feet onto the mat. Inhale slowly sweeping the arms upward until the palms are pressed together above the head and the arms are fully extended and locked at the elbows

3 Exhale as you bend your knees, remaining conscious of your body alignment. At the same time, lower your arms, bringing your hands into the prayer position in front of the chest.

Useful tip As you lower, bend the knees until they are in line with the feet.

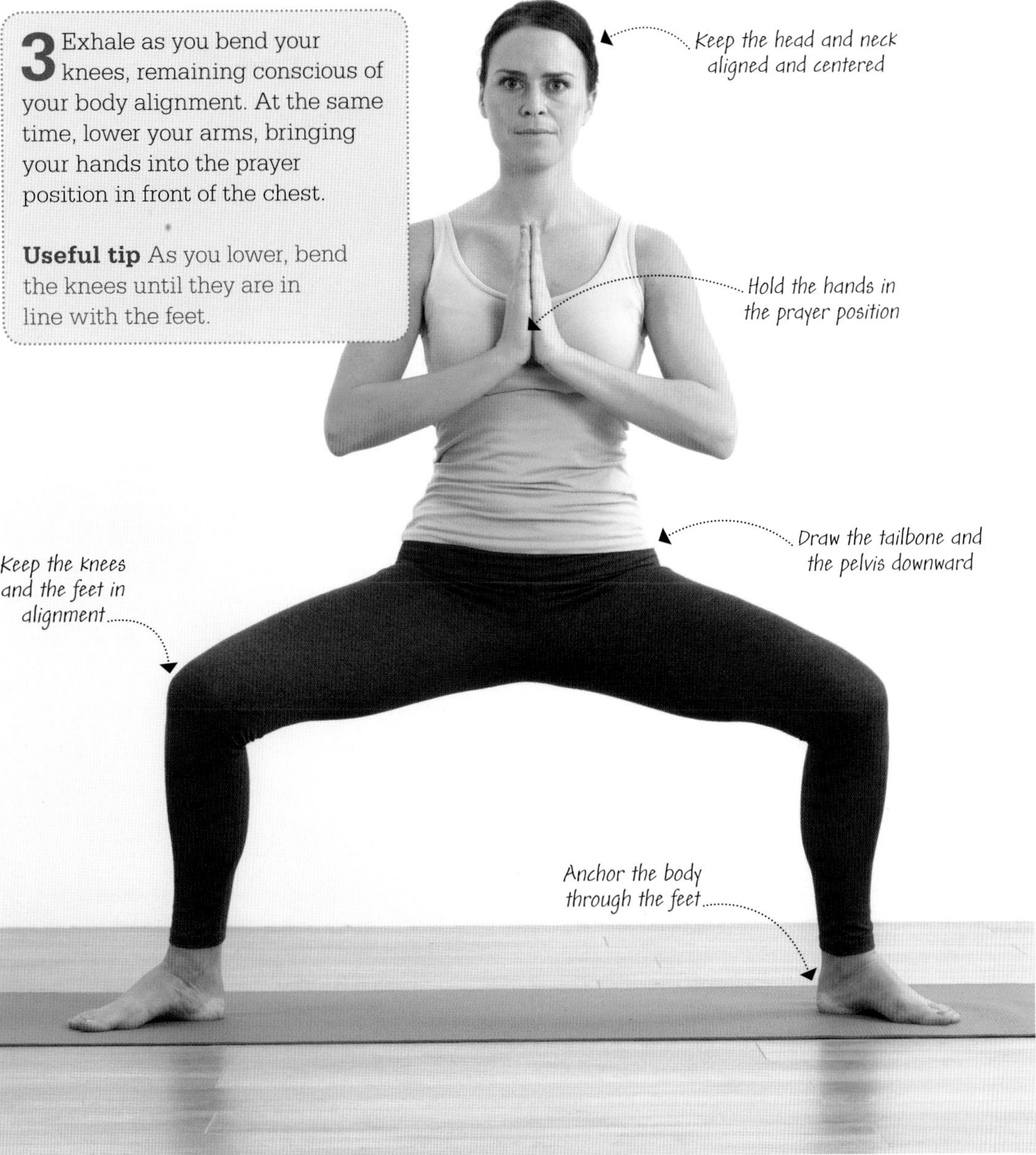
Keep the head and neck aligned and centered
Hold the hands in the prayer position
Draw the tailbone and the pelvis downward
Keep the knees and the feet in alignment
Anchor the body through the feet

Take care...

A common tendency is for the torso to lean forward. To prevent this from happening, reduce the flexion at the knees and bring the spine into an erect position.

Avoid tilting the head forward or sideways to check body alignment. Focusing the mind on alignment and concentrating on your balance will enable you to center yourself.

Warrior Lunge

Strengthen Ankles and Legs • **Develop** Poise

This energizing pose gives a strong stretch to your "quads," the muscles at the front of your thighs, as well as a gentle stretch to your lower back.

1 Start by kneeling on all fours with your wrists aligned with the shoulders and your knees with the hips. Point the toes away from the body. Reduce the lumbar curve and draw the navel toward the spine to flatten the back.

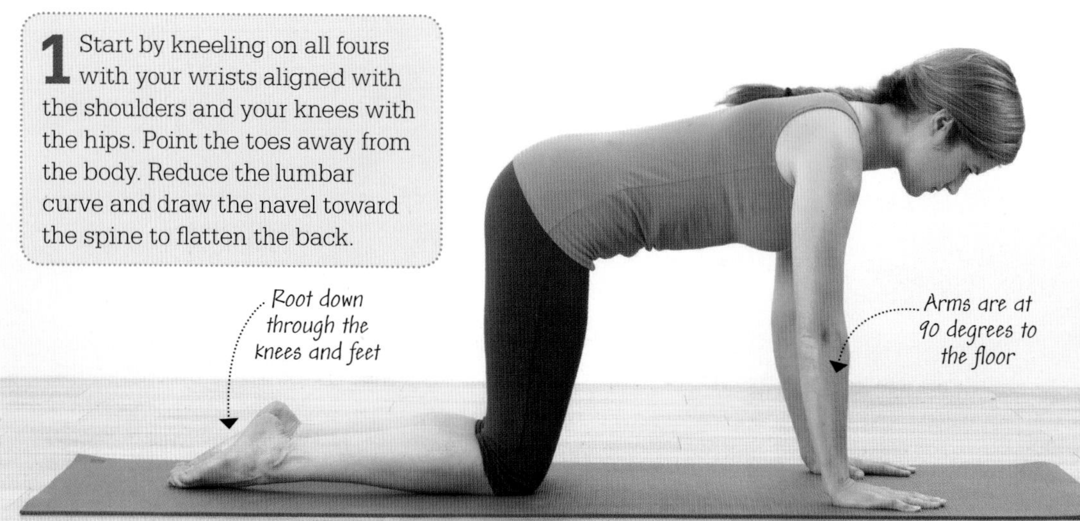
Root down through the knees and feet
Arms are at 90 degrees to the floor

2 As you exhale, bring your right foot forward and place beside the right hand. As you do, lean your torso forward at a 45-degree angle, nestling the right side of your abdomen into the right thigh.

Useful tip Anchor through your left foot and knee and stretch the left leg quads to assist positioning.

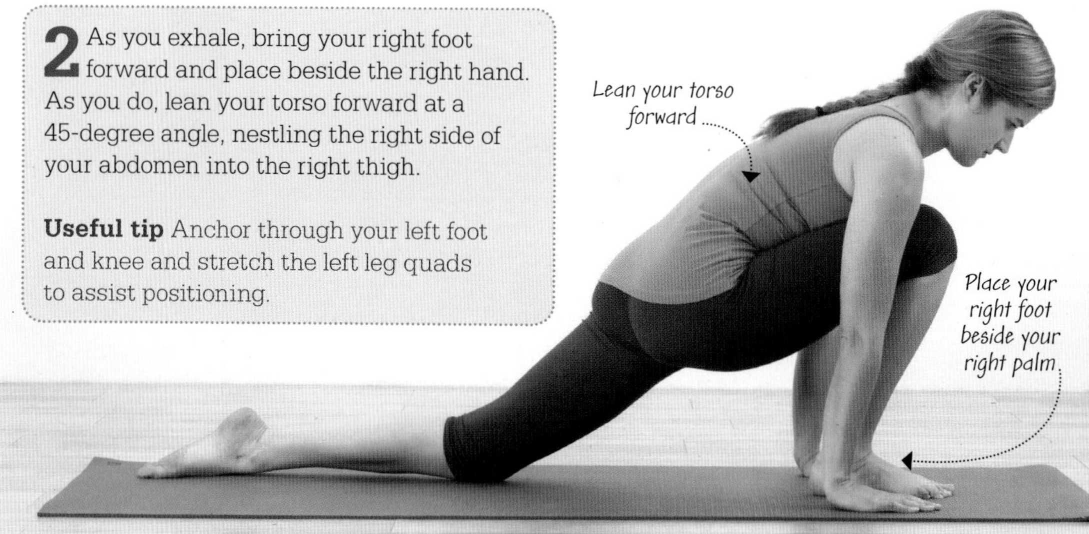
Lean your torso forward
Place your right foot beside your right palm

1 2 3

3 Raise up slightly by shifting your hand position and pressing your fingers onto the mat. Lift your left knee off the floor, turn your toes in, bearing the weight through the flexed toes.

Useful tip Spread the weight of your body evenly through the feet and fingers.

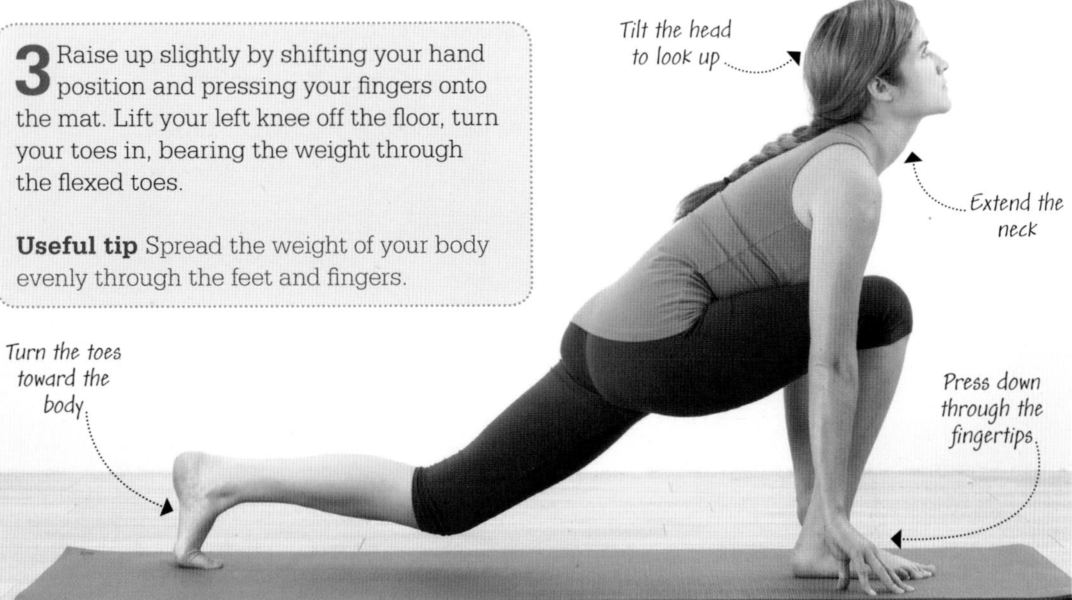

Tilt the head to look up
Extend the neck
Turn the toes toward the body
Press down through the fingertips

4 Raise the fingers off the floor and bring both hands to rest on your right knee. Look forward and straighten your torso. Hold for five breaths. Exhale to release and return to kneeling on all fours. Repeat on the other side.

Useful tip Draw your pelvis down with each exhalation, increasing the stretch in the legs.

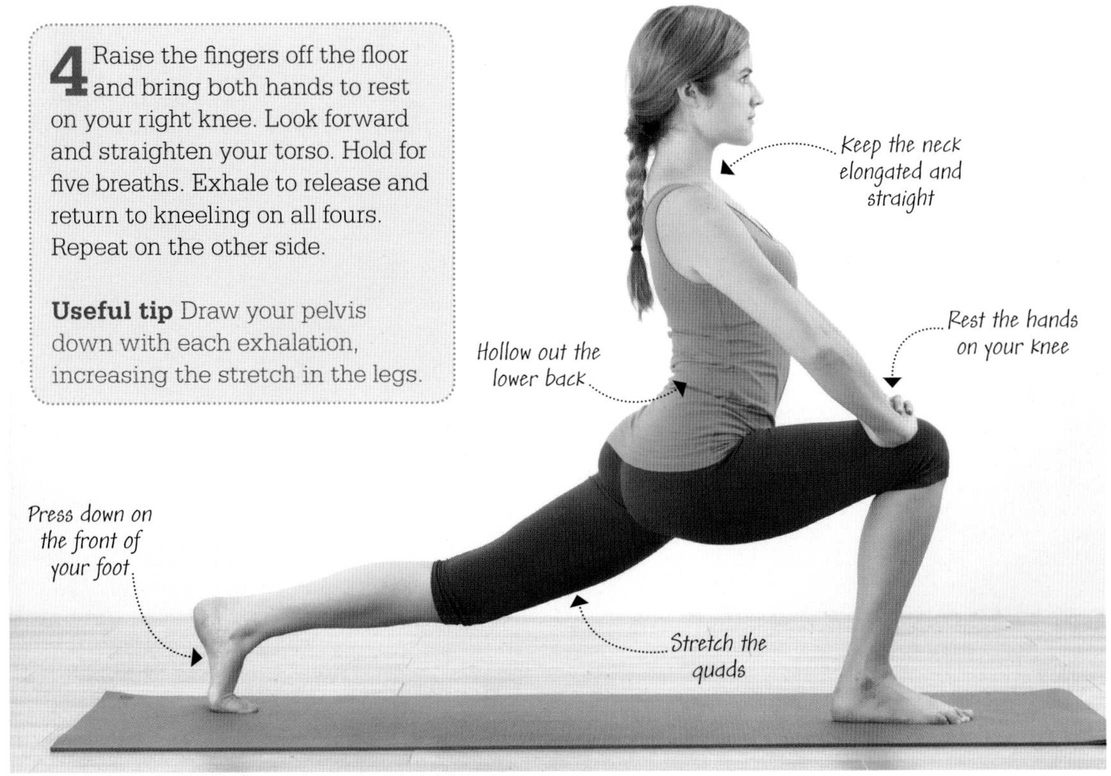

Keep the neck elongated and straight

Rest the hands on your knee

Hollow out the lower back

Press down on the front of your foot

Stretch the quads

Wide Forward Bend

Tone Legs • **Improve** Circulation

This wide-standing forward bend pose stretches the hamstrings and widens the groin. By increasing the blood flow to the brain, this pose invigorates the mind.

1 Stand with your feet about 3ft (1m) apart, hands on hips, and feet facing forward. Firm your stance by engaging the leg muscles and pressing your feet firmly into the floor. Align your head, neck, and torso while looking straight ahead.

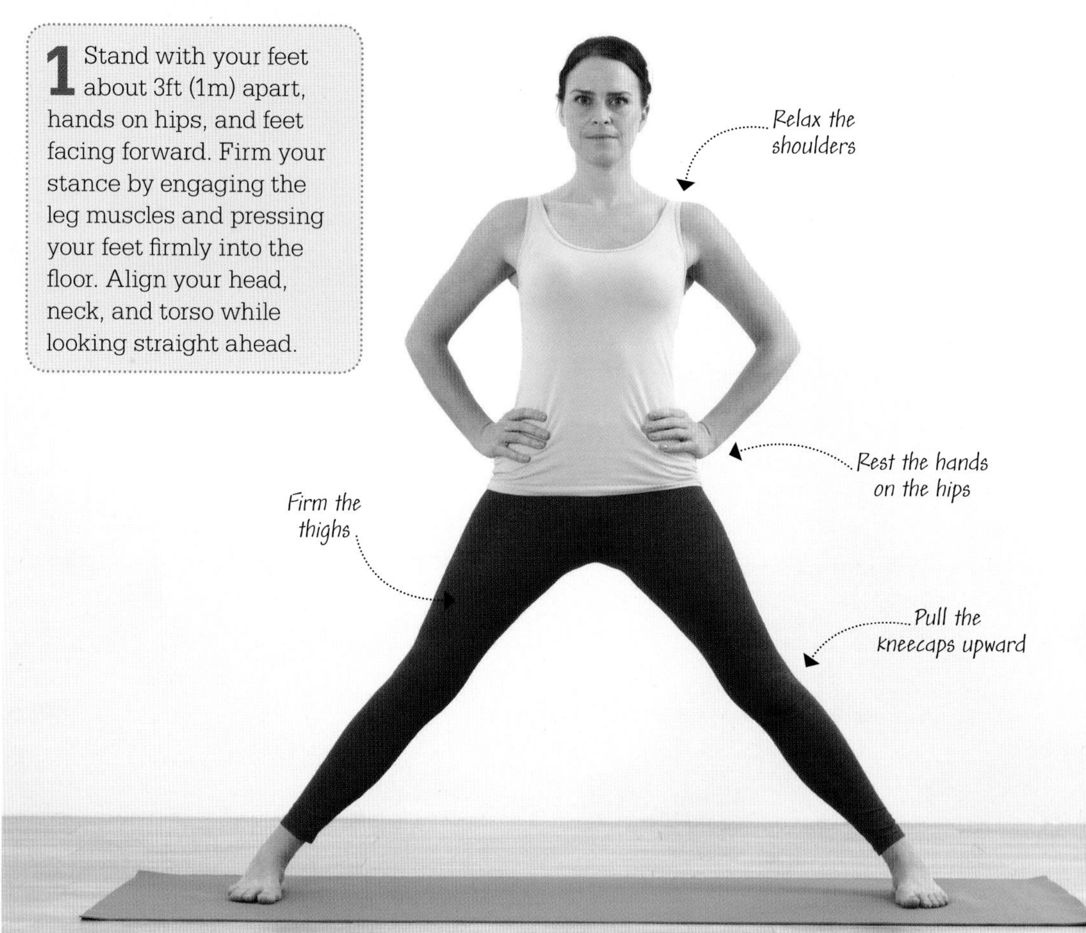
Relax the shoulders
Rest the hands on the hips
Firm the thighs
Pull the kneecaps upward

Take care...

There is a tendency to bend from the waist rather than from the hips, creating a rounded back. If this occurs, then bend the knees slightly to allow hip flexion.

Stiffness in the back often results in one shoulder being lower than the other. To level the shoulders, work on releasing tension from your shoulders and upper back.

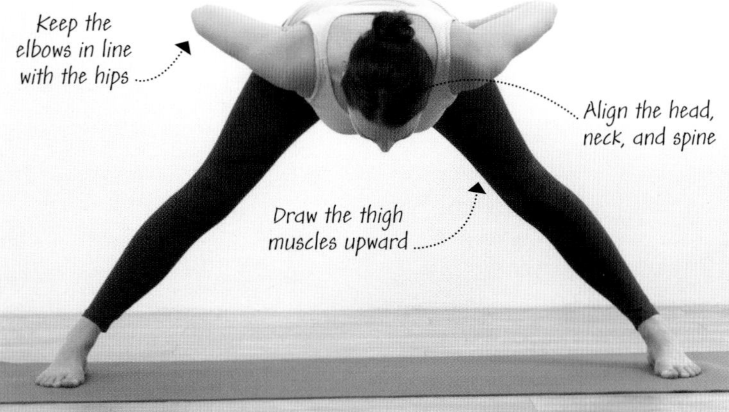
Keep the elbows in line with the hips
Align the head, neck, and spine
Draw the thigh muscles upward

2 As you exhale, slowly bend forward from the hips, keeping the back straight and aligned with the neck until your upper body is at a right angle to your legs. If you have a back problem, bend your knees slightly.

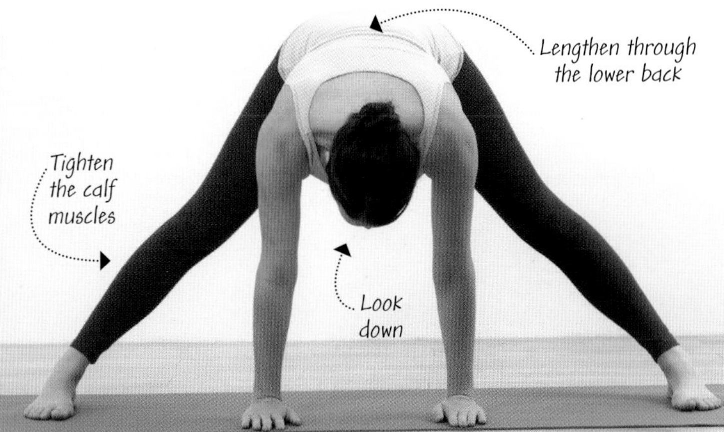
Lengthen through the lower back
Tighten the calf muscles
Look down

3 Exhale again, bringing your palms to rest on the floor directly below the shoulders, keeping the head and neck aligned. Look down. Inhale, pressing the palms down and lengthen through the arms and back.

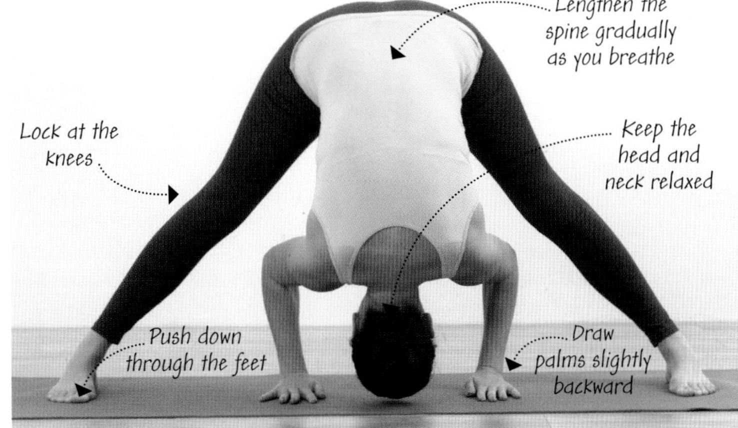
Lengthen the spine gradually as you breathe
Lock at the knees
Keep the head and neck relaxed
Push down through the feet
Draw palms slightly backward

4 Exhale again, bending the arms and lowering the head farther down. Relax the neck. With each exhalation, draw the head farther down, allowing gravity to lengthen your spine. Hold for a few breaths. To release from the pose, reverse the movements.

Cow Arms

Promote Physical Equilibrium • **Stretch** Shoulders

This pose works on both arms simultaneously and in doing so enhances postural awareness and upper-body flexibility.

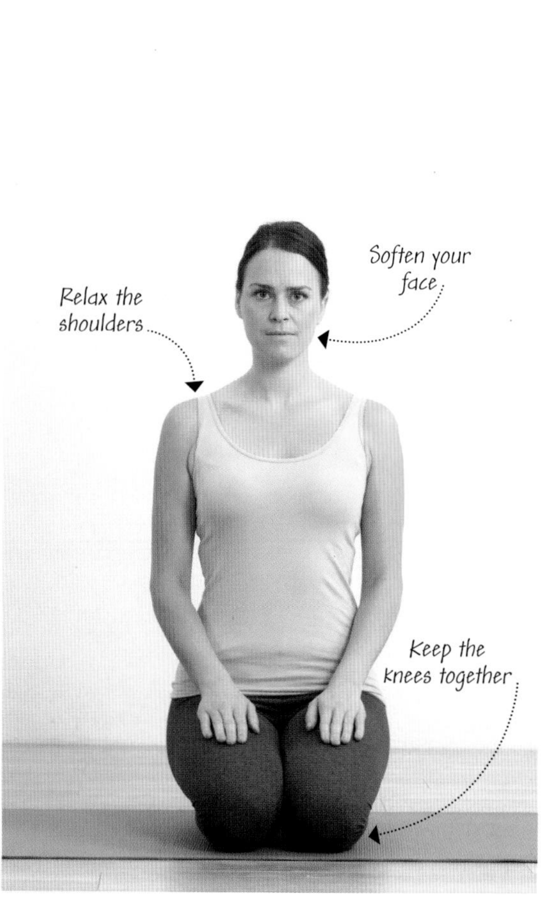
Relax the shoulders
Soften your face
Keep the knees together

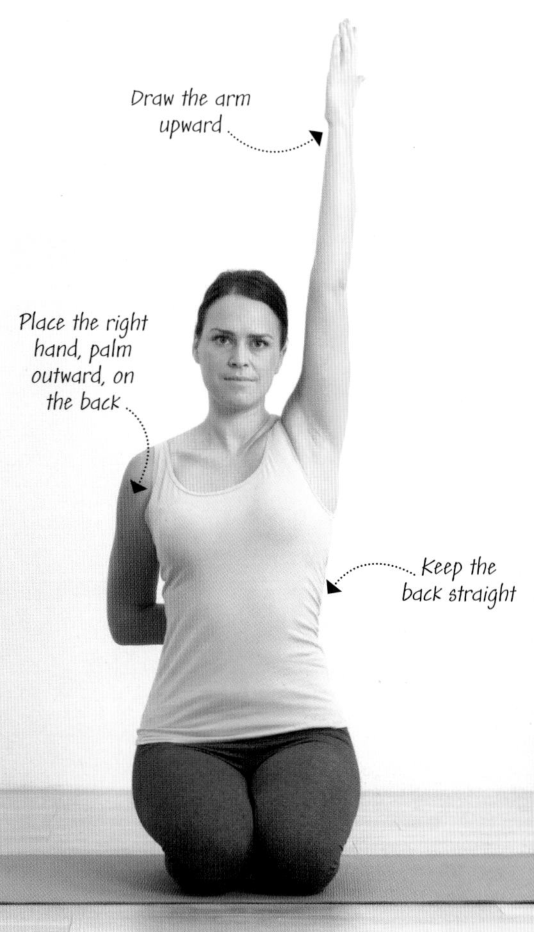
Draw the arm upward
Place the right hand, palm outward, on the back
Keep the back straight

1 Kneel on the mat, sitting on your heels, with your toes pointing away from your body. Rest the hands on your thighs. Look forward and soften the muscles of the face. Relax your shoulders as you breathe in and out.

2 Inhale to raise your left arm straight up. Work the stretch along the left side of your body and lengthen through to the fingertips. Fold your right arm at the waist so that the right hand is on your back, with the palm facing away from the body.

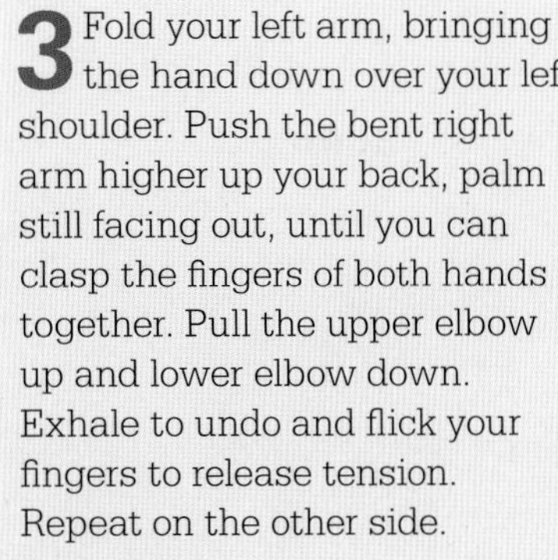

3 Fold your left arm, bringing the hand down over your left shoulder. Push the bent right arm higher up your back, palm still facing out, until you can clasp the fingers of both hands together. Pull the upper elbow up and lower elbow down. Exhale to undo and flick your fingers to release tension. Repeat on the other side.

Remember Point the right elbow up and left elbow down for an effective diagonal stretch to the upper back.

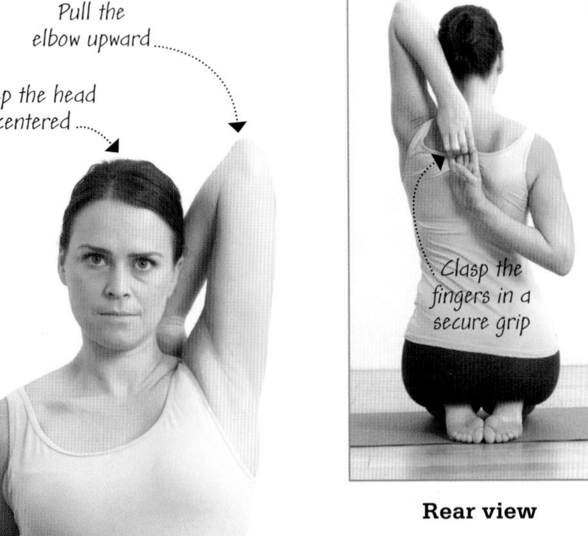
Pull the elbow upward
Keep the head centered
Breathe in a gentle rhythm
Clasp the fingers in a secure grip

Rear view

Make it easier

If you are not able to link your fingers, then use a resistance band to assist the pose. Hold the band firmly in your left hand and bend the left arm as in Step 3. Bring the right hand behind your back and feel for the end of the band, taking a firm hold. Work on gradually edging both hands along the band, bringing them closer together.

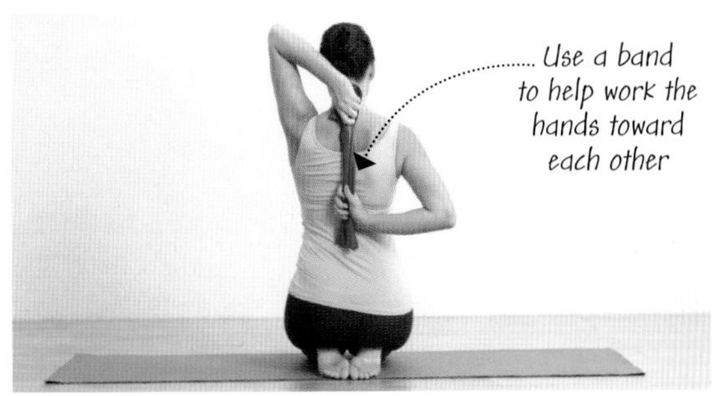
Use a band to help work the hands toward each other

Cat

Stretch Spine • **Restore** Energy

The Cat pose provides a gentle massage to the abdominal organs and the spine while relieving stress by stretching the back, torso, and neck.

1 Begin on all fours with your wrists aligned with the shoulders and your knees with the hips. Point the toes away from the body. Flatten your back by reducing the lumbar curve and drawing the navel up to the spine.

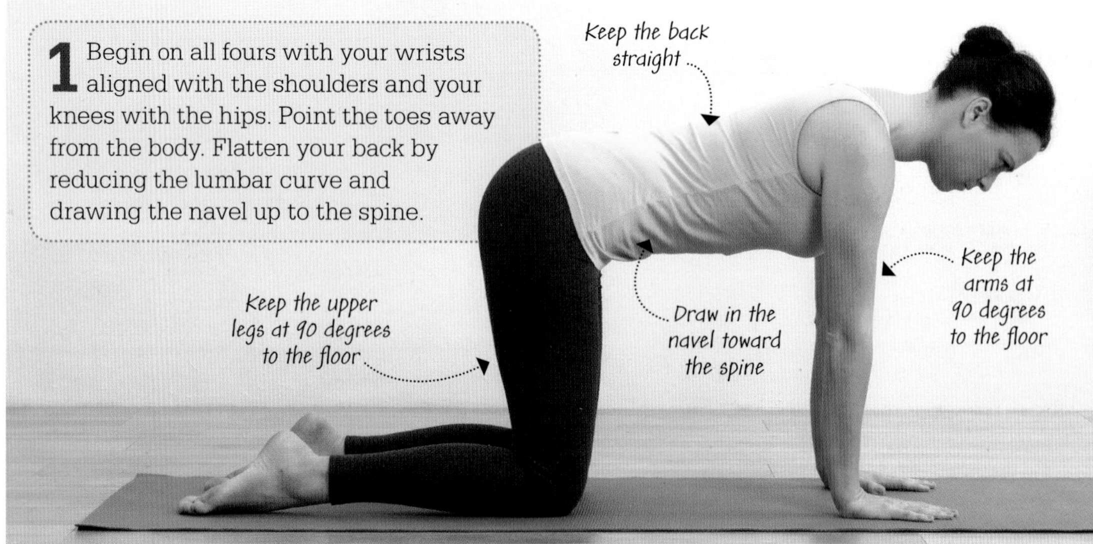
Keep the back straight
Keep the arms at 90 degrees to the floor
Keep the upper legs at 90 degrees to the floor
Draw in the navel toward the spine

3 Exhale as you lower the tailbone and raise the abdomen, arching your spine in an upward direction. Make sure that your hands and knees are in their original position. Let your head drop between your arms toward the floor, but don't force your chin against your chest.

Useful tip It may be beneficial to rest in the Child's Pose (see pp.62–63) after doing this.

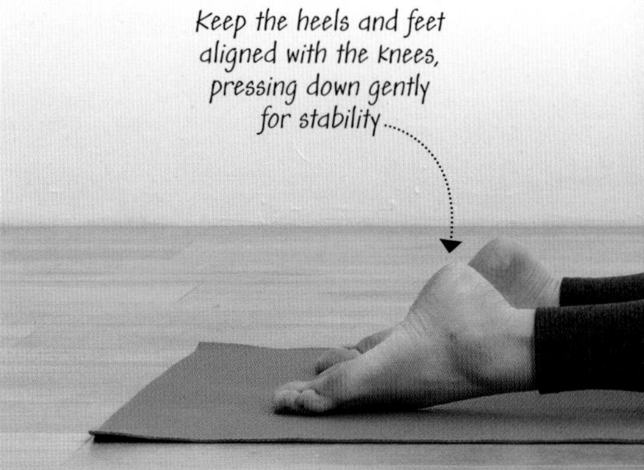
Keep the heels and feet aligned with the knees, pressing down gently for stability

2 Inhaling, arch the spine downward by pulling the tailbone upward and pushing out the chest. Raise your chin and look upward.

Help! If you feel pain in your knees, place a folded towel beneath them.

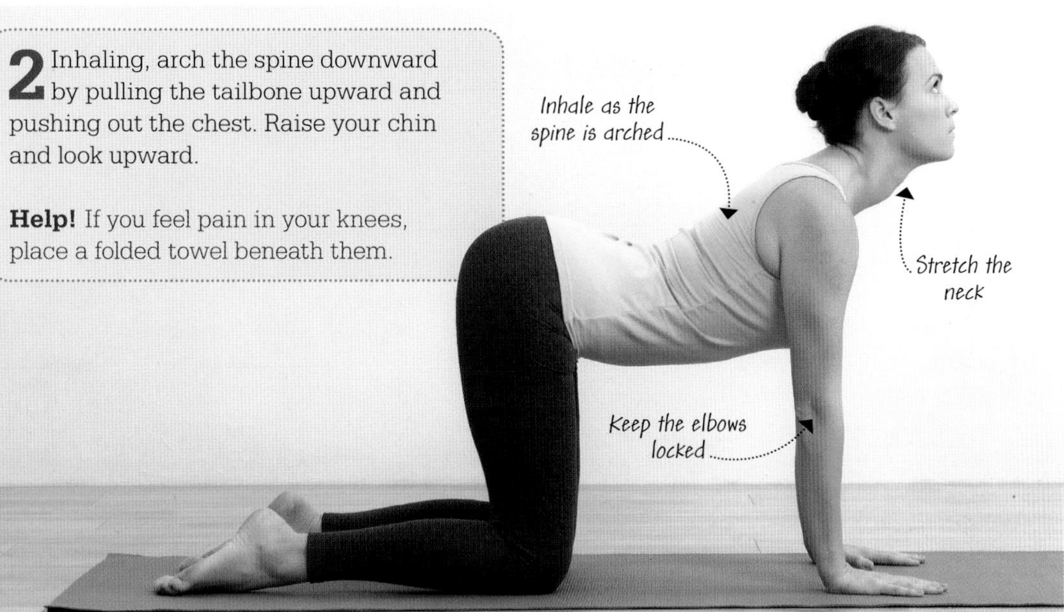
Inhale as the spine is arched
Stretch the neck
Keep the elbows locked

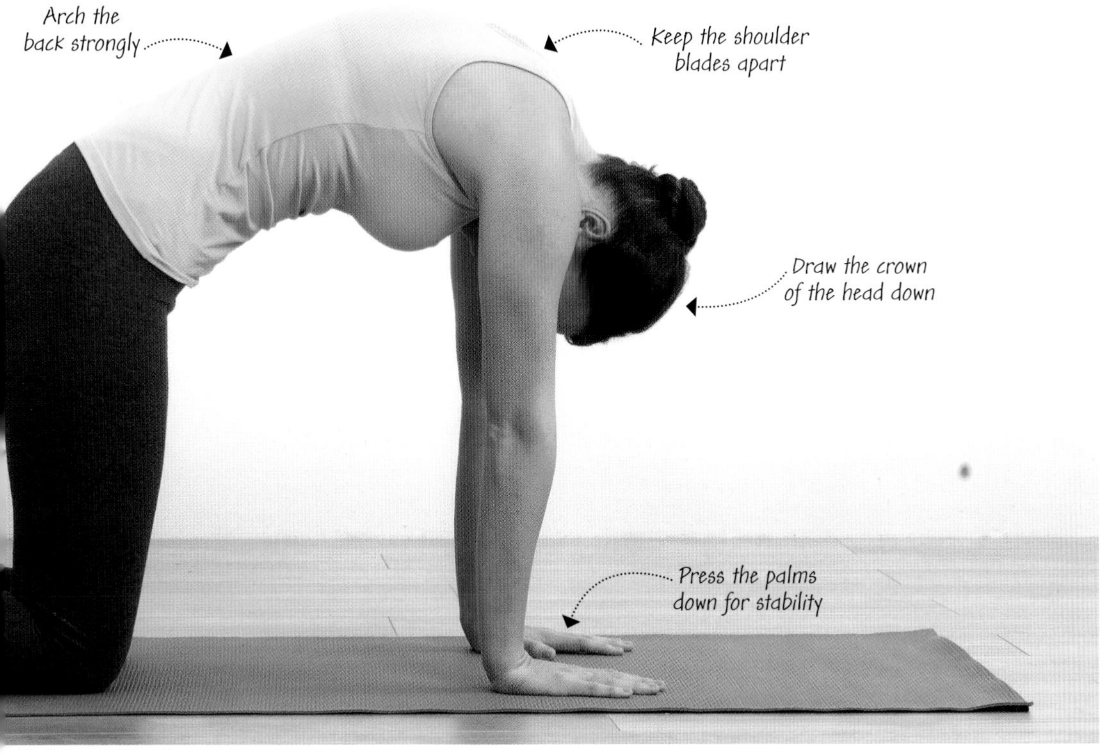

Arch the back strongly

Keep the shoulder blades apart

Draw the crown of the head down

Press the palms down for stability

Cat Balance

Promote Balance • **Stabilize** Hips and Shoulder Joints

Although many balancing postures are done from a standing position, this posture, done on the floor, develops your core and strengthens the arm and leg muscles.

1 Begin on all fours, with your wrists aligned with the shoulders and your knees with the hips. Point the toes away from the body. Keep your weight even through the palms, knees, and feet. Flatten your back by reducing the lumbar curve and drawing the navel toward the spine.

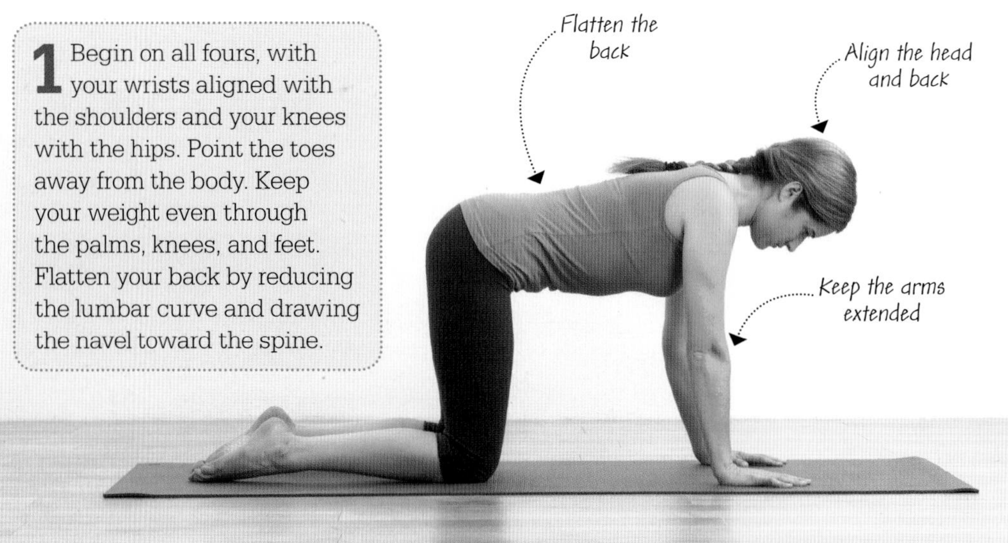
Flatten the back
Align the head and back
Keep the arms extended

2 As you inhale, tighten the abdominal muscles while raising the right arm in line with the body and keeping the shoulders level. As you exhale, lower your arm back to the floor. Repeat with the left arm. Repeat five times with each arm.

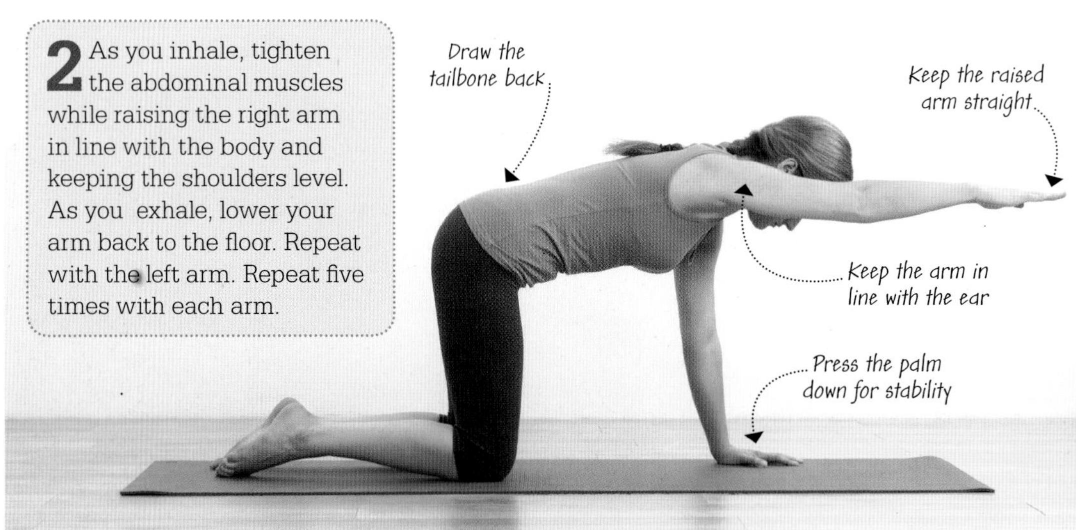
Draw the tailbone back
Keep the raised arm straight
Keep the arm in line with the ear
Press the palm down for stability

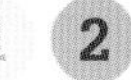

3 Return to the starting position. Inhale, pulling in the abdomen once more and raise and extend your right leg, with the ankle aligned with your shoulders. Lower your leg on exhalation and repeat, using the other leg. Repeat five times with each leg.

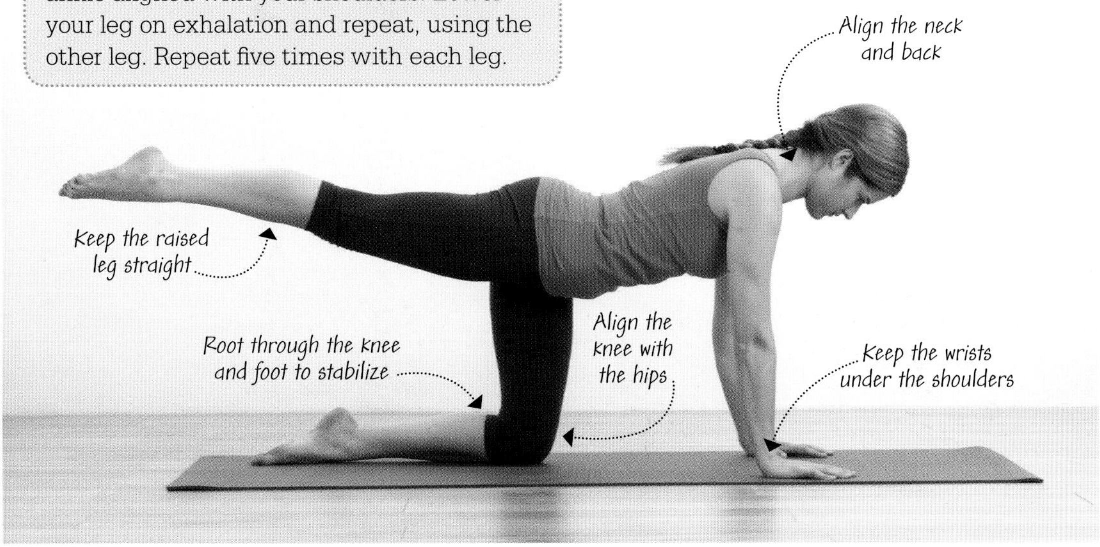

Align the neck and back
Keep the raised leg straight
Root through the knee and foot to stabilize
Align the knee with the hips
Keep the wrists under the shoulders

4 Return to your starting position. Inhale as you extend your left leg and right arm simultaneously. Hold for five breaths before repeating with the opposing limbs. Repeat five times, alternating your limbs.

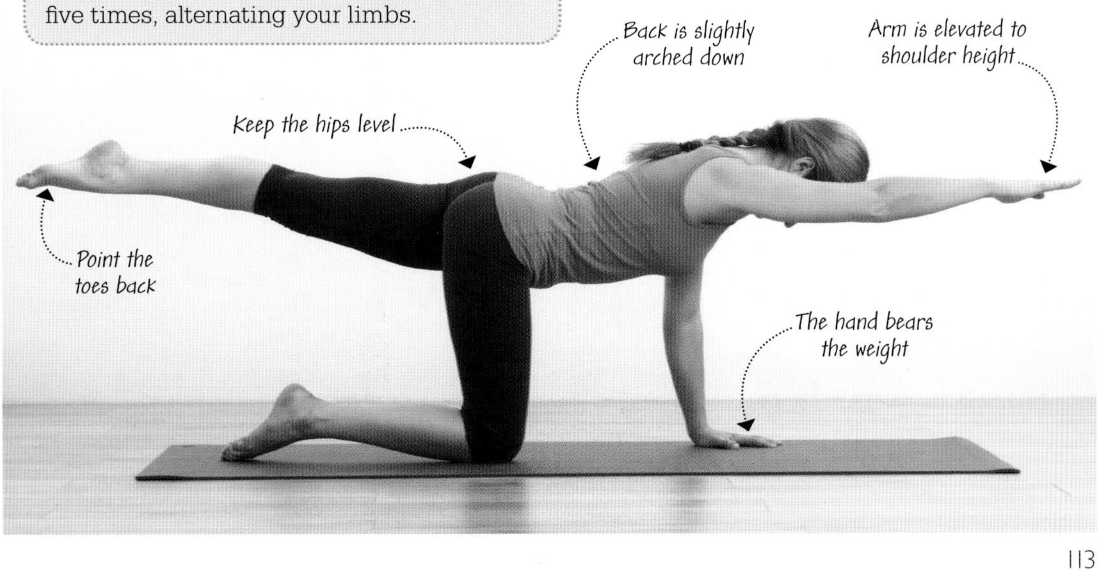

Back is slightly arched down
Arm is elevated to shoulder height
Keep the hips level
Point the toes back
The hand bears the weight

Extended Sitting Stretch

Strengthen Spine • **Tone** Legs and Arms

This pose extends the spine, arms, and legs simultaneously and prepares the body for the other sitting stretch poses.

1 Sit with your legs stretched out straight and the palms resting flat on your thighs. The feet are together with your big toes touching. Work on straightening your back and opening the chest.

Help! If you cannot maintain a straight back, then practice sitting against a wall so that the length of the back is supported by the wall.

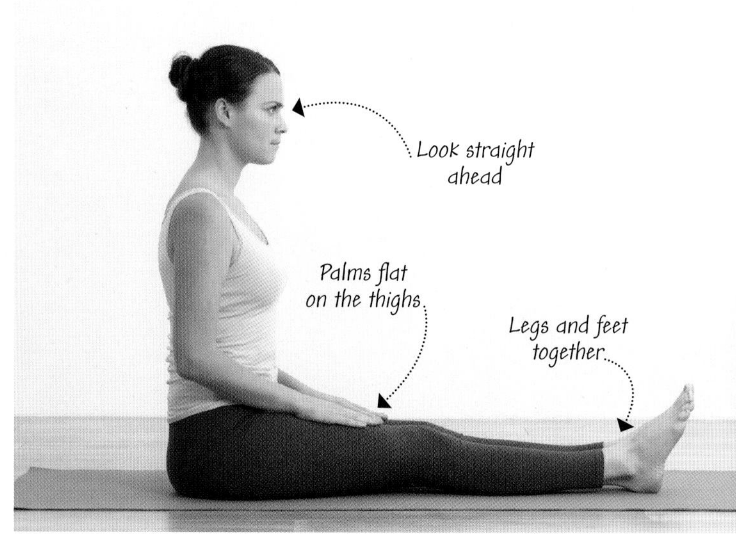
Look straight ahead
Palms flat on the thighs
Legs and feet together

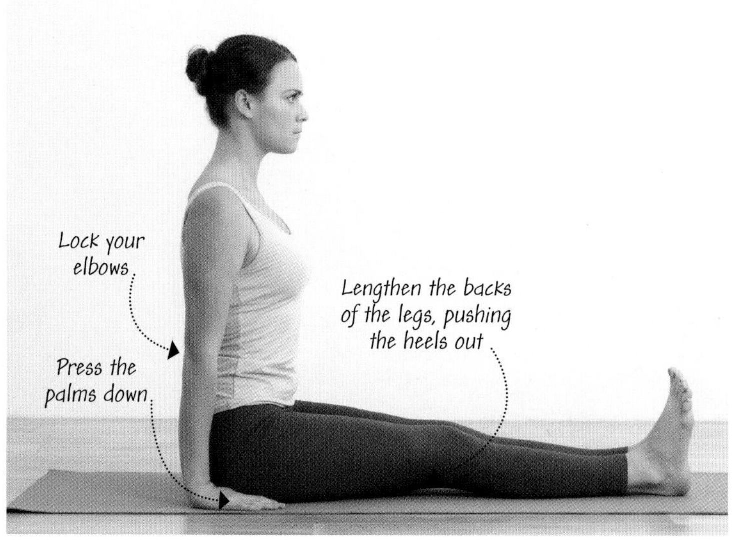
Lock your elbows
Press the palms down
Lengthen the backs of the legs, pushing the heels out

2 Place your arms beside your hips. Lock the elbows and press your palms down on the floor. Extend the backs of your legs, pushing the heels out and flexing the toes toward your torso. Inhale deeply to lift the sternum and expand the chest

Useful tip Use the downward pressure through the arms and palms to help you to lengthen your back.

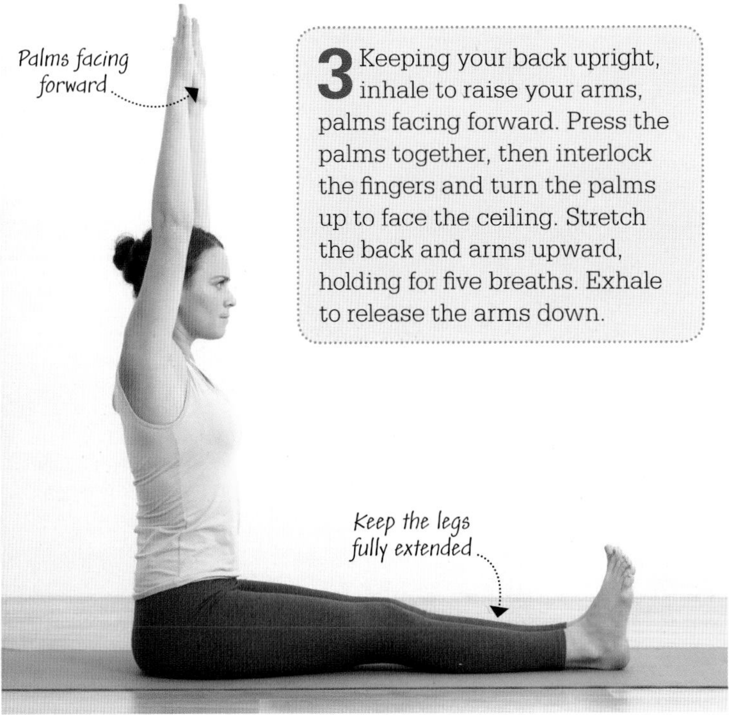
Palms facing forward
Keep the legs fully extended

3 Keeping your back upright, inhale to raise your arms, palms facing forward. Press the palms together, then interlock the fingers and turn the palms up to face the ceiling. Stretch the back and arms upward, holding for five breaths. Exhale to release the arms down.

Take it further

An alternative position is to cross the right wrist with the left wrist and rotate your arms and wrists to press the palms together. This twist helps to lengthen the spine.

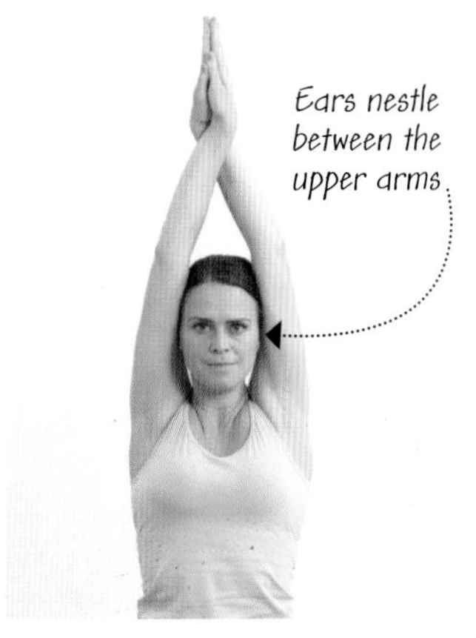
Ears nestle between the upper arms

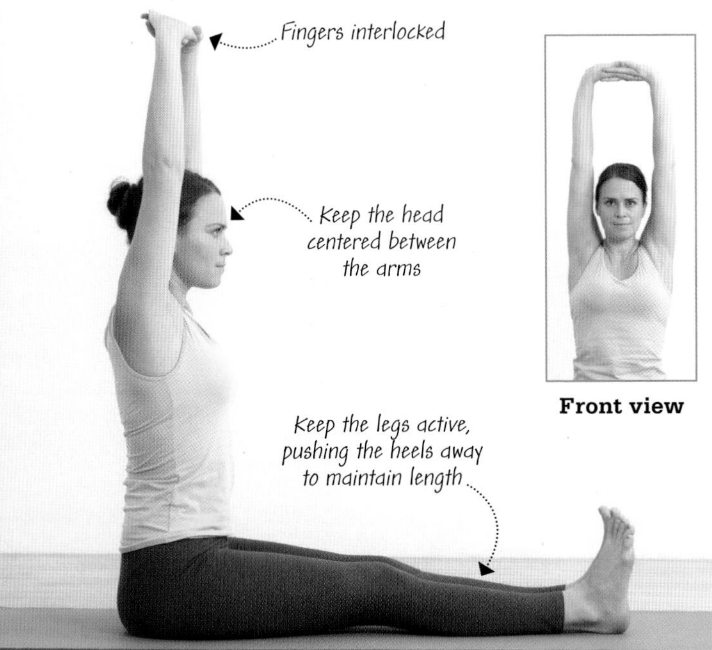
Fingers interlocked
Keep the head centered between the arms
Keep the legs active, pushing the heels away to maintain length

Front view

4 Raise the arms and interlock the fingers again, this time so that the thumb that was on top becomes the one underneath. Again, keeping your fingers interlocked, turn the palms to face the ceiling. Stretch your back and arms upward, holding for five to ten breaths. Release and lower the arms.

Useful tip To ensure that your arms are at 90 degrees to the floor, check that your ears are nestled between the upper arms.

Sitting Forward Stretch

Strengthen Lower Back • **Stretch** Hamstrings

This therapeutic posture calms the mind, massages the abdominal organs, and gives a good stretch to both the hamstring muscles and the spine.

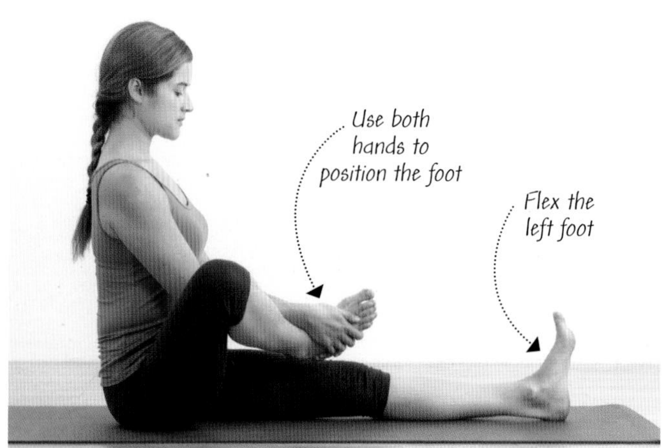
Use both hands to position the foot
Flex the left foot

1 Sit with your legs straight, and extended out in front. Inhale, bend your right knee and use both hands to clasp the right foot to help position the heel toward the groin.

Remember Keep the left leg extended with heel pushed out and toes curled toward the body.

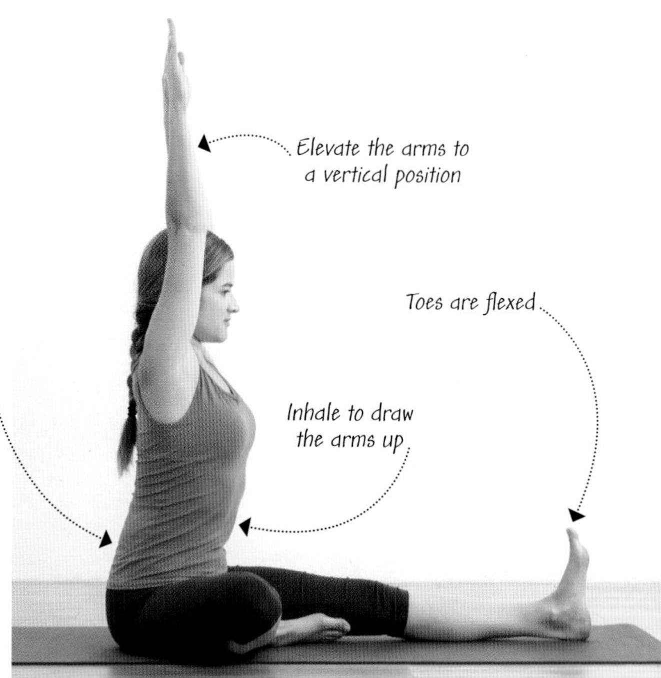
Elevate the arms to a vertical position
Lengthen the lumbar vertebrae
Toes are flexed
Inhale to draw the arms up

2 With the sole of the right foot against the left leg, inhale to raise both arms up straight with your palms facing forward.

Useful tip If your bent knee is off the ground, you could support it with a cushion.

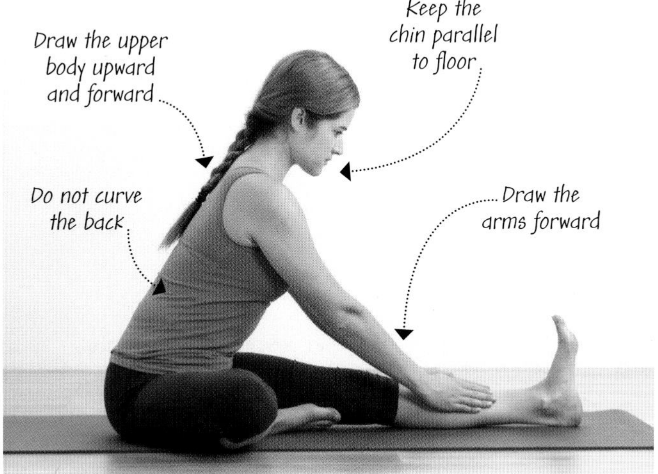
Draw the upper body upward and forward
Keep the chin parallel to floor
Do not curve the back
Draw the arms forward

3 On exhalation, bring your arms down, resting them on the calf of your extended leg as you hinge forward from the waist. Breathe in as you stretch through the spine.

Useful tip Keep your back straight and keep your gaze on a point straight in front of you.

4 As you exhale, try to bring your torso closer to your extended leg by lengthening forward and, if possible, clasping your left ankle or foot with your hands. Breathe in slowly as you return to sitting. Repeat on the other side.

Useful tip Use your exhalations to lengthen the spine and lean forward a little more.

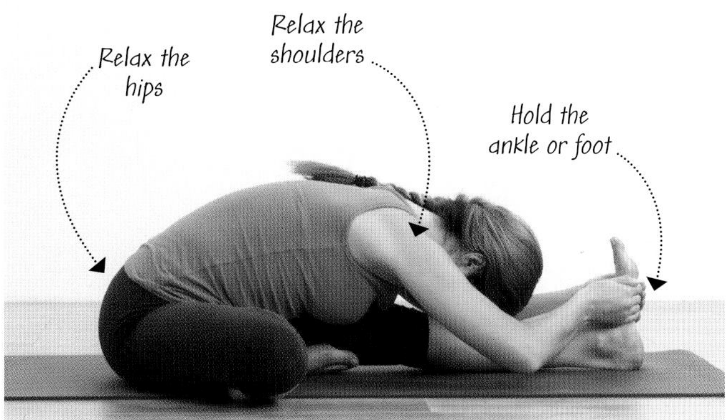
Relax the hips
Relax the shoulders
Hold the ankle or foot

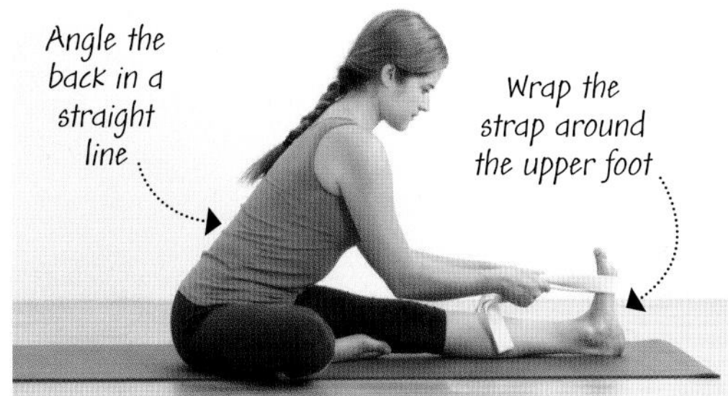
Angle the back in a straight line
Wrap the strap around the upper foot

Make it easier

Wrap a strap around your foot and hold it with both hands, keeping your sitting bones grounded and lengthening from the base of your spine. Keep lengthening the spine evenly and work on moving your hands a little farther along the strap as you exhale. Drop the strap if you have extended forward enough and are able to hold the feet comfortably. Repeat on the other side.

Chair Twist

Release Neck and Shoulder Tension • **Stretch** Spine

This spinal twist is a simple yet effective way of incorporating yoga into your daily life. The exercise can be done easily either in the office or at home—all you need is a standard chair and a few spare minutes.

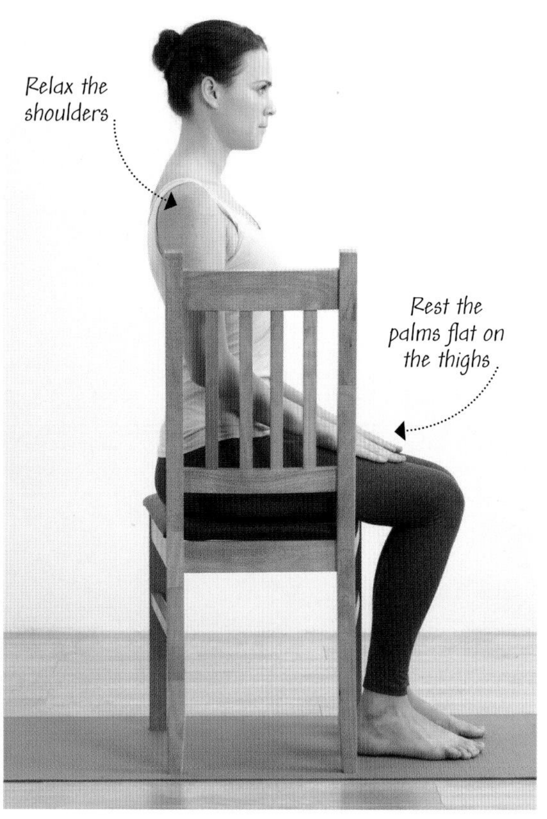
Relax the shoulders
Rest the palms flat on the thighs

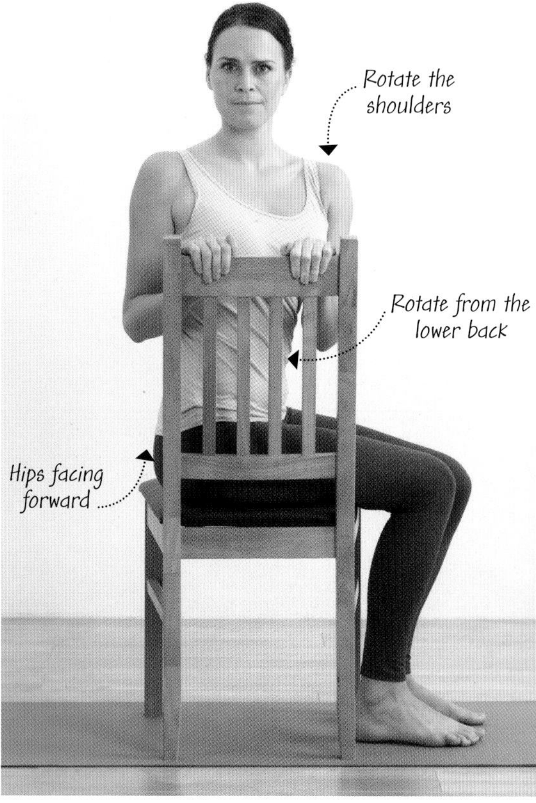
Rotate the shoulders
Rotate from the lower back
Hips facing forward

1 Sit sideways on a standard chair so that the backrest is next to your arm and your feet are flat on the floor. Keeping a straight back, rest your hands on your thighs and look ahead. Focus on relaxing the shoulders.

2 Grasp the backrest of the chair with both hands and lift up your chest. On exhalation, start to twist from the lower back, following the direction of your arms toward the rear of the chair.

3 Stretching the spine upward, rotate the trunk, shoulders, and neck. Turn your head to the right as far as is comfortable, and raise your right arm. Relax the shoulders and face muscles. Hold for five to ten breaths then exhale and release. Repeat on the other side.

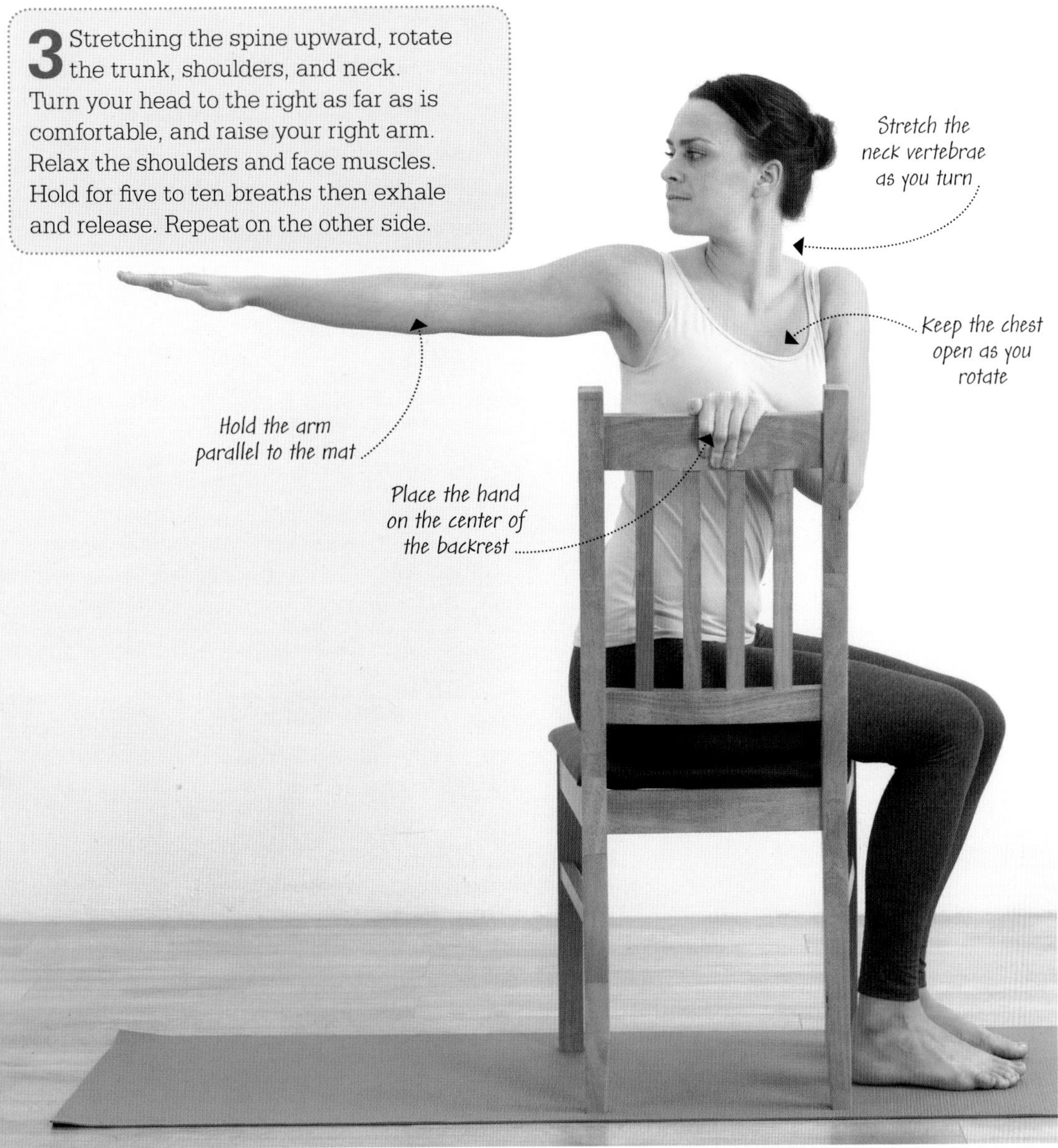
Stretch the neck vertebrae as you turn
Keep the chest open as you rotate
Hold the arm parallel to the mat
Place the hand on the center of the backrest

Take care...

Stiffness in the neck can result in an incomplete twist. With each exhalation, gently work the twist from your waist, up the back, and finally along the neck and head. Make the movements slow and purposeful, rotating to a comfortable level.

Avoid hunching the shoulders toward the ears, and prevent flexing at the wrist by lengthening through the whole stretched arm, drawing the fingertips toward the wall.

Half Spinal Twist

Strengthen Back and Thighs • **Improve** Posture

This pose involves a lateral twist along the complete length of the spine. It is designed to increase the flexibility of the spine and therefore benefit overall posture. It can also help to release tension in the body.

1 Start in a seated position with your legs extended. Straighten your arms behind you with your palms on the mat and fingers pointing away from your body. Breathe from the abdomen.

Draw the shoulders back
Focus on your breath
Palms facing away from the body
Feet are vertical

Take care...

Avoid leaning your trunk at an angle as it should be at 90 degrees to the floor. Adjust the position of the rear hand to keep the trunk upright.

People with lower back stiffness have a tendency to twist from the waist upward. If you experience discomfort in the lower back in Step 3, then reduce the twist, rotating 45–60 degrees instead of 90 degrees.

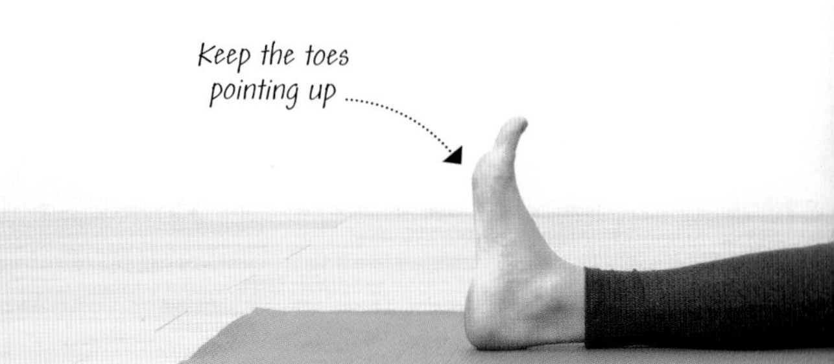
Keep the toes pointing up

2 Bring your left foot to the mat over your right leg, adjacent to your right calf. Inhale as you lift your right arm straight upward, palm open and fingers extended.

Remember Keep your hips even and your sitting bones in contact with the floor throughout the pose.

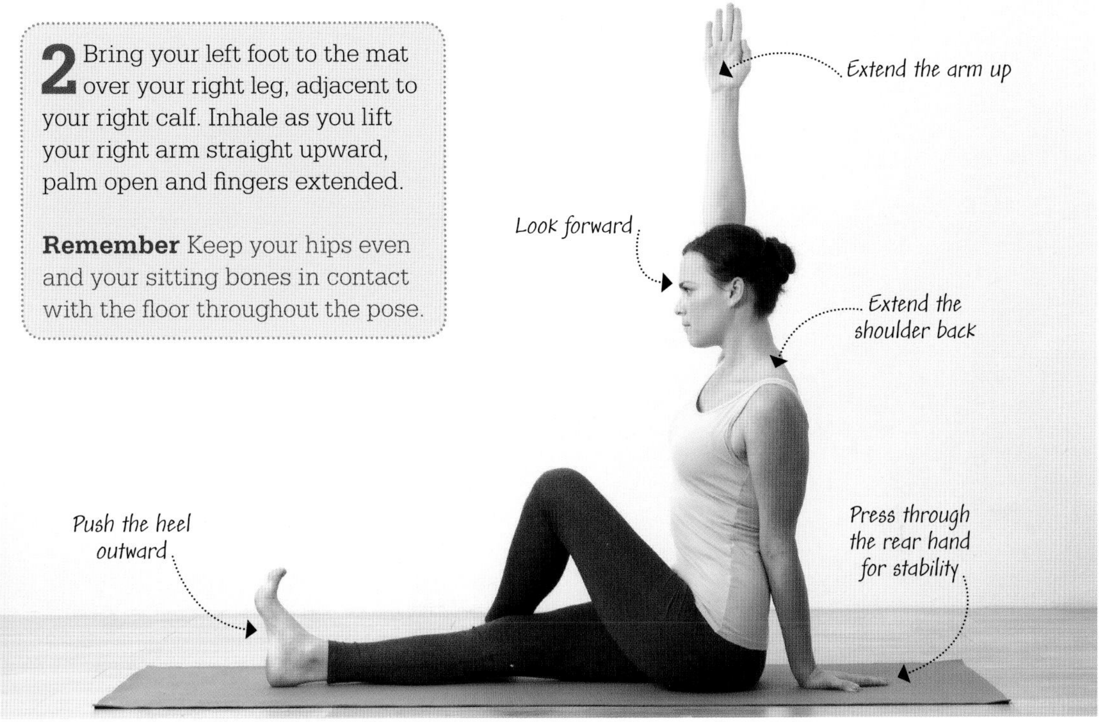

Extend the arm up

Look forward

Extend the shoulder back

Push the heel outward

Press through the rear hand for stability

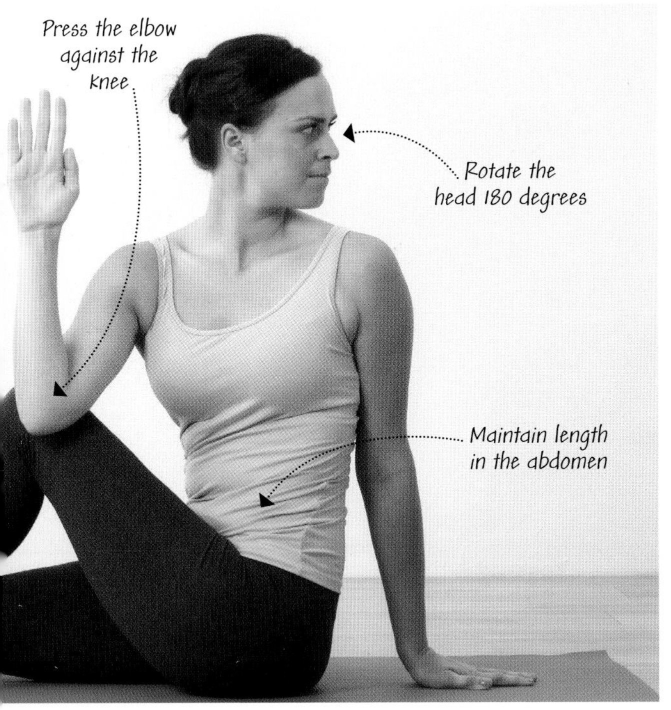
Press the elbow against the knee
Rotate the head 180 degrees
Maintain length in the abdomen

3 On exhalation, bring the right arm across the left knee, palm facing forward. Lift upward from the waist then twist until you are looking over your shoulder. Breathe slowly via the abdomen.

Useful tip Ground the buttock bones to ensure you twist without pinching the lower back.

Crossed Leg Forward Bend

Release Hips and Outer Thighs • **Relieve** Tension

This cross-legged forward bend has three main benefits: It calms and quietens the mind, improves digestion, and relieves tension in the lower back.

1 Begin in a cross-legged position with your right ankle in front of the left. Root down with your sitting bones and hinge forward from the waist, putting your palms flat on the floor in front of you. Exhale and lean forward, keeping your back straight.

Useful tip To get the feet farther back under the thighs, lift the knees up slightly, hold your toes and slide the feet back a fraction more toward the torso.

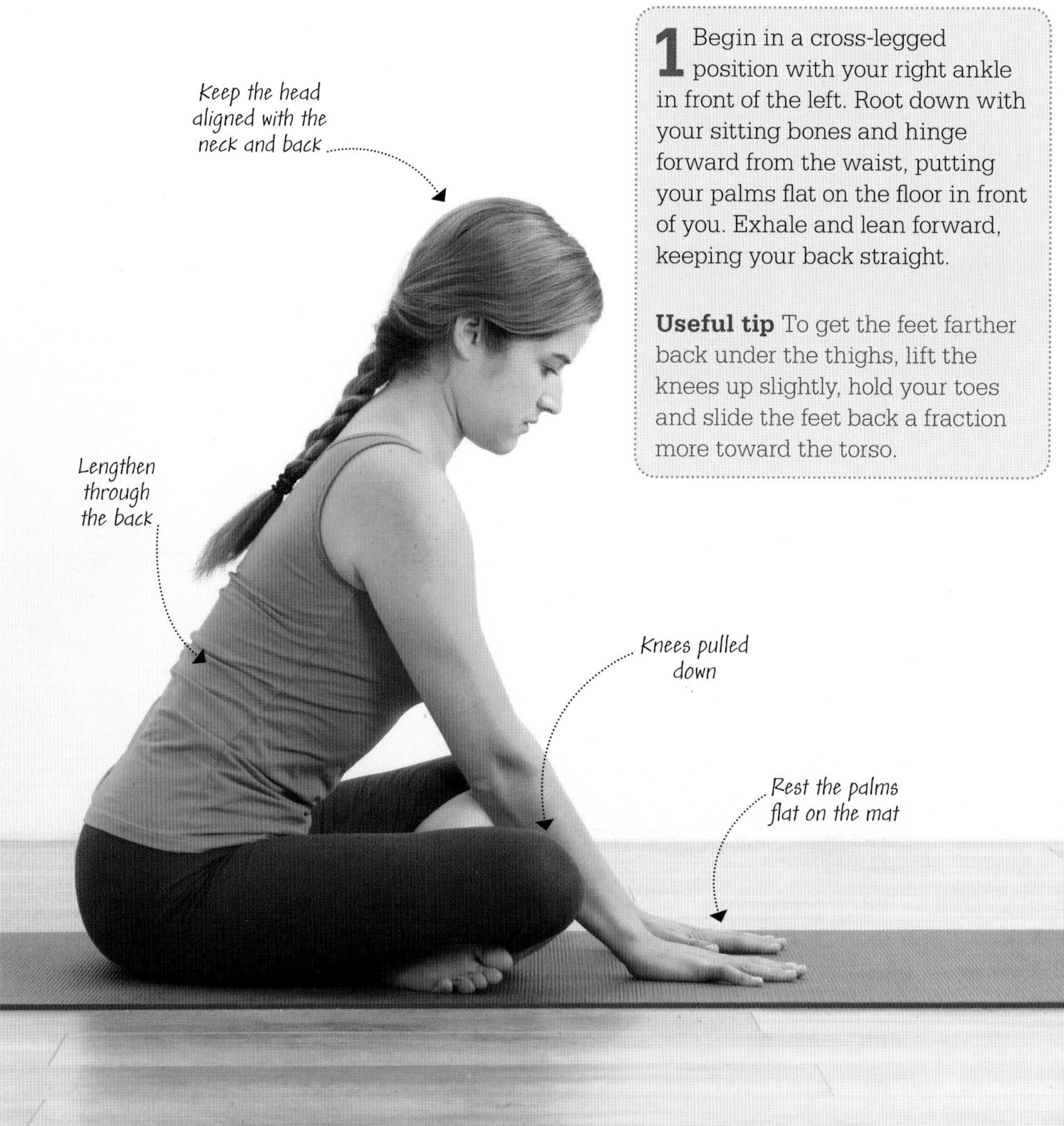
Keep the head aligned with the neck and back
Lengthen through the back
Knees pulled down
Rest the palms flat on the mat

2 Rooting down through your sitting bones, stretch your torso and arms, placing your palms farther away from you. On exhaling, try to inch forward. Hold for five to ten breaths, then release. Reverse the cross of your legs and repeat the stretch.

Useful tip Practice floor sittings in your leisure hours to develop flexibility in the knees, so that cross-legged sitting feels natural.

Take care...

As you try to get the head closer to the floor, the front foot tends to slip forward. To avoid this, try sitting on a blanket and keeping your feet on the mat.

Avoid flexing the neck in order to get the forehead closer to the floor. The back, neck, and head should remain aligned.

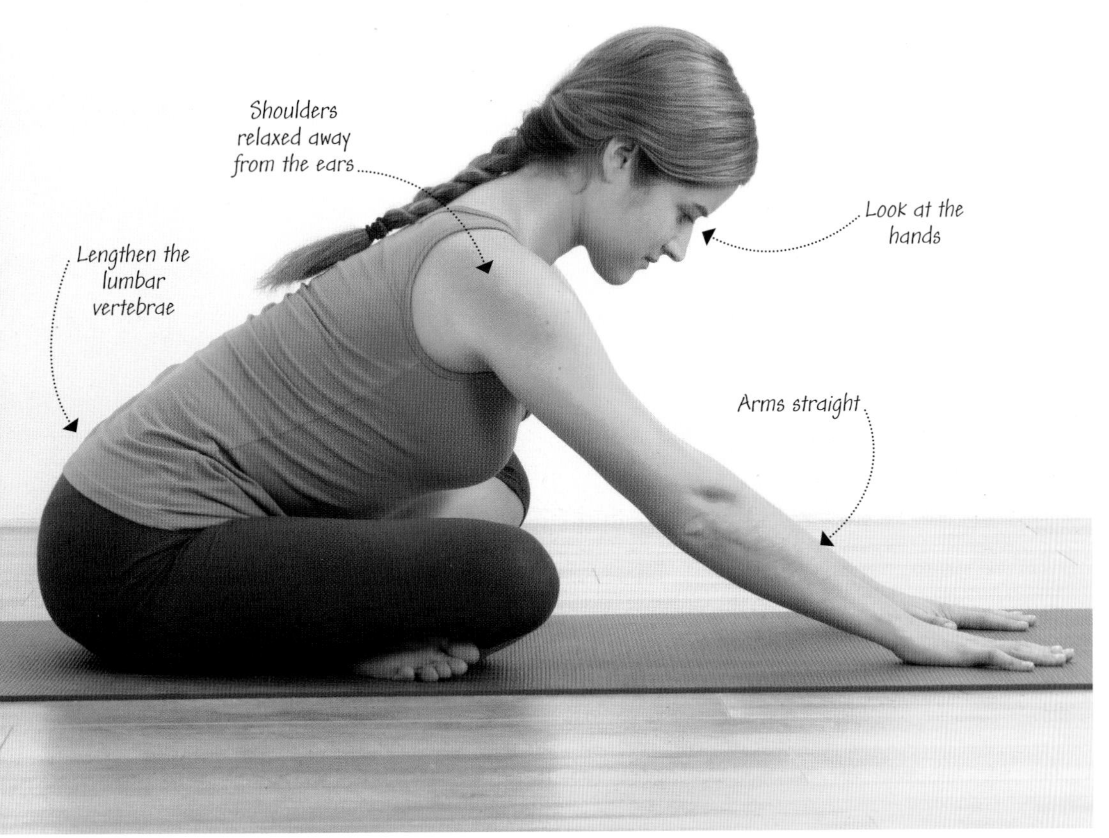
Shoulders relaxed away from the ears
Look at the hands
Lengthen the lumbar vertebrae
Arms straight

Bridge

Strenthen Spine • **Revitalize** Body

This pose promotes relaxation and can help reduce stress. In addition to stretching the spine, it is also a good posture to do if your feet are feeling tired.

1 Lie on your back with your knees fully bent and feet flat on the floor. Extend and relax your arms alongside your body with the palms facing the floor.

Useful tip If you look down the side of your body, you should be able to see the outer edges of your feet parallel to the mat.

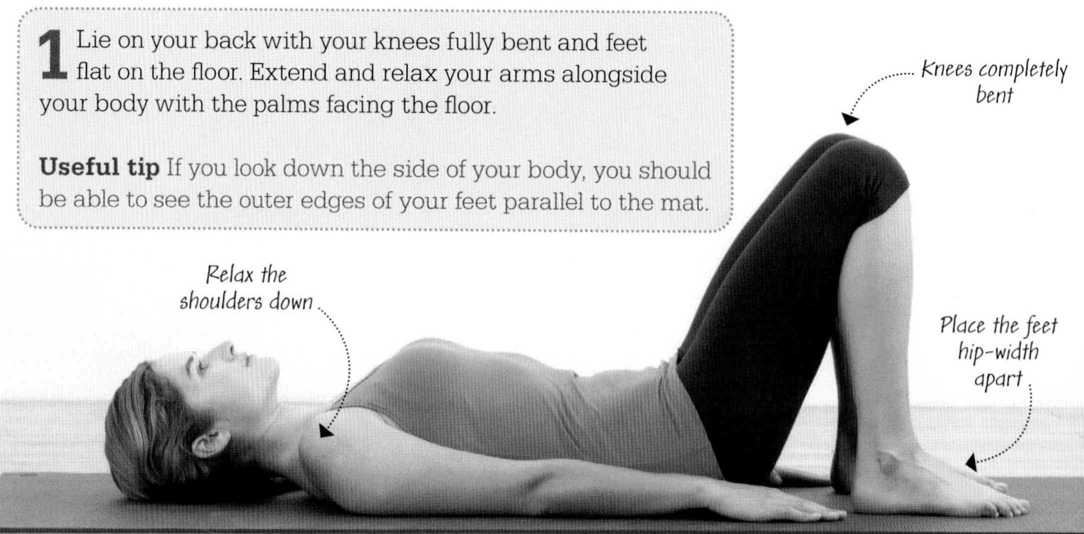
Knees completely bent
Relax the shoulders down
Place the feet hip-width apart

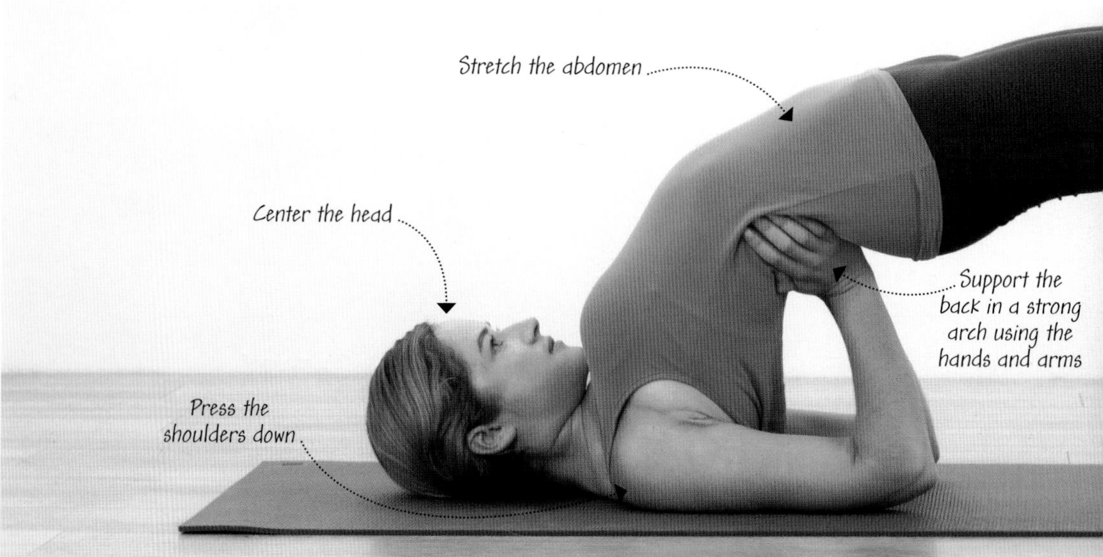
Stretch the abdomen
Center the head
Support the back in a strong arch using the hands and arms
Press the shoulders down

2 Edge the hands to the feet and either hold the heels or grasp each ankle. Plant your feet firmly. Inhale as you push your hips upward, lifting the lower back clear of the floor to arch the spine. Your shoulders will support the weight of the upper body.

Useful tip Work on drawing your chest toward the chin by lifting your hips higher and arching your back a little more.

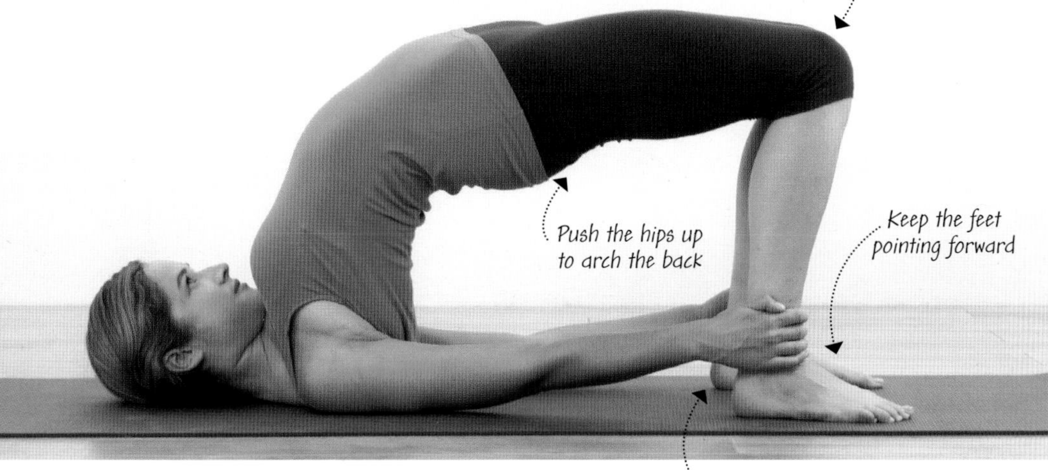
Keep the leg muscles engaged to lift the hips
Push the hips up to arch the back
Keep the feet pointing forward
Keep the feet hip-width apart

Keep the legs apart

Lower legs are vertical to the floor

3 Maintaining your position, release your ankles and bend your elbows as you slide your hands up the back as near as possible to the shoulder blades. Take a few deep breaths in this position before releasing by lowering your hands, followed by your hips and back.

Remember Your hands should be firmly underneath your back, with fingers outward and thumbs inward. Press down with the upper arms and use your hands to gently arch the back farther to a comfortable level.

Bridge Variations

Strengthen Legs • **Revitalize** Brain

This pose takes the weight off your legs, allowing you to gently work the hamstring muscles of each leg individually, lessening the chance of strain or injury.

Start in the Bridge Pose, making sure you are anchored correctly at the feet and shoulders. Take several deep breaths and edge your feet forward so that the lower legs are angled at about 45 degrees to the floor.

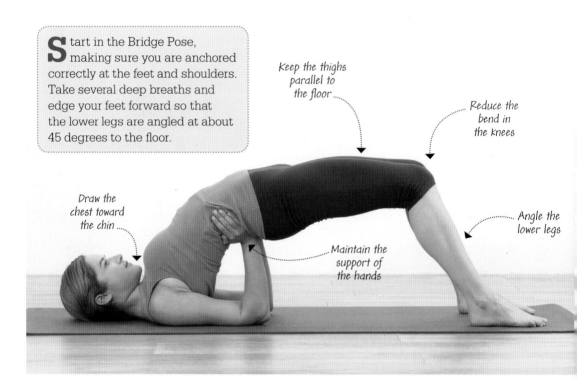

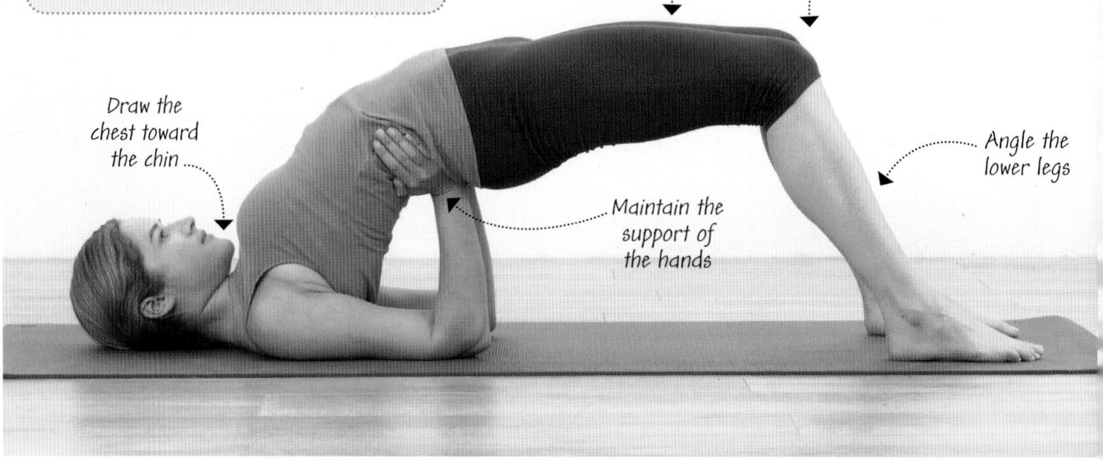

Keep the thighs parallel to the floor

Reduce the bend in the knees

Draw the chest toward the chin

Angle the lower legs

Maintain the support of the hands

What not to do

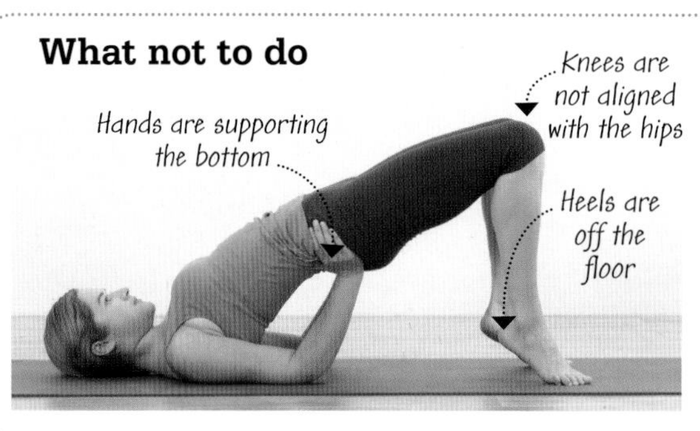
Hands are supporting the bottom
Knees are not aligned with the hips
Heels are off the floor

Take care...

Don't allow your heels to rise off the floor or to be placed at an angle. Focus on pressing your feet flat on the mat.

Make sure your hands are supporting the small of your back and not lower down at your bottom.

Avoid tilting the head and lifting the neck off the floor.

More of a challenge Single Leg Lift

Begin to raise your left foot, extending upward and pointing your toes. Continue to raise your foot until your leg is perpendicular to the floor. Take five full breaths before releasing upon exhalation, and then repeat with the other leg.

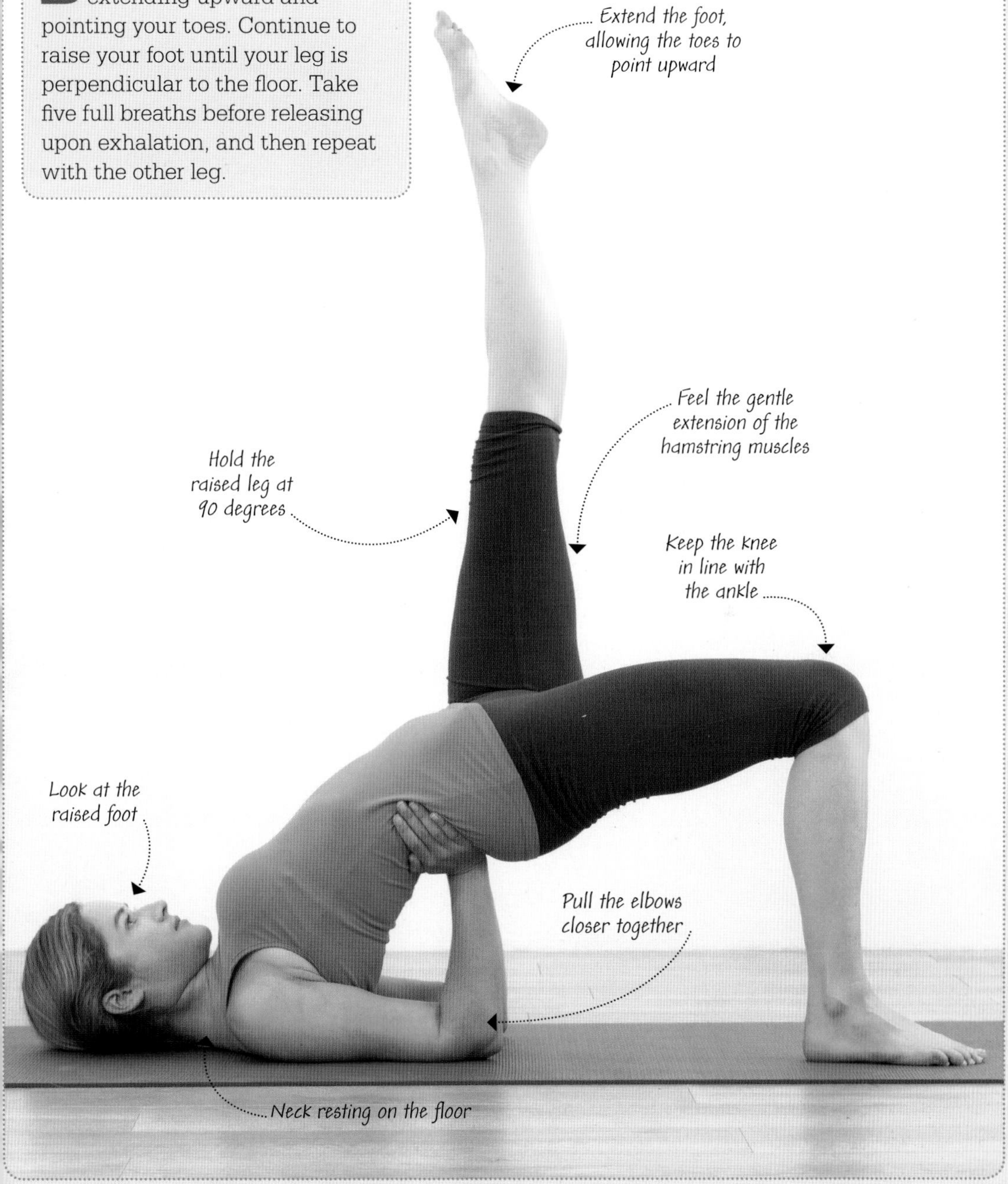

Extend the foot, allowing the toes to point upward

Feel the gentle extension of the hamstring muscles

Hold the raised leg at 90 degrees

Keep the knee in line with the ankle

Look at the raised foot

Pull the elbows closer together

Neck resting on the floor

Half Shoulder Stand with Wall

Improve Circulation • **Promote** Youthfulness

The inverted postures reverse the flow of blood, increasing the supply of blood to the face and brain, as well as the heart and other organs. These postures are particularly restorative.

1 Place your mat at right angles to the wall. Fold a blanket so the width of the fold is the length of your lower back, and place it adjacent to the wall. Sit on the blanket with your left shoulder next to the wall, legs bent, and hands clasped over your shins.

Remember Your shoulders, arms, and hips should gently touch the wall, but your feet should slightly away from the wall, so that the body is aligned.

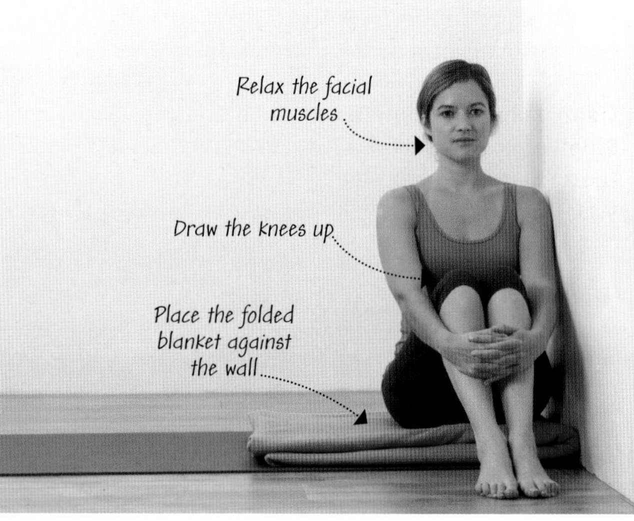
Relax the facial muscles
Draw the knees up
Place the folded blanket against the wall

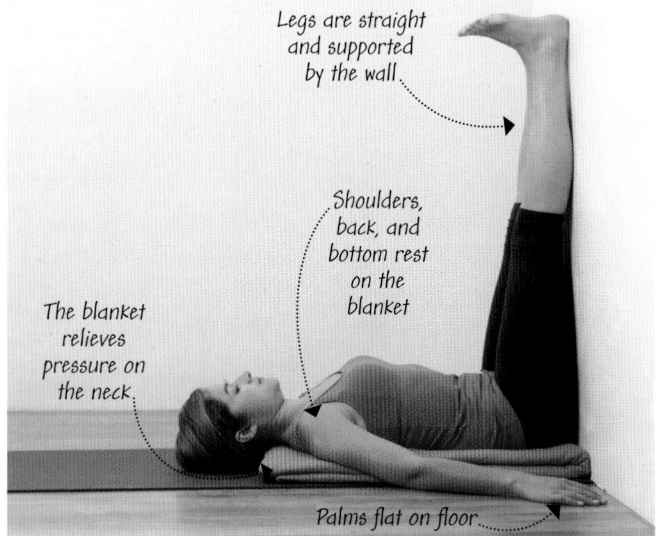
Legs are straight and supported by the wall
Shoulders, back, and bottom rest on the blanket
The blanket relieves pressure on the neck
Palms flat on floor

2 Swiveling your body through 45 degrees, lay your upper body down on the mat. At the same time, swing your legs upward until your legs and hips are resting against the wall, with your feet together.

Useful tip Press the full length of your legs up against the wall and have your feet parallel to the mat.

3 Bend your knees so that your feet are flat against the wall. Pushing off from your feet, raise your torso and bring your hands onto the small of your back.

Useful tip Pull your elbows closer together, and press down through the shoulders as you prepare to take your feet off the wall.

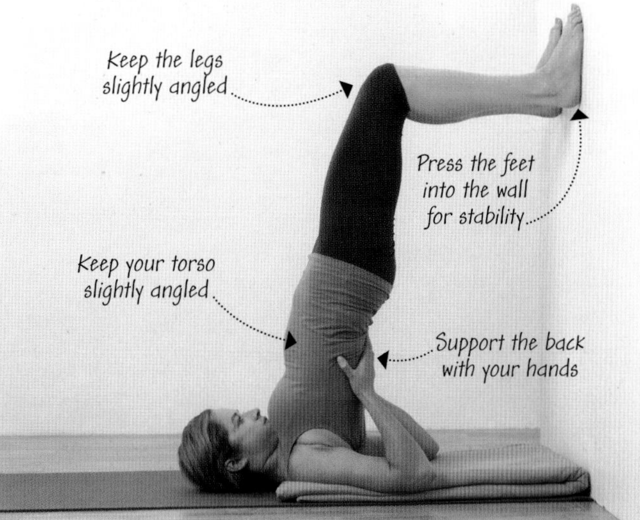
Keep the legs slightly angled
Press the feet into the wall for stability
Keep your torso slightly angled
Support the back with your hands

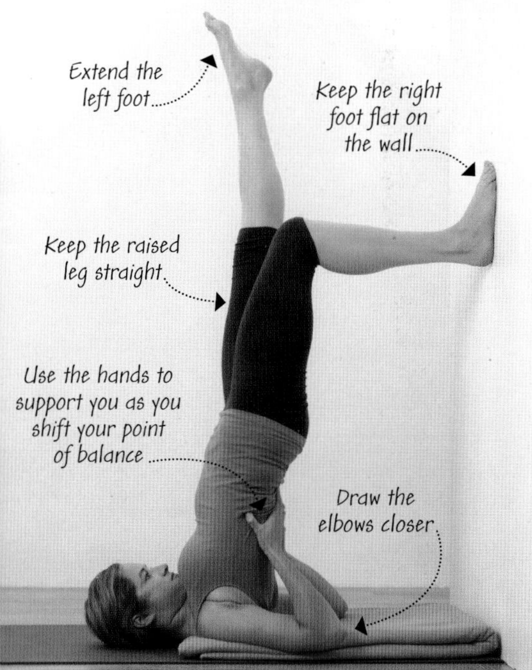
Extend the left foot
Keep the right foot flat on the wall
Keep the raised leg straight
Use the hands to support you as you shift your point of balance
Draw the elbows closer

4 Adjust your position so that your back is as straight as possible. Now raise one leg until it is pointing straight upward.

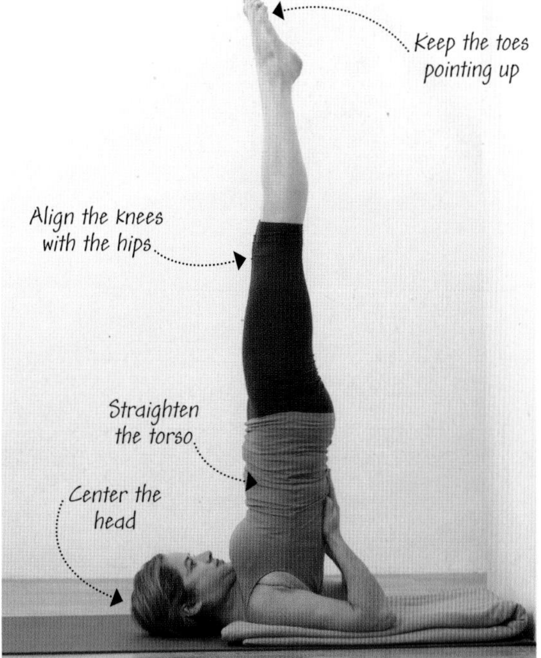
Keep the toes pointing up
Align the knees with the hips
Straighten the torso
Center the head

5 Bring your other leg into the same position, adjusting the position of your hands so they provide adequate support.

Take care...

Moving your feet off the wall can often make your body wobble. Press down through the shoulders and arms for better support. Slowing the movements and activating your core will help your stability during this transition.

There is a tendency to have the legs tilted as it is often difficult to get the legs 90 degrees to the floor. Draw your elbows closer together to get better leverage for pressing your hands to support and lengthen the lower back.

Misalignment of the elevated part of the body can cause the neck and arm muscles to become overengaged. You can avoid straining your neck and elbows by centering your weight evenly over your shoulders and aligning your hips, knees, and feet.

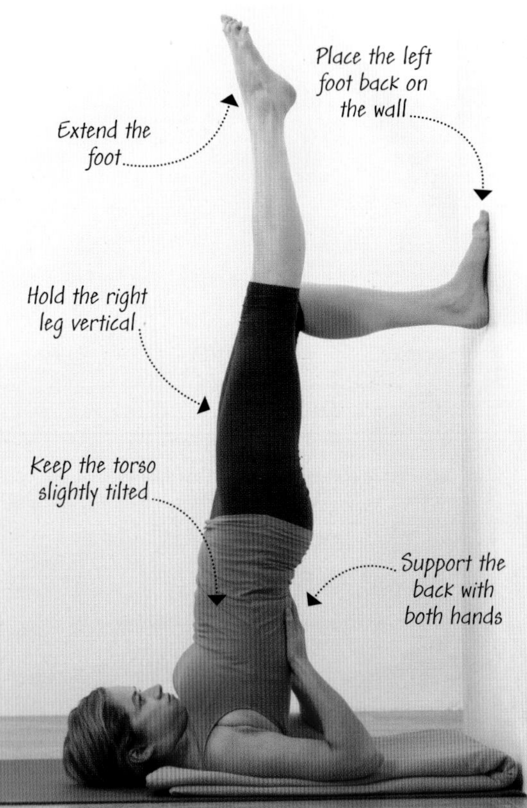
Extend the foot
Place the left foot back on the wall
Hold the right leg vertical
Keep the torso slightly tilted
Support the back with both hands

Press both feet against wall

Slightly tilt the upper legs

Lower legs parallel to the floor

The torso follows the tilt of your legs

6 Start to release the posture by bending your left knee, and bringing your foot to rest against the wall once more. Use your hands and arms to help you keep your balance and give support to your back.

7 Bringing your other leg into the same position and with your arms still supporting your back, gradually lower your spine back to the floor in a controlled move.

8 Once your back is flat on the floor, straighten your legs up against the wall with your feet a little apart. Extend your arms along the floor at a 45-degree angle to your body. Gently close your eyes and feel the nourishing effects of the pose. Take several relaxing breaths in this position.

Useful tip Allow the floor and wall to take the full weight of the body and ease away any tension that you can feel.

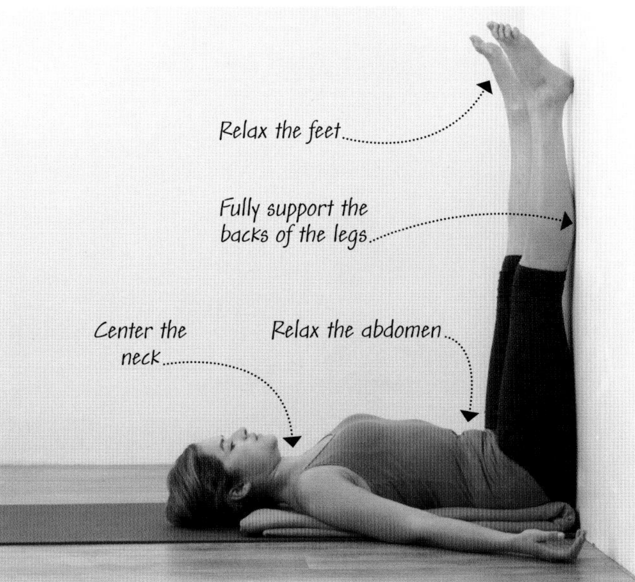
Relax the feet
Fully support the backs of the legs
Center the neck
Relax the abdomen

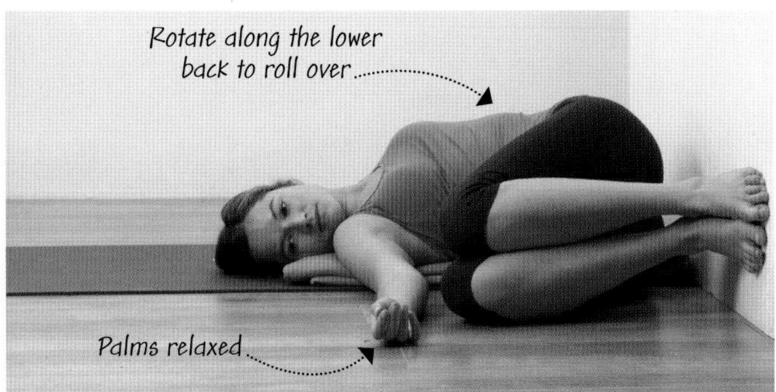
Rotate along the lower back to roll over
Palms relaxed

9 As you exhale, bend your knees over the chest, and stretch along the lower back through the hips to roll the bent legs sideways until your knees reach the floor. Remain in this position for a few breaths, then move into a sitting position.

Make it easier

After the active use of the legs in the Half Shoulder Stand with Wall, these variations provide a gentle counter-stretch for the muscles of the legs.

Bend the knees toward the chest and draw your feet down, keeping the soles of your feet flat against the wall (see right).

Bend the knees toward the chest. Then move the knees wide apart until the soles of the feet are pressed together and resting against the wall.

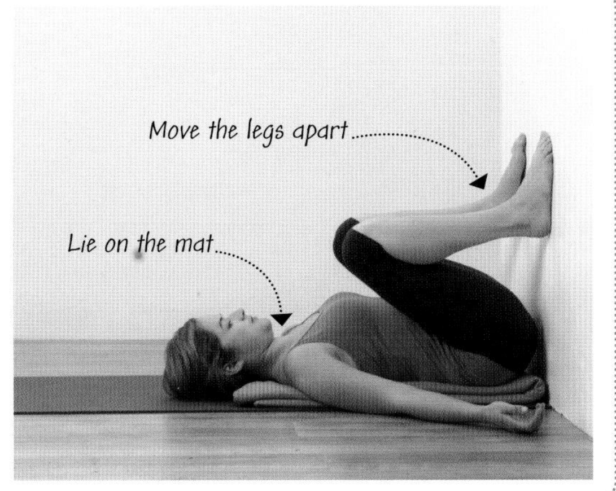
Move the legs apart
Lie on the mat

15-Minute Twisting Sequence

1 **Mountain Pose**
pp.44–45

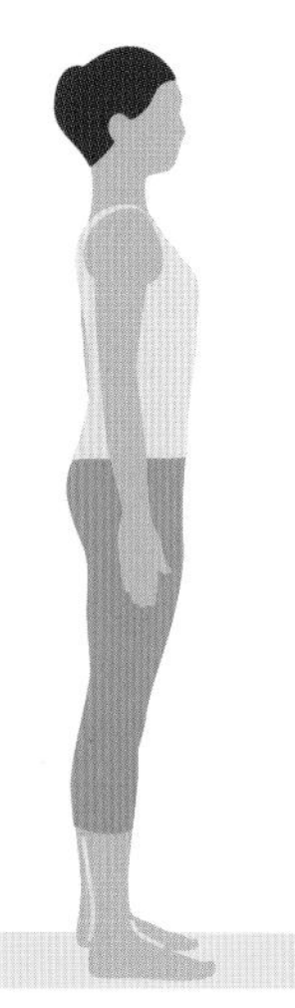

2 **Standing Arm Stretches**
pp.46–47

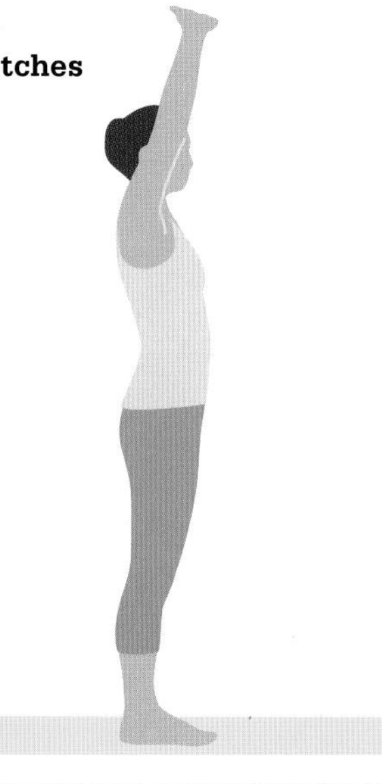

5 **Child's Pose**
pp.62–63

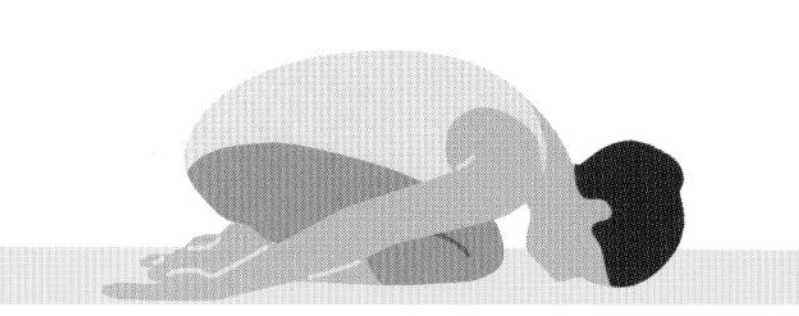

6 **Half Spinal Twist**
pp.120–121

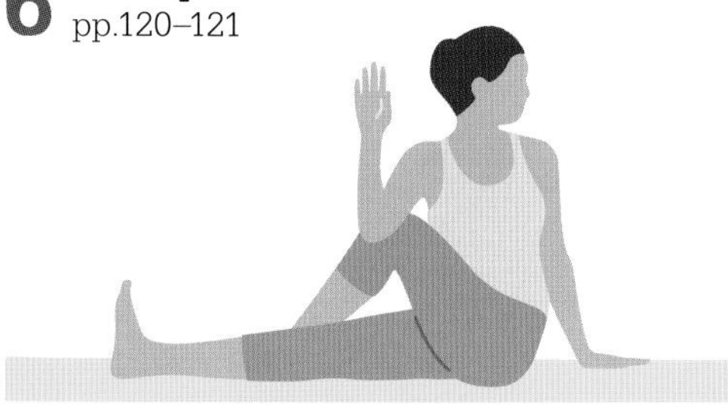

8 **Cobbler**
pp.74–75

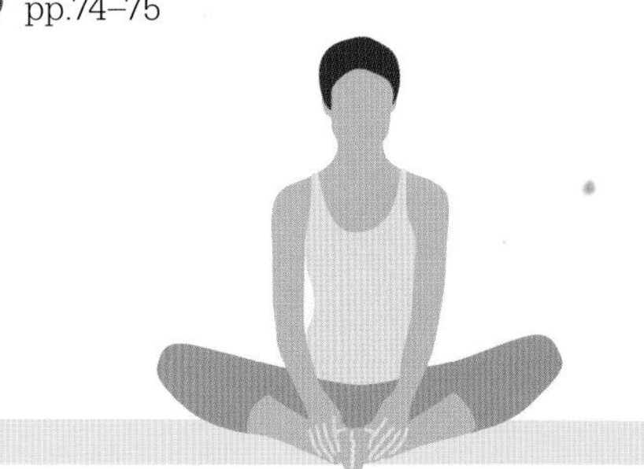

9 **Crossed Leg Forwards Bend**
pp.122–123

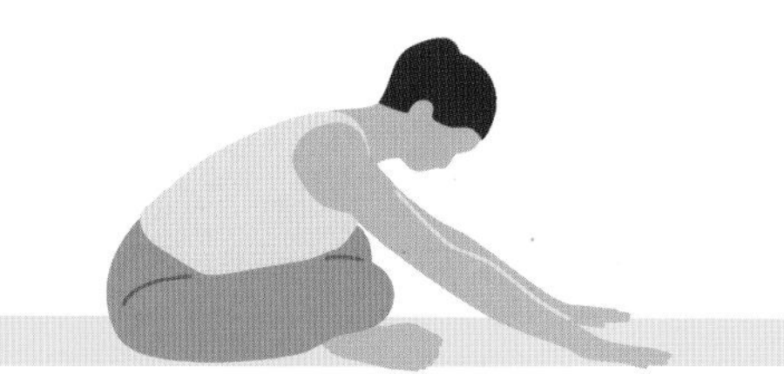

3 Chair Twist
pp.118–119

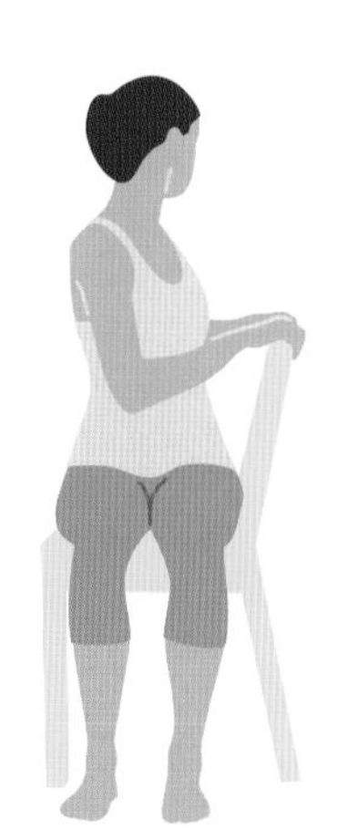

4 Eagle
p.97

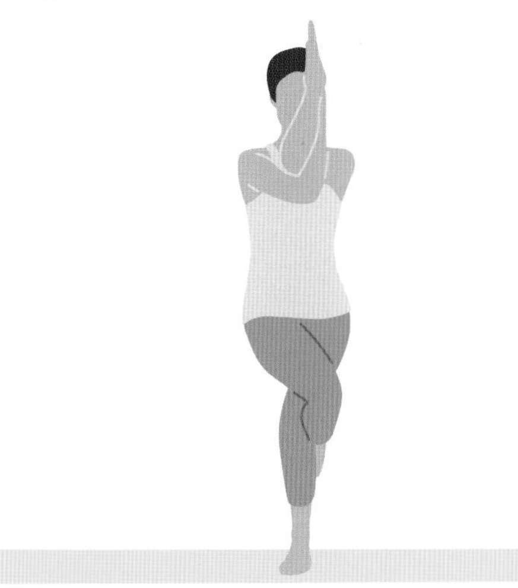

7 Easy Floor Twist
pp.72–73

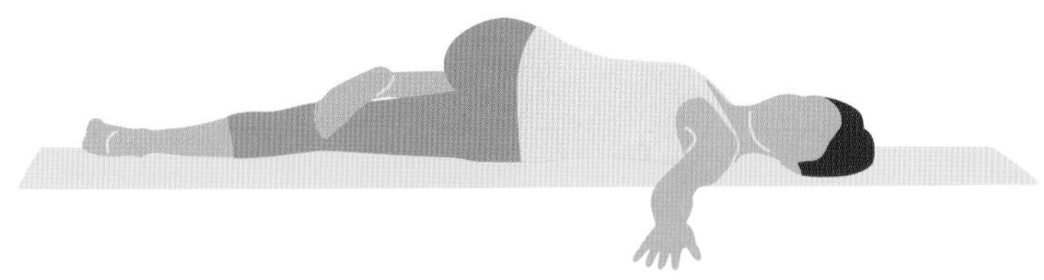

10 Corpse and Final Relaxation pp.78–81

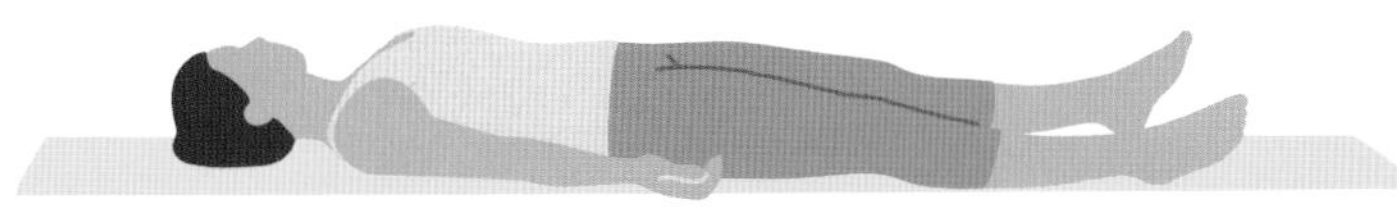

15-Minute Starting Inversion Sequence

1 **Mountain Pose** pp.44–45

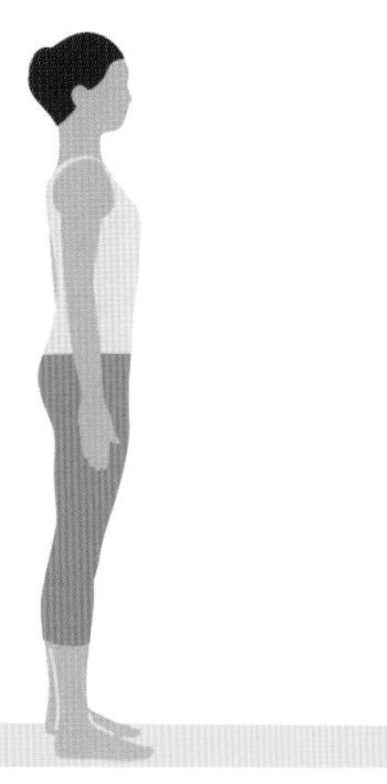

2 **Standing Forward Bend** pp.52–53

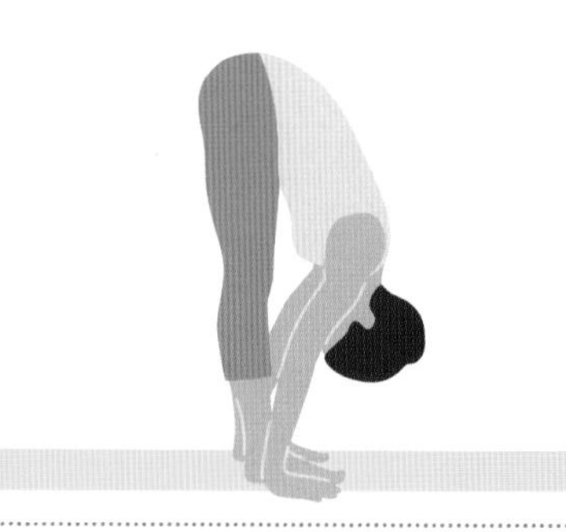

5 **Downward Facing Dog** pp.56–57

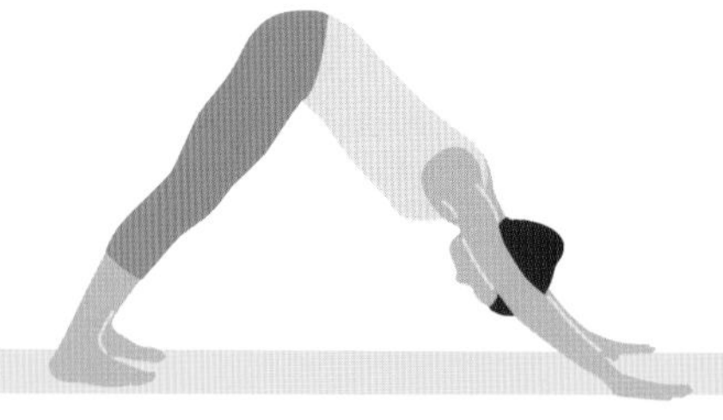

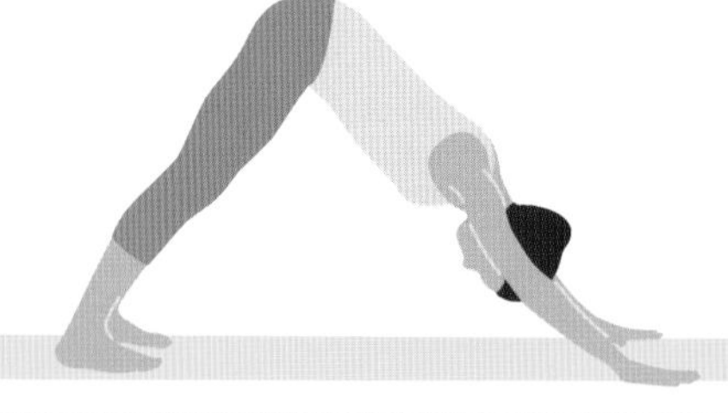

6 **Child's Pose** pp.62–63

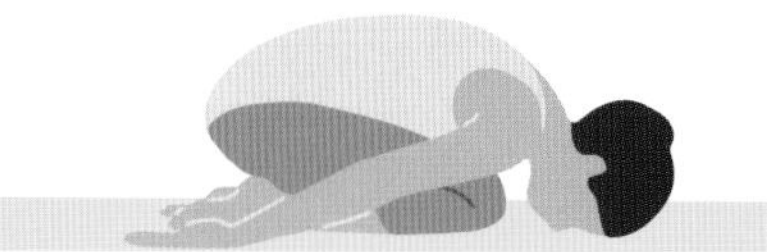

9 **Half Shoulder Stand with Wall** pp.128–131

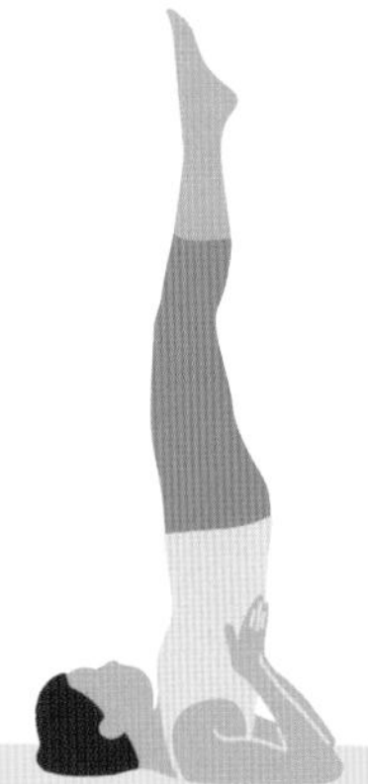

3 Wide Forward Bend pp.106–107

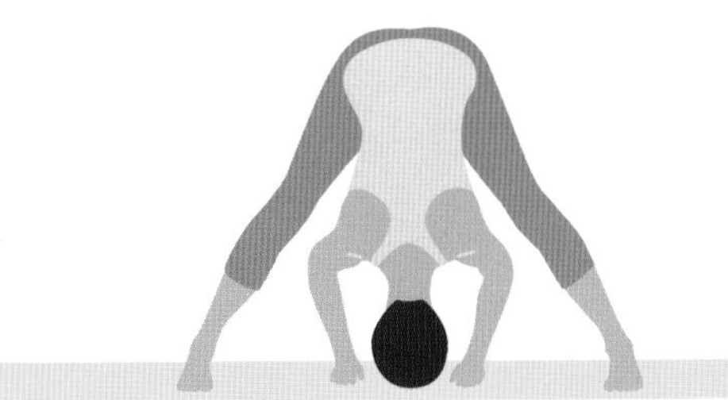

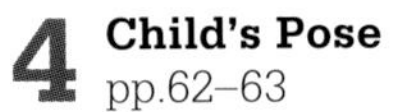

4 Child's Pose pp.62–63

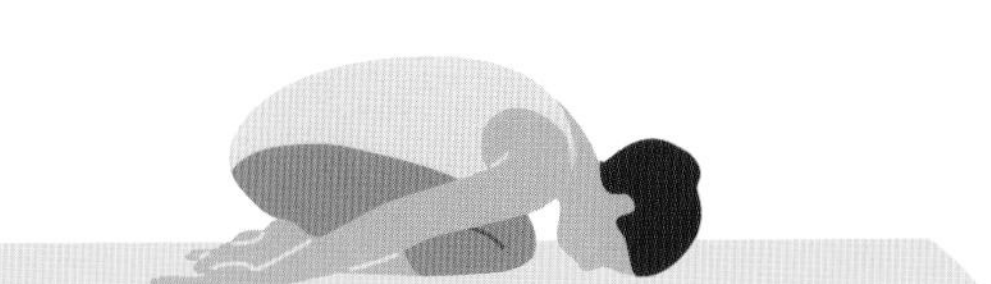

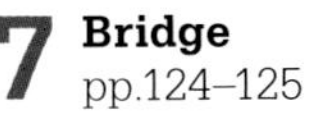

7 Bridge pp.124–125

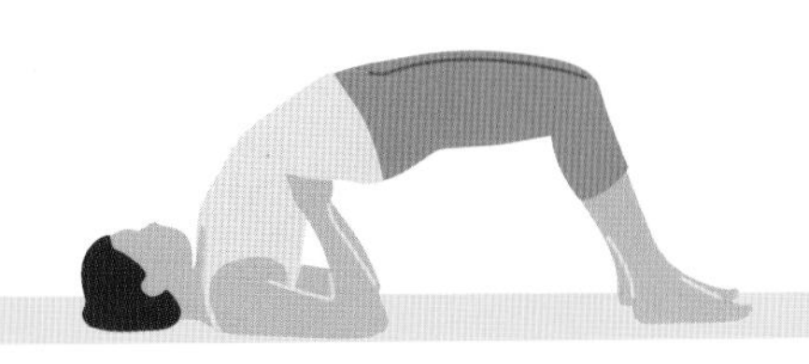

8 Leg Raise 1 p.48

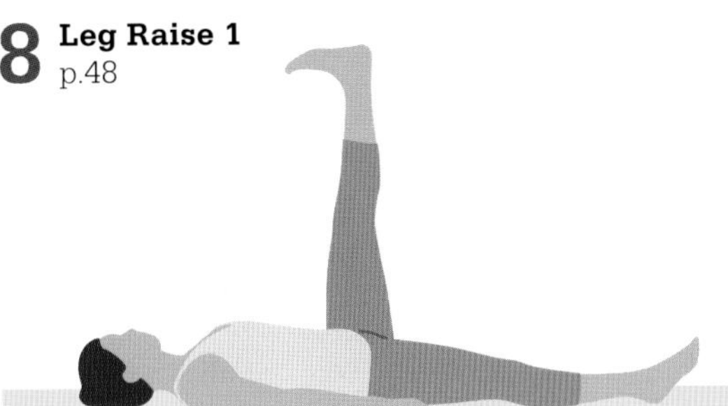

10 Corpse and Final Relaxation pp.78–81

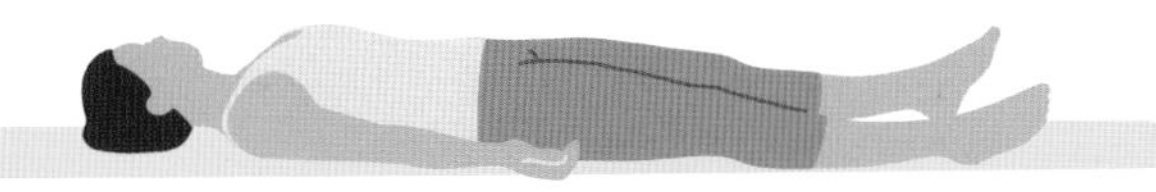

30-Minute Simple Standing Sequence

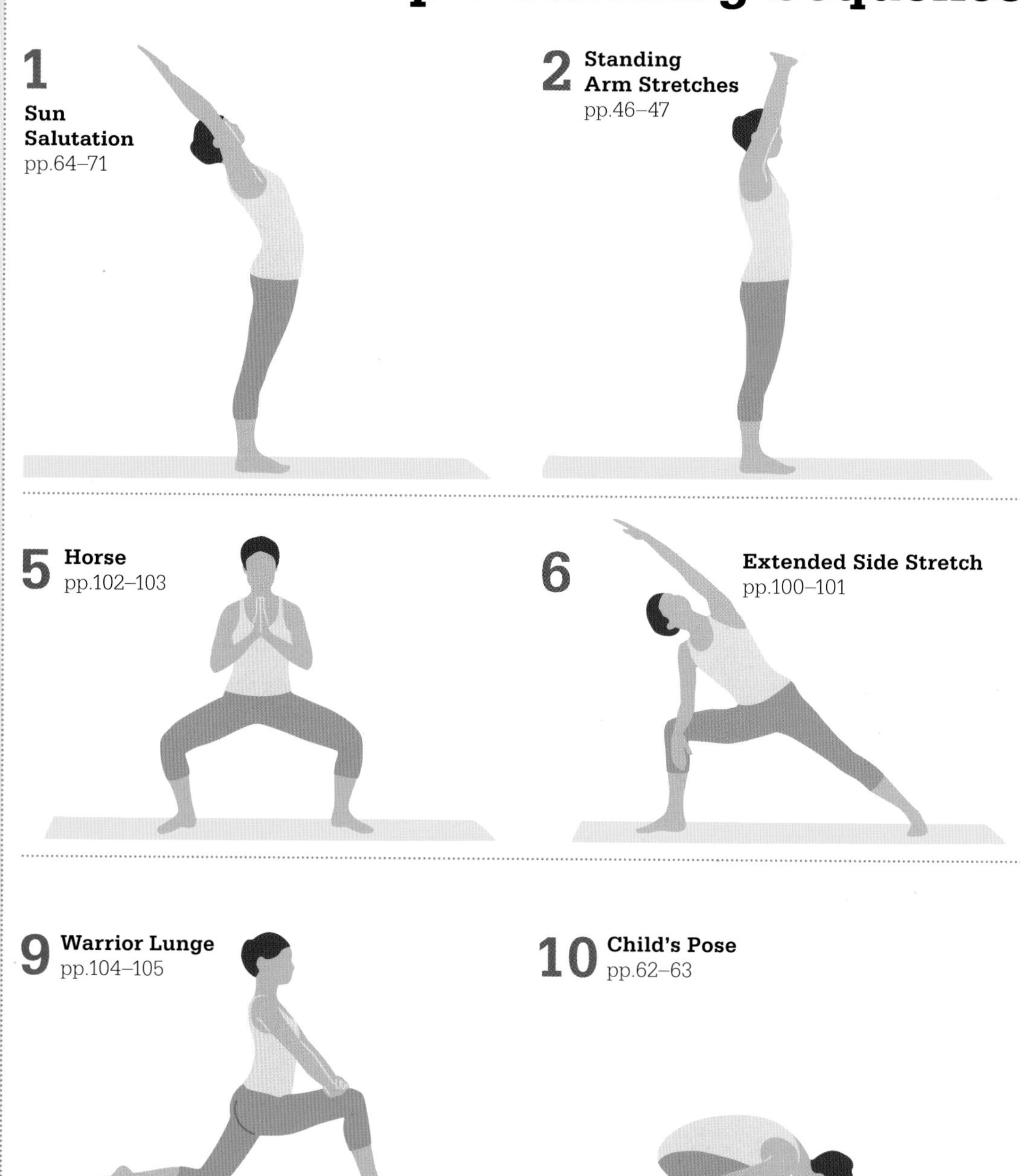
1
Sun
Salutation
pp.64–71
2 Standing
Arm Stretches
pp.46–47
5 Horse
pp.102–103
6
Extended Side Stretch
pp.100–101
9 Warrior Lunge
pp.104–105
10 Child's Pose
pp.62–63

3 **Tree Pose** pp.94–95

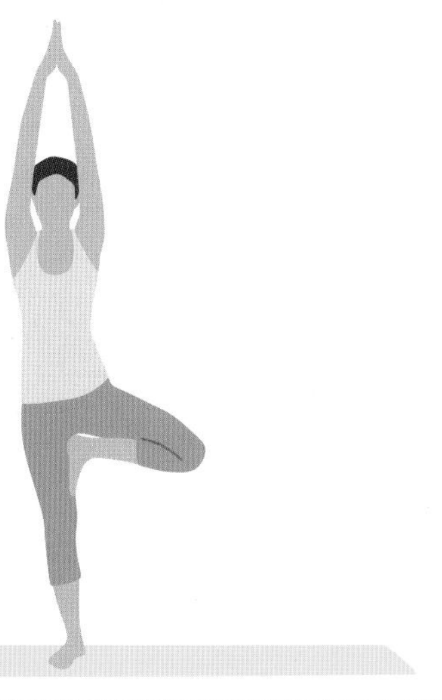

4 **Triangle** pp.50–51

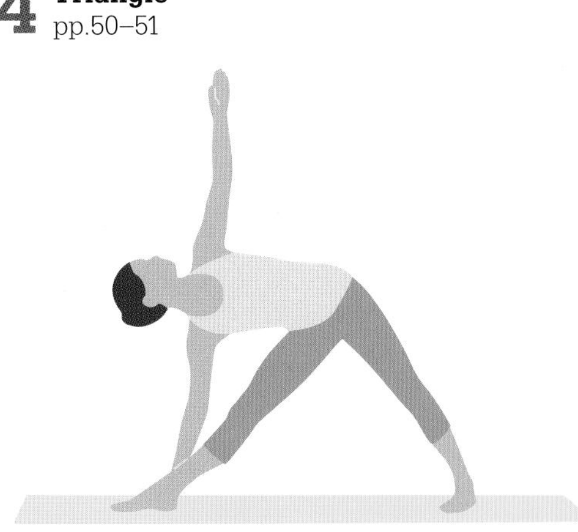

7 **Wide Forward Bend** pp.106–107

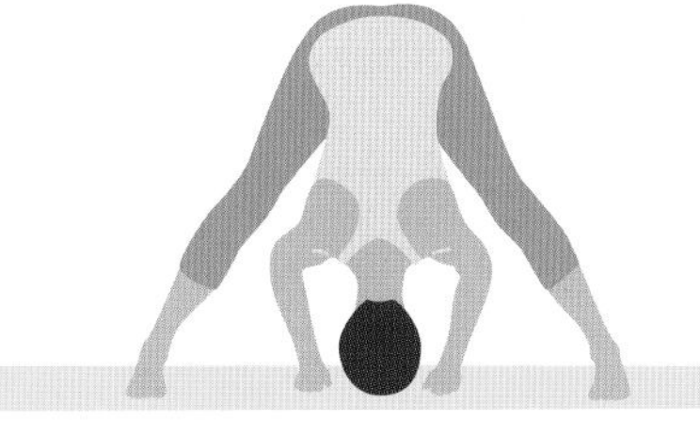

8 **Child's Pose** pp.62–63

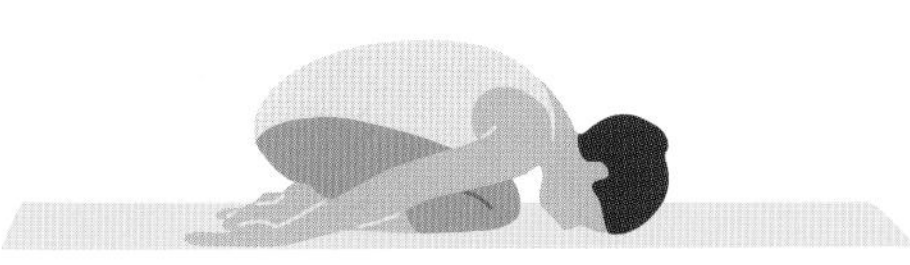

11 **Crossed Leg Forward Bend** pp.122–123

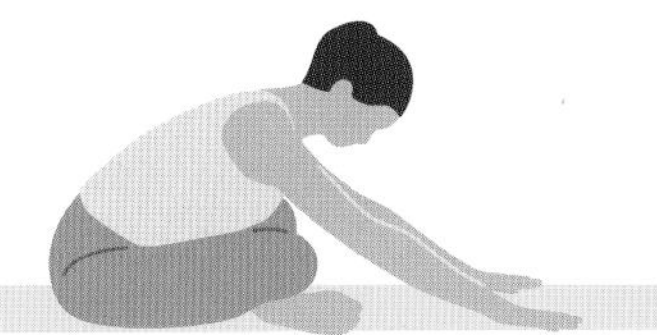

12 **Corpse and Final Relaxation** pp.78–81

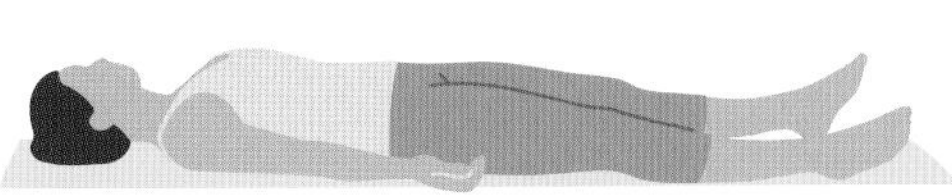

45-Minute Sequence

1 Sun Salutation x **2**
pp. 64–71

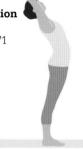

2 Extended Side Stretch
pp.100–101

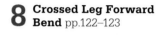

3 Warrior 2
pp.98–99

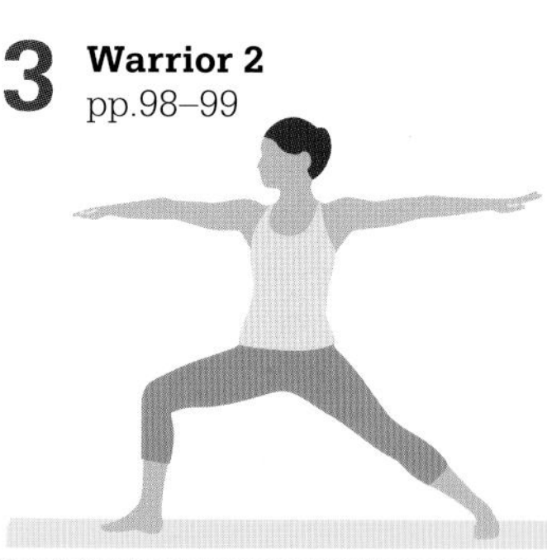

7 Sitting Forward Stretch
pp.116–117

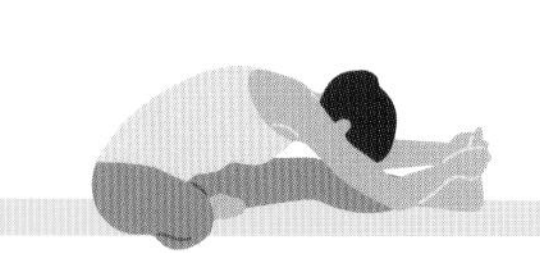

8 Crossed Leg Forward Bend pp.122–123

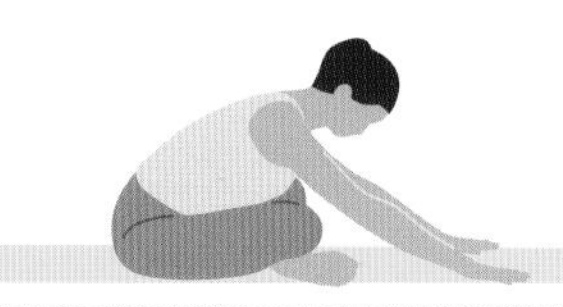

9 Half Spinal Twist
pp.120–121

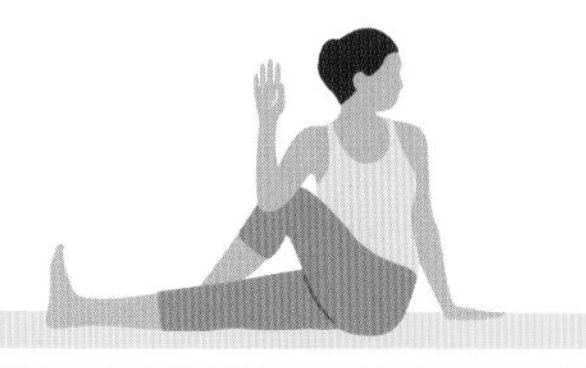

13 Child's Pose
pp.62–63

14 Bridge
pp.124–125

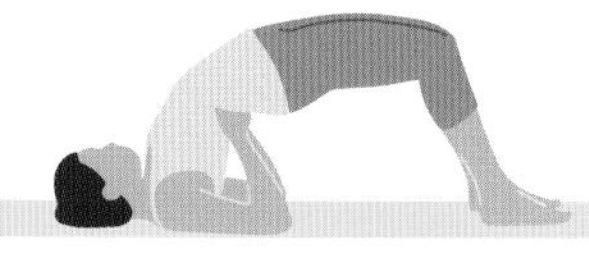

15 Half Shoulder Stand with Wall
pp.128–131

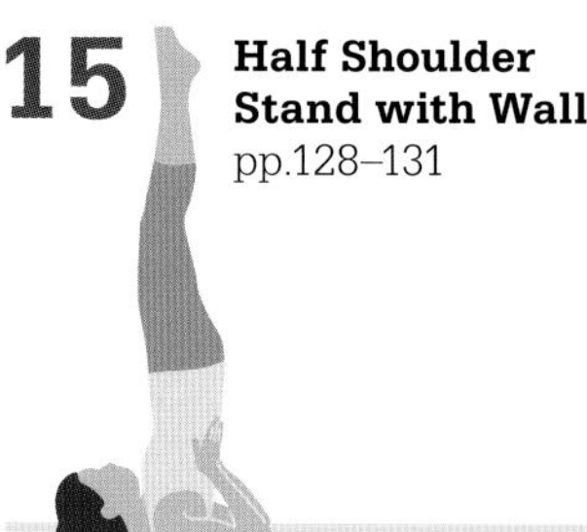

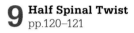

19 Corpse and Final Relaxation pp.78–81

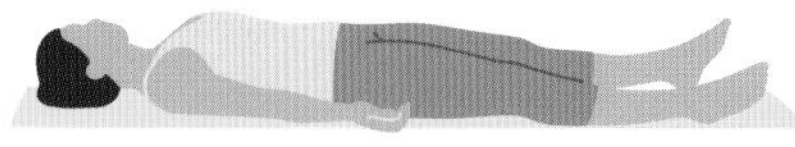

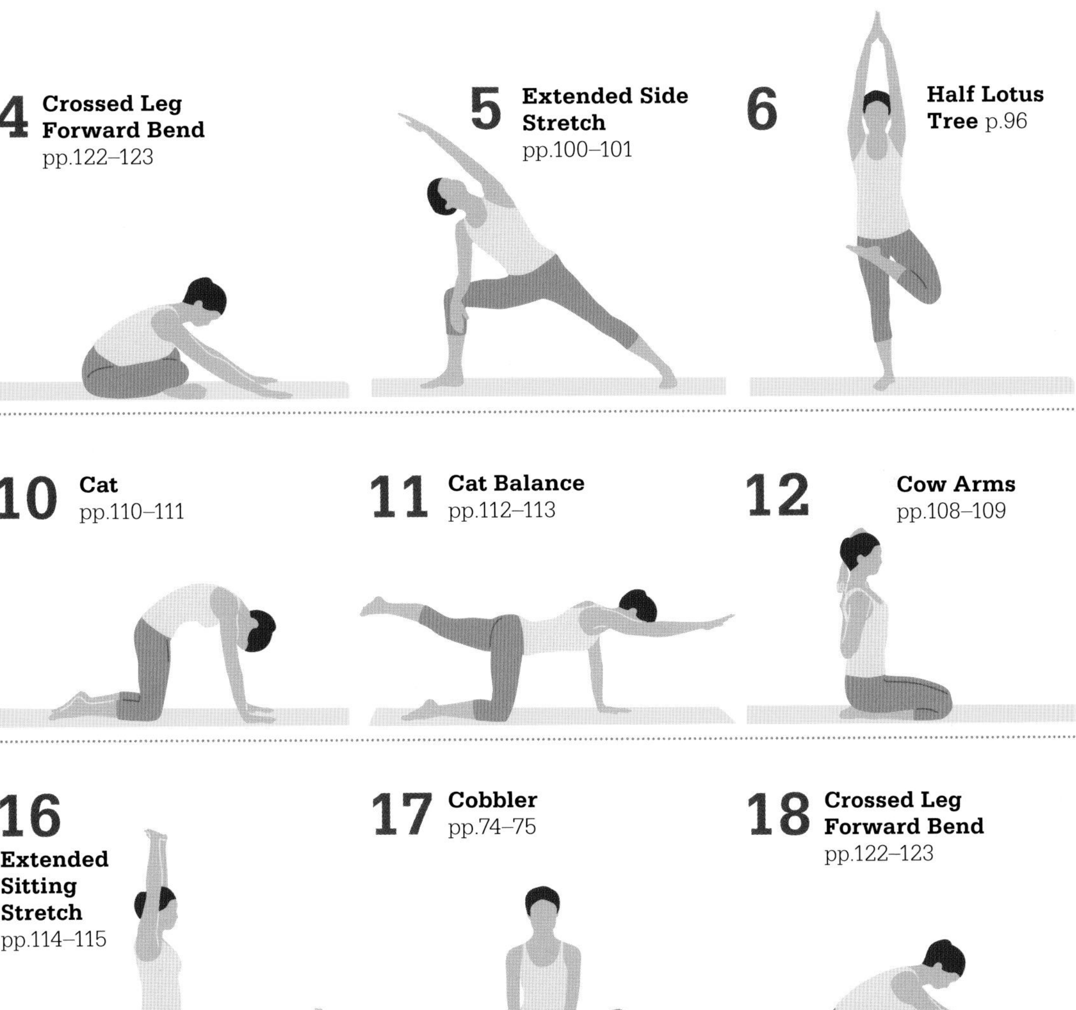
4 Crossed Leg Forward Bend pp.122–123
5 Extended Side Stretch pp.100–101
6 Half Lotus Tree p.96
10 Cat pp.110–111
11 Cat Balance pp.112–113
12 Cow Arms pp.108–109
16 Extended Sitting Stretch pp.114–115
17 Cobbler pp.74–75
18 Crossed Leg Forward Bend pp.122–123

Assess your progress

Now is a good time to review what you have learned so far and to assess your overall progress. By this point, you'll have familiarized yourself with the five principles underpinning yoga, as well as breathing techniques, warm-up exercises, and level 1 and level 2 postures.

Memorizing postures

Once you are familiar with the first- and second-level sequences described in this book, try to follow them from memory. This should help you to understand the logic behind the inclusion of each posture and how to regulate your breath during practice.

Revisit the steps and tips

- **As you practice more** and learn to listen to your body, you should begin to trust your instincts to tell you whether a posture feels right or wrong. Acquiring and then honing these instincts provides you with the means to correct yourself if you are doing some part of the posture incorrectly. Because all parts of the body are connected, a fault in the positioning of one limb will adversely impact on the posture by distorting the shape of the rest of your body.
- **To ensure you are aligning** the poses correctly, practice in front of a mirror. Study the hints and tips in each section, as they provide guidelines for starting positions and descriptions of correct alignment, as well as advice on breathing correctly. If you have any concerns about pain or discomfort that you experience with a posture, consult a medical practitioner.

Revisit the poses

- **Check the pose** step-by-step images—some of them detail common faults.
- **Check your alignment**, using a mirror if you can. Remember a misplaced limb can impact adversely on your whole body.
- **Assess** how your yoga instinct is developing.
- **Continue to revisit pose details** in the book, looking closely at the steps. The annotations also give you valuable tips.
- **Constantly refresh your memory** of each yoga pose's requirements.
- **Consult a medical practitioner** if you experience continued pain or discomfort from a posture.
- **Reread the hints and tips** as they'll provide guidelines for starting positions.

Moving at your body's pace

Over time, regular practice should also help you to build up an increasingly clear and accurate picture of your own physical state and of your level of conditioning. Being aware of your own physical strengths and shortcomings gives you yet another way to judge how you perform poses. This awareness will enable you to moderate your approach to the postures, using your developing intuition and understanding of the concepts of "good" and "bad" pain. In addition to limiting how far into a posture you go, you will also be in a better position to know how and when to use blocks, bolsters, cushions, furniture, and other supports in a safe and effective manner.

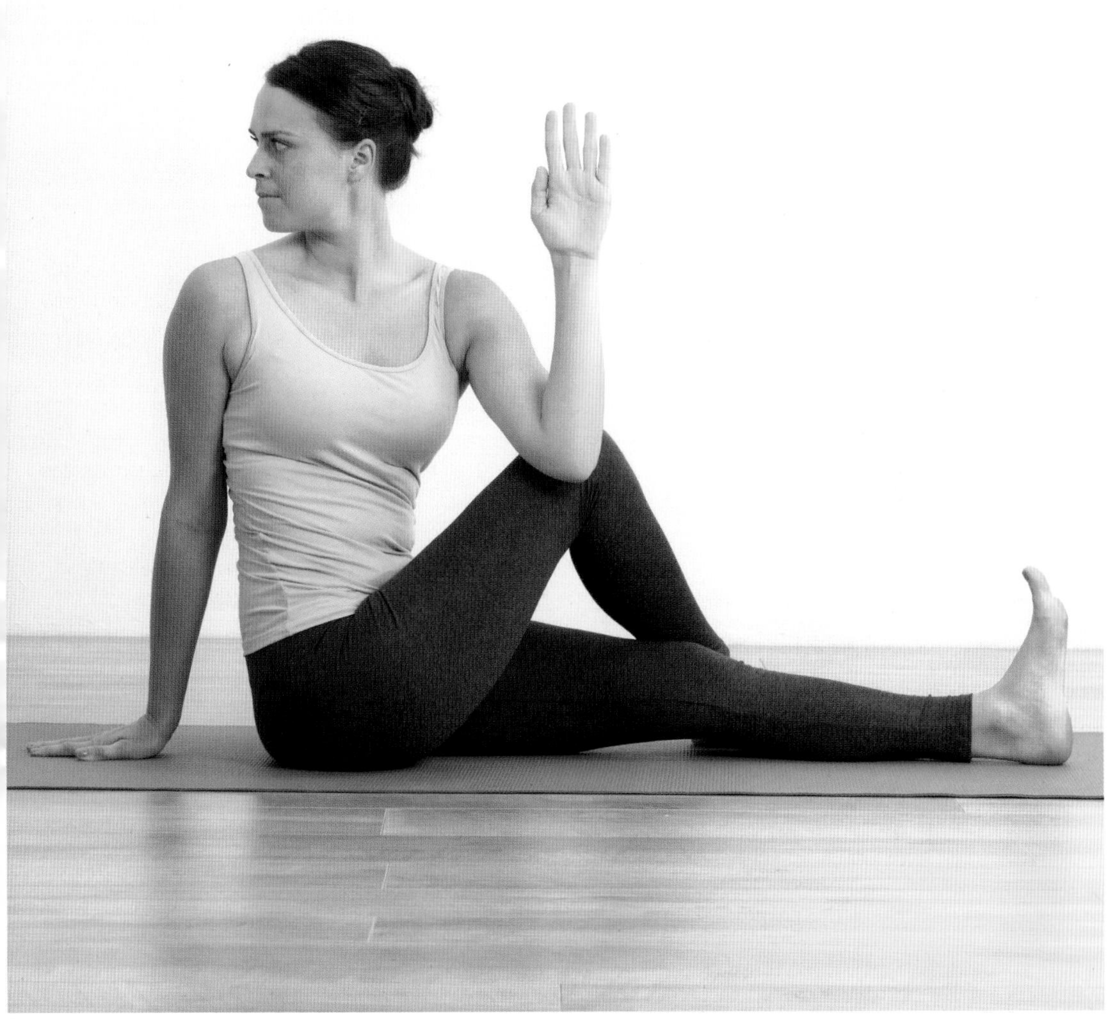

Review your yoga journal

It is generally accepted that the practice of yoga can bring latent emotions to the surface, some of which will inevitably be negative and self-critical. Writing about these emotions in a yoga context gives you a way to express them in a private and safe environment. Releasing these emotions from your body and confining them to paper is a way of liberating yourself from the bad habits and attitudes that are often the result of negative emotions trapped in the body. Conversely, it is equally important to try and record any feelings of joy and positivity that yoga has brought into your life. As time passes, you should be able to look through your yoga journal and see both how your practice has progressed and how you have developed yourself in terms of reaching your full potential.

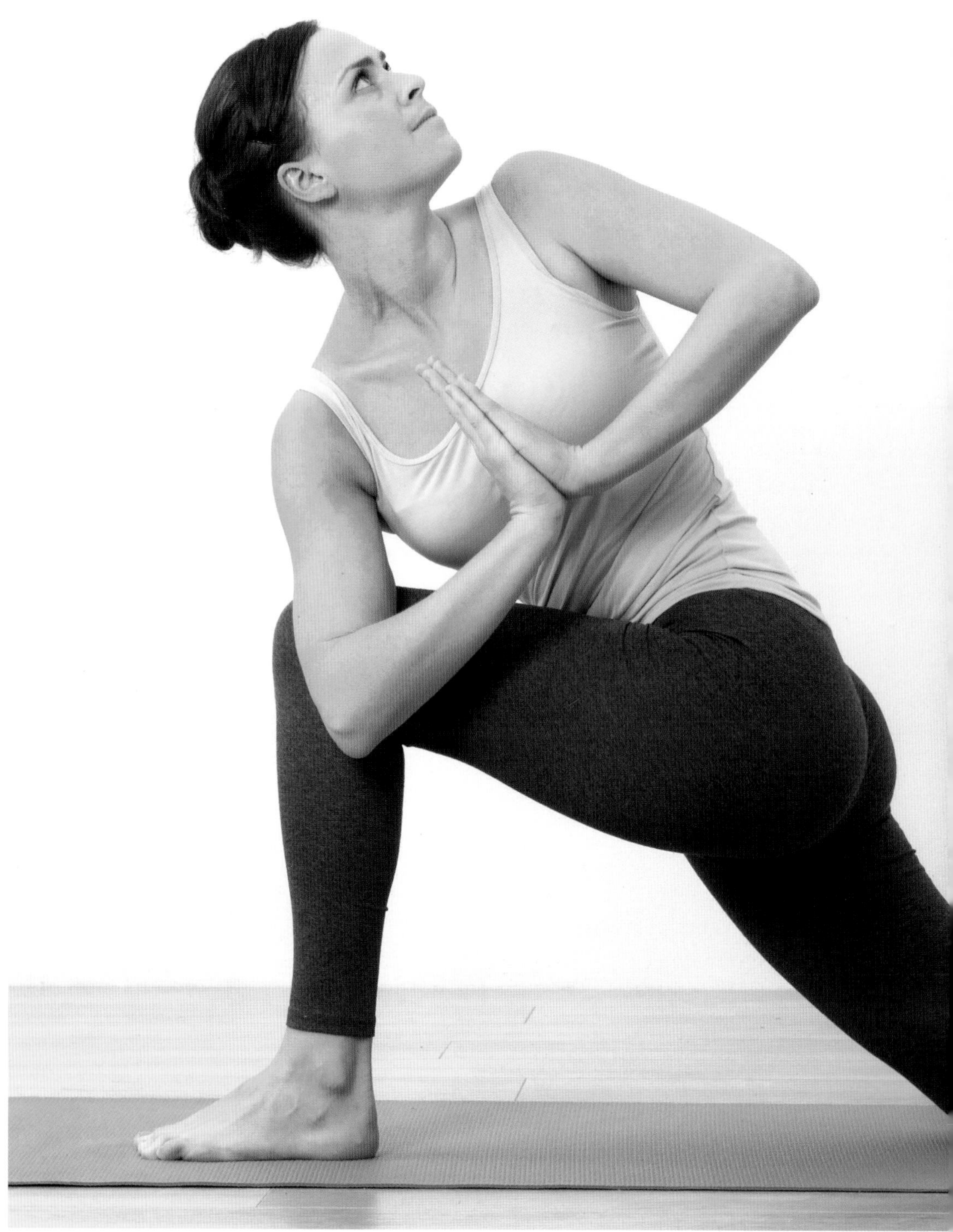

3

Take It Further

Continue to build on your achievements by reviewing and consolidating what you have learned so far. Increase your knowledge of the discipline of yoga, thinking about positive ways in which you could improve the way you practice. This will help to ensure that all your future practice is based on firm foundations and correct principles. Yoga requires you to constantly revisit and review what you already know, and this will show that improvement is always possible.

Self-awareness

Any practice of yoga, no matter how basic, should lead to an increase in self-awareness. Developing physical and mental self-awareness provides you with a powerful tool for assessing progress because yoga is all about getting to know yourself better, accepting the way you are, and embracing the path of self-development.

How to develop awareness

Some of the areas of physical and mental development to pay particular attention to are noted on these pages. Incorporating these elements into your practice should have the effect of empowering you, so you approach new postures with anticipation rather than trepidation, knowing that you have equipped yourself to take control of your own learning process.

1. Be alignment aware

Postures such as the Mountain Pose (see pp.44–45) are designed to get you thinking consciously about the alignment of your body. The fact that you have become increasingly conscious of misalignment, and make the necessary corrective adjustments, indicates that you have already made significant progress. Because the mountain pose simply involves standing, it bridges the gap between practice and everyday life. Whenever you find yourself standing in a line, you have the opportunity to refine and perfect the art of standing correctly through practicing this pose. The result of this is that you should be feeling more centered and steady on your feet.

2. Keep a positive attitude

In the past, you may have refused to acknowledge a physical problem by deliberately ignoring or hiding it in the hope that it would go away. Yoga practice can get you to change these patterns of behavior by helping you to accept that you suffer from a problem. More importantly, it will also reveal to you that it is within your power to take positive steps to alleviate the problem. Over time, yoga will help you develop a positive attitude toward your body and a greater sense of honesty in dealing with its inevitable problems.

3. Monitor your breath

To increase awareness of performing postures correctly, and at the correct level, you need to monitor your breath. Ragged or uneven breathing indicates that you are pushing yourself too hard and need to take a step back and reassess what you are doing. In your daily life, recognizing shallow breathing caused by stress, and consciously making an effort to breathe more deeply, will cause stress to affect you less. You can quantify this by comparing your reactions to negative events or behavioral patterns before and after starting yoga.

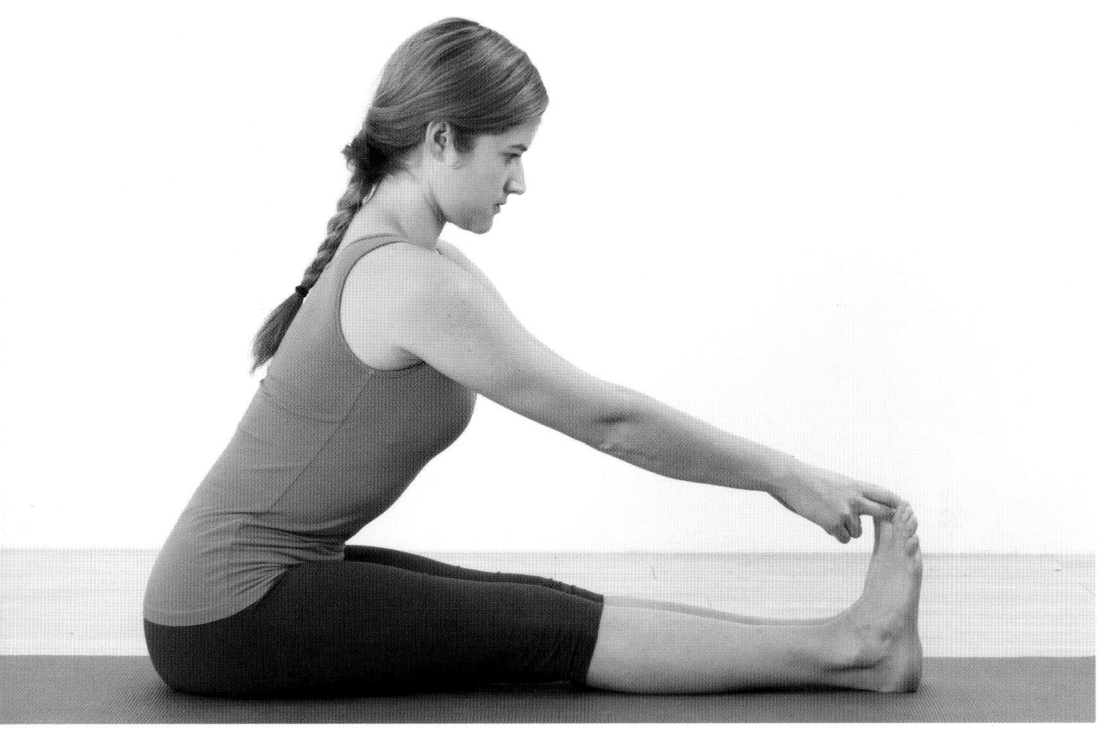

4. Tell "good" from "bad" pain

Learn to distinguish between "good" and "bad" pain by listening to your body. Letting your body tell you when you are in danger of exceeding your limitations will help prevent injury. Yoga challenges us to use previously neglected parts of the body, and you may experience some stiffness and soreness in your muscles and joints. The nature of "bad" pain is that it is generally sudden, sharp, and intense. By the time you experience it, the damage will already have been done. "Good" pain, on the other hand, manifests itself more gradually and is part of the process of readjustment your body is making. You have the chance to pull out of the posture before you damage yourself. By taking things slowly and taking care of yourself with proper nutrition and rest, you should be able to use the sensations of "good" pain to gauge your progress and gradually improve your physical condition over time.

5. Strengths and weaknesses

Learn to recognize your physical strengths and weaknesses, and how these are shaped by your daily routine and habits. For example, you may realize your hamstrings are short as result of cycling to your workplace on a daily basis. Incorporating some simple leg stretches before and after cycling will help balance the muscles being used. Building up this mental picture of your physical strengths and weaknesses will prove invaluable in developing a safe and effective home practice.

Warrior 1

Strengthen Lower Back • **Increase** Lung Capacity

This set of movements is designed to strengthen not just the whole body but also the mind. The lower part of the body should be firmly grounded, allowing the upper body to move in a controlled and purposeful manner.

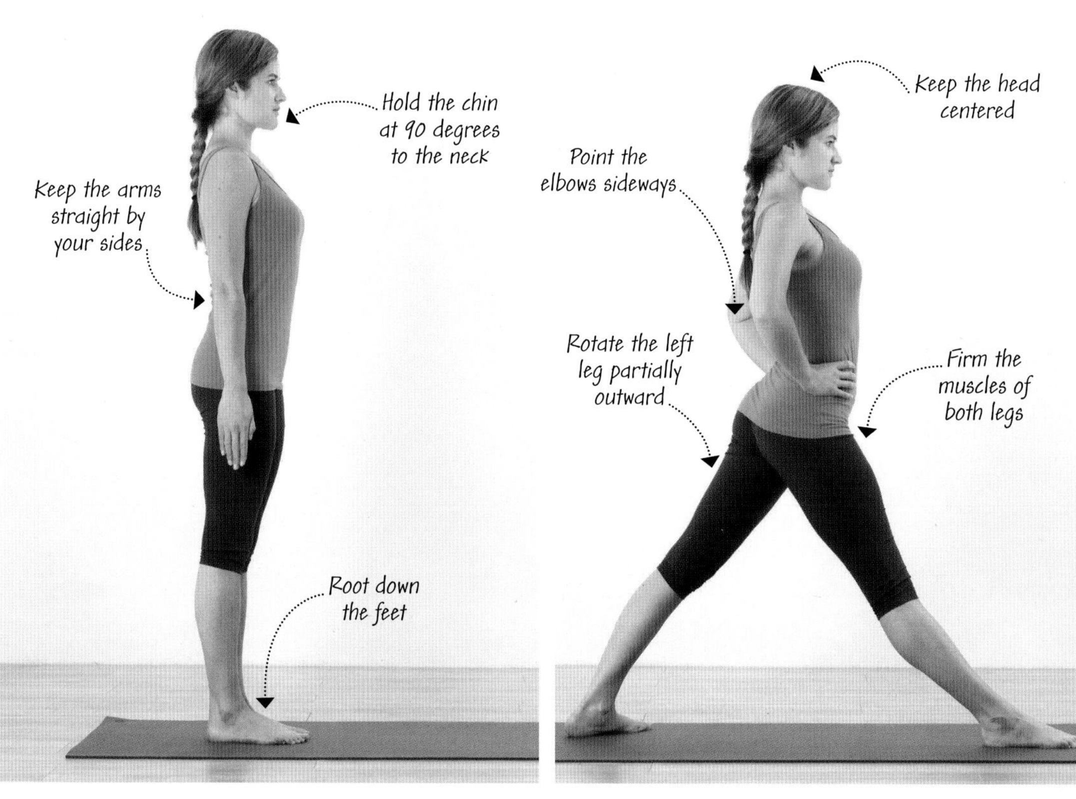
Hold the chin at 90 degrees to the neck
Keep the arms straight by your sides
Root down the feet
Keep the head centered
Point the elbows sideways
Rotate the left leg partially outward
Firm the muscles of both legs

1 Start in the Mountain Pose with your hands by your sides and feet together. Focus on lengthening your spine and breathe in a gentle rhythm.

Useful tip Imagine that your tailbone is being weighted down and your head is being pulled up.

2 Exhaling, step forward with your right foot as far as you comfortably can, with your hips facing forward and your knees locked. The rear foot is angled at about 60 degrees. Inhale deeply.

Useful tip Use your hands to check that your hips are facing forward.

3 As you inhale, bend your right knee forward until it is directly above your ankle. Raise both arms up straight to bring the palms together. Keep the heel of your left foot in contact with the floor. Tilt your head backward and look at your hands. Take five breaths. Exhale to release, returning the hands to the hips and straightening the right leg. Step back to return to the Mountain Pose. Repeat steps 1, 2, and 3 with the left leg forward.

Make it easier

You can vary the hand position in Warrior 1. Interlock all the fingers except the index fingers, which point upward. This hand position will help you stabilize the arms and lengthen the back slightly more.

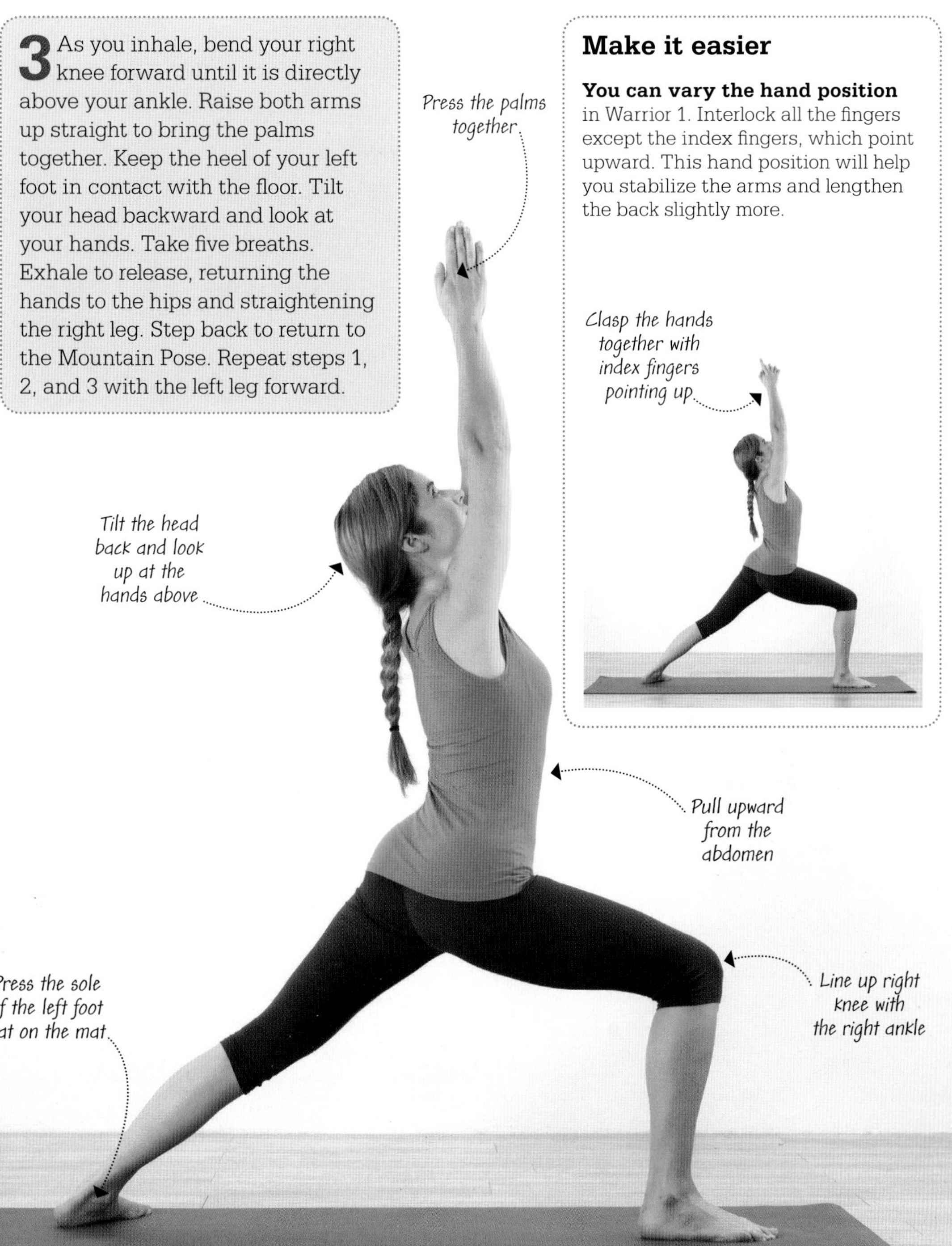
Press the palms together
Clasp the hands together with index fingers pointing up
Tilt the head back and look up at the hands above
Pull upward from the abdomen
Line up right knee with the right ankle
Press the sole of the left foot flat on the mat

Lunge Twist

Tone Legs • **Stretch** Spine

This pose gives a strong extension to the upper legs, toning and strengthening the muscles, as well as improving the flexibility of the spine.

1 Kneel on all fours with your feet behind you. Your arms should be shoulder-width apart and your fingers spread out, with the middle finger pointing straight ahead. Look down at your fingers.

Take care Reduce excessive curving of the back by drawing your navel inward.

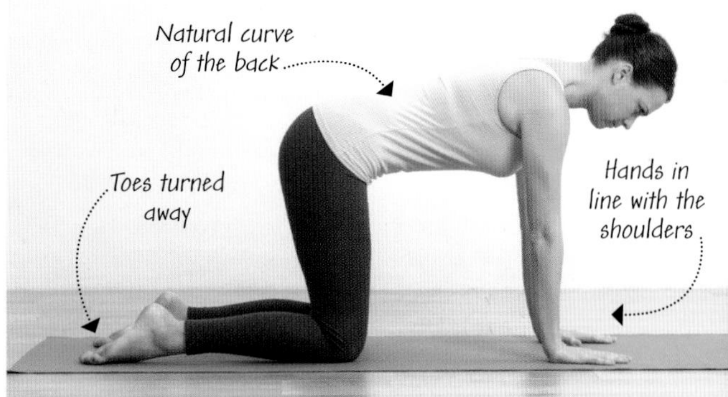
Natural curve of the back
Toes turned away
Hands in line with the shoulders

2 Inhale to extend the right leg out in front, lifting the torso upright and bringing the right knee to align vertically with the right ankle. Rest both hands on your right knee.

Useful tip Firm the leg muscles. Press through the feet to give stability to the body.

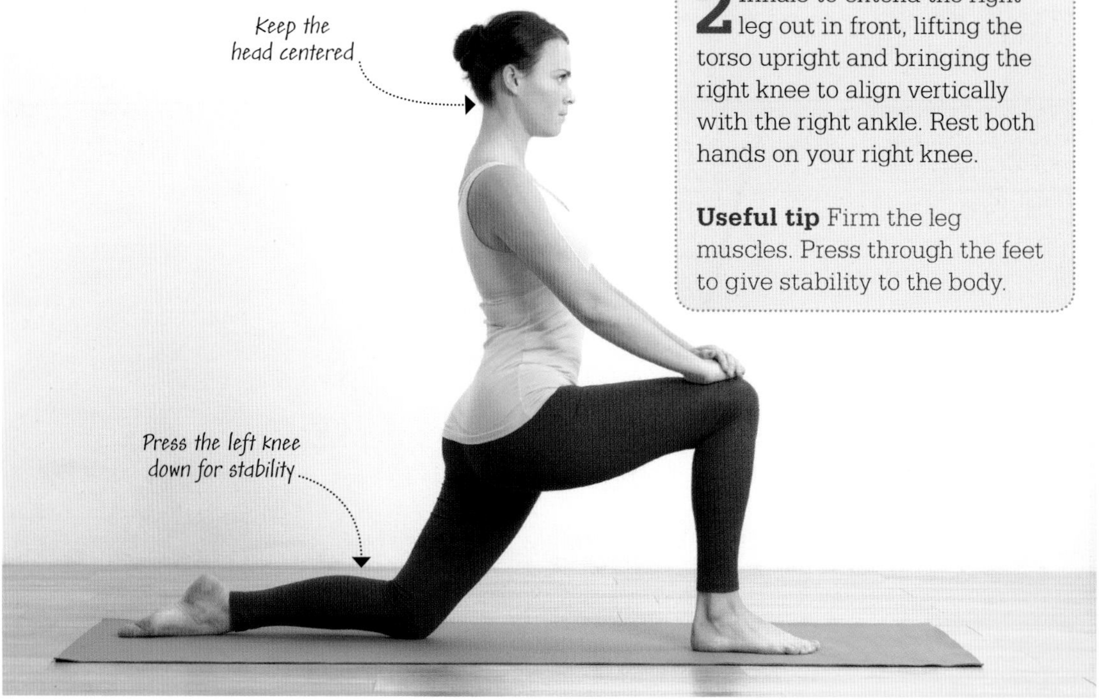

Keep the head centered

Press the left knee down for stability

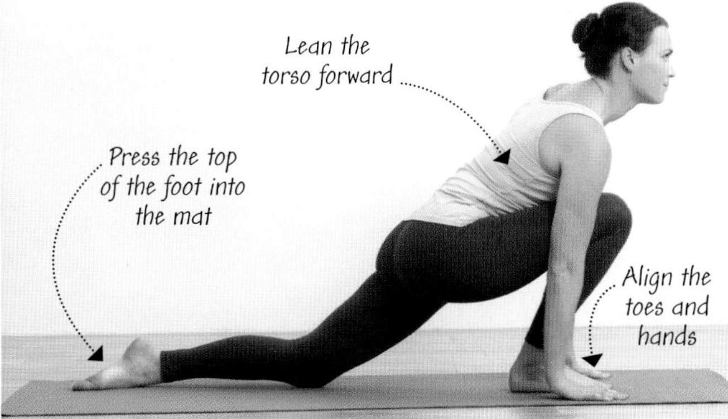
Lean the torso forward
Press the top of the foot into the mat
Align the toes and hands

3 Maintaining the position of both feet, inhale to lean forward, increasing the bend at the knee and bringing your hands to rest on the mat alongside your feet—glance down to make sure they align, but then look straight ahead. Try to lengthen through your spine, feeling the stretch in your legs as you push forward.

4 As you exhale, press into the mat with your left hand before extending your right arm upward, opening your palm and pointing your fingers at the ceiling. Rotate your head until you are looking at your raised hand. Hold for five breaths. Release from the pose by lowering your right hand to the mat. Take your right leg backward, stretching it, before returning to the all-fours position. Center yourself and repeat on the left side.

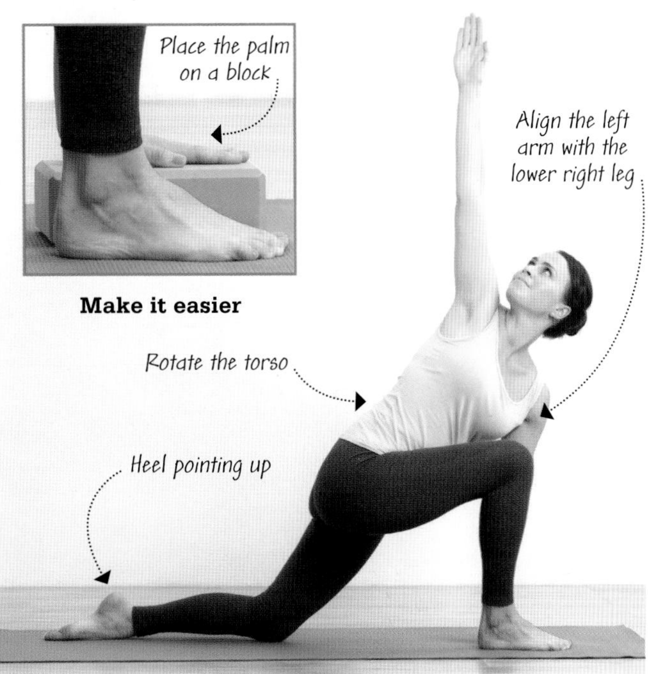
Place the palm on a block
Align the left arm with the lower right leg
Rotate the torso
Heel pointing up

Make it easier

More of a challenge

This is a variation of step 4. Bring your left arm over the right knee and lower the right arm to bring the palms together in the prayer position. Turn your head to look up, so that the chin is over the right shoulder. As you exhale, work on opening the chest and rotating the trunk a little more. Hold for five breaths and repeat on the other side.

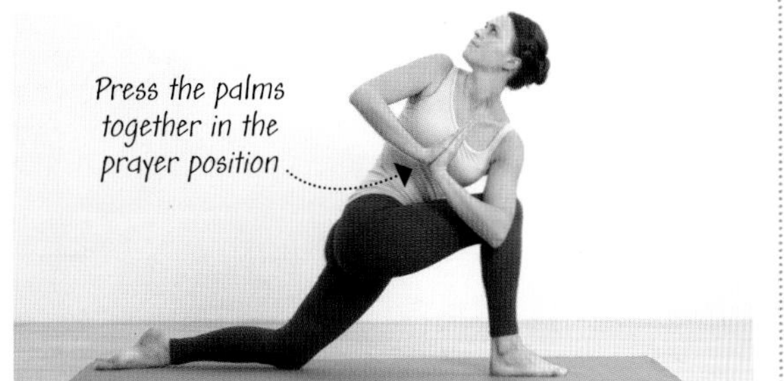
Press the palms together in the prayer position

Half Moon Pose

Develop Body Awareness • **Release** Hips

This advanced balancing posture targets the legs, buttocks, and hips. Mastering this pose will bring improved balance and strengthen the legs and spine.

1 Stand with your legs apart and your arms at shoulder height. Your right foot should be parallel to the mat and your left foot facing forward. Ensure the block is placed about 4–6in (10–15cm) away in line with the right foot. Look in the direction of that foot.

Help! Practice the pose against a wall if you find it difficult to maintain your balance.

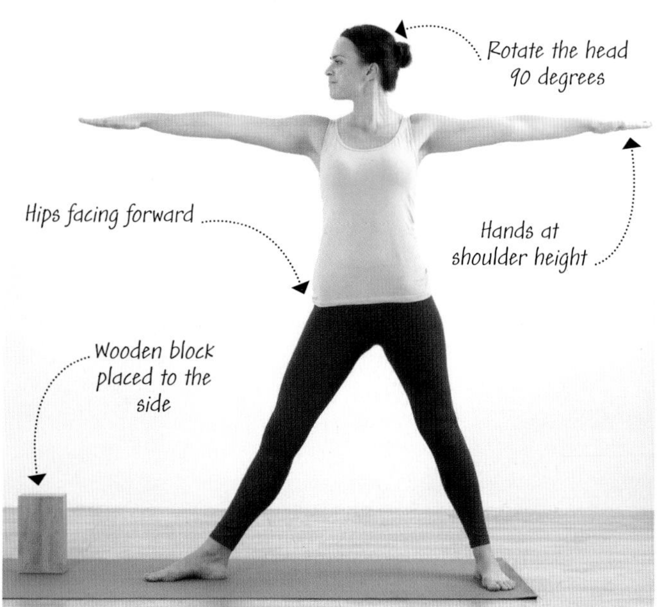
Rotate the head 90 degrees
Hips facing forward
Hands at shoulder height
Wooden block placed to the side

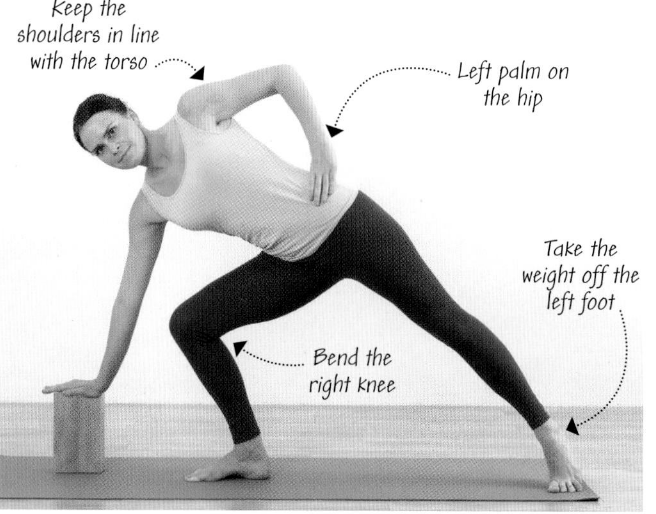
Keep the shoulders in line with the torso
Left palm on the hip
Take the weight off the left foot
Bend the right knee

2 On exhalation, bend your right knee and lower your right hand onto the block, tilting your left foot as you go. Place your left hand on your left hip. Feel the hip bone and use it as a guide to keep the hips in line with the torso.

Useful tip Pull your left foot slightly inward as you reach down for the block.

3 Start lifting your left leg upward by straightening your right leg and locking at the knee. Keep raising the left leg until it is parallel to the ground, rotating the left hip upward and back.

Useful tip Steady your head and fix your eyes on a spot in front of you to help keep your balance.

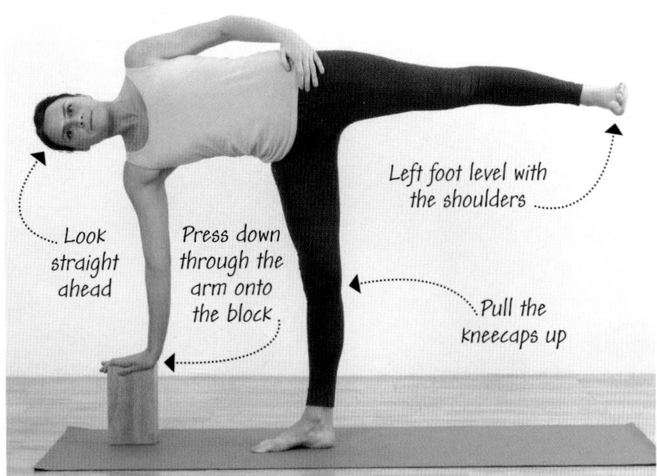
Left foot level with the shoulders
Look straight ahead
Press down through the arm onto the block
Pull the kneecaps up

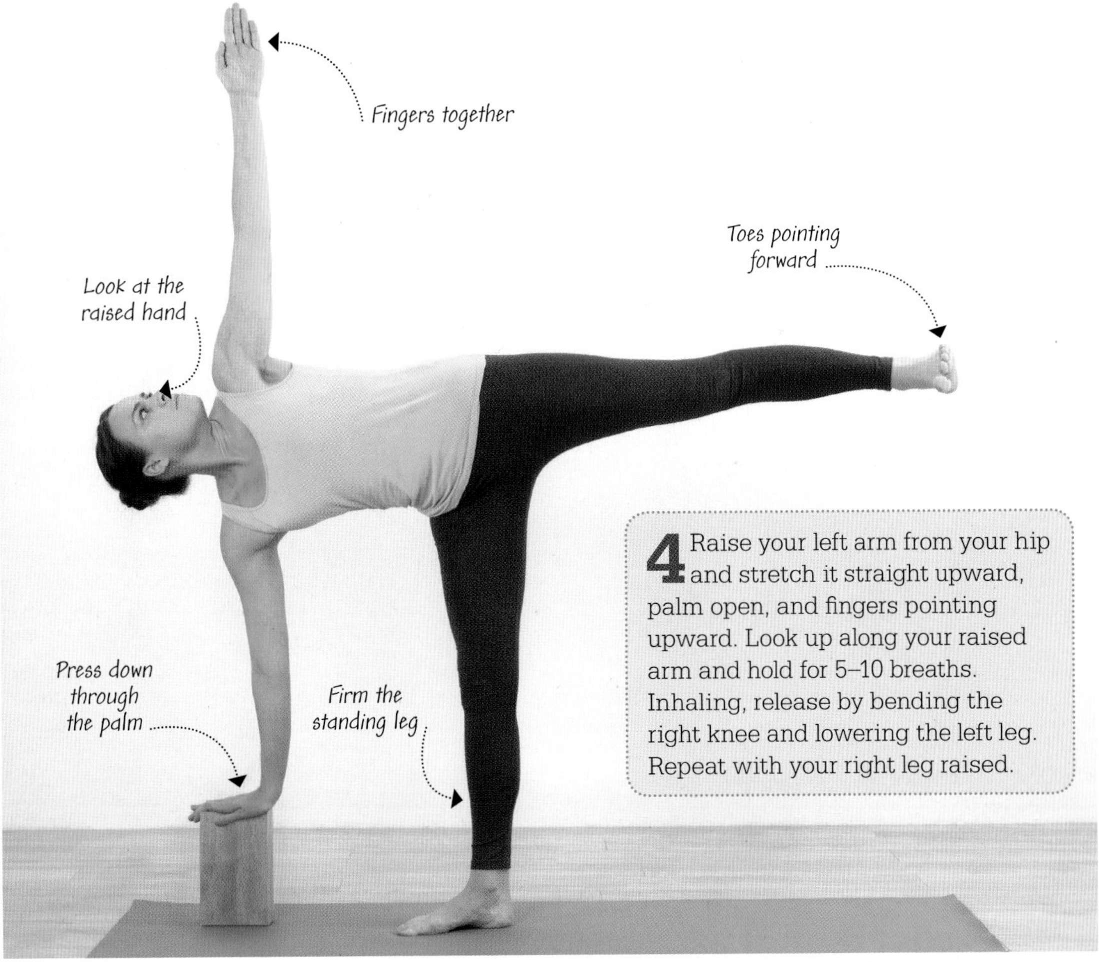

Fingers together

Toes pointing forward

Look at the raised hand

Press down through the palm

Firm the standing leg

4 Raise your left arm from your hip and stretch it straight upward, palm open, and fingers pointing upward. Look up along your raised arm and hold for 5–10 breaths. Inhaling, release by bending the right knee and lowering the left leg. Repeat with your right leg raised.

Locust

Strengthen Core and Spine • **Calm** Mind

This position is great for relieving stress and improving posture. In addition, the Locust helps strengthen the core muscles and the spine.

1 Start in a resting position with your feet relaxed, soles upward, and big toes touching. Place your arms along the sides of your body with palms facing upward. Rest your head on one cheek, breathing evenly and gently.

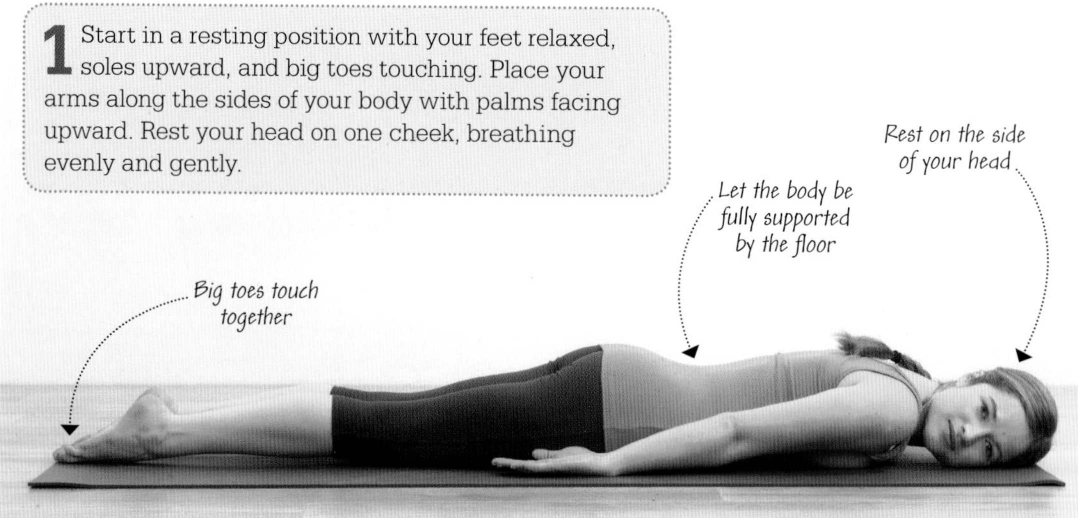
Rest on the side of your head
Let the body be fully supported by the floor
Big toes touch together

2 Inhaling, turn your neck to bring your forehead against the mat and stretch both arms toward your feet. On exhalation, lift your head and then your upper torso and arms off the mat. Take 5–8 breaths before inhaling and lowering back to the mat.

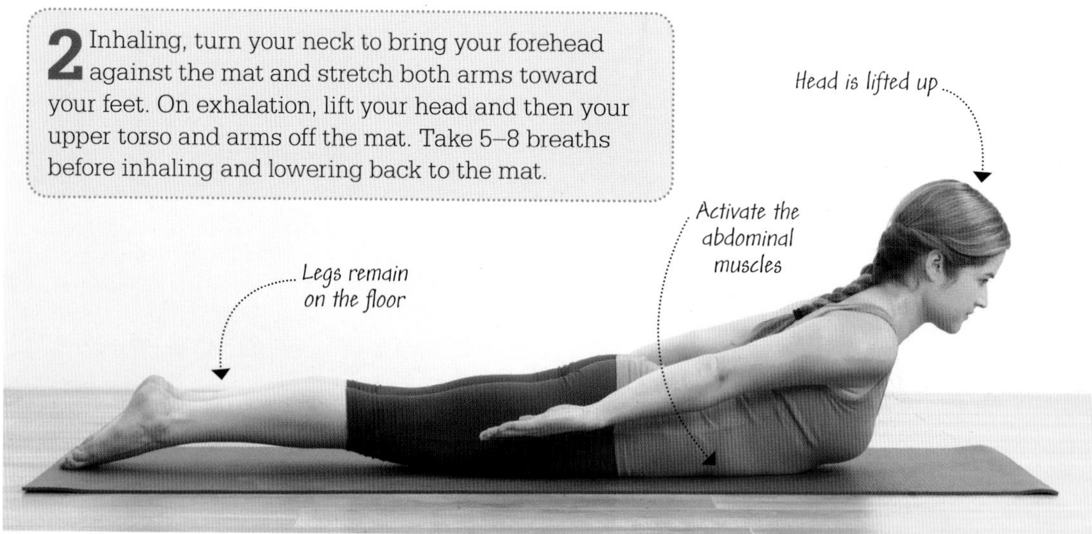
Head is lifted up
Activate the abdominal muscles
Legs remain on the floor

3 Repeat but as you exhale, deepen the pose by raising the arms farther and pulling the shoulder blades together. Raise your head and look straight forward.

Useful tip Press the hips and legs into the floor to give stability to the lifted upper body.

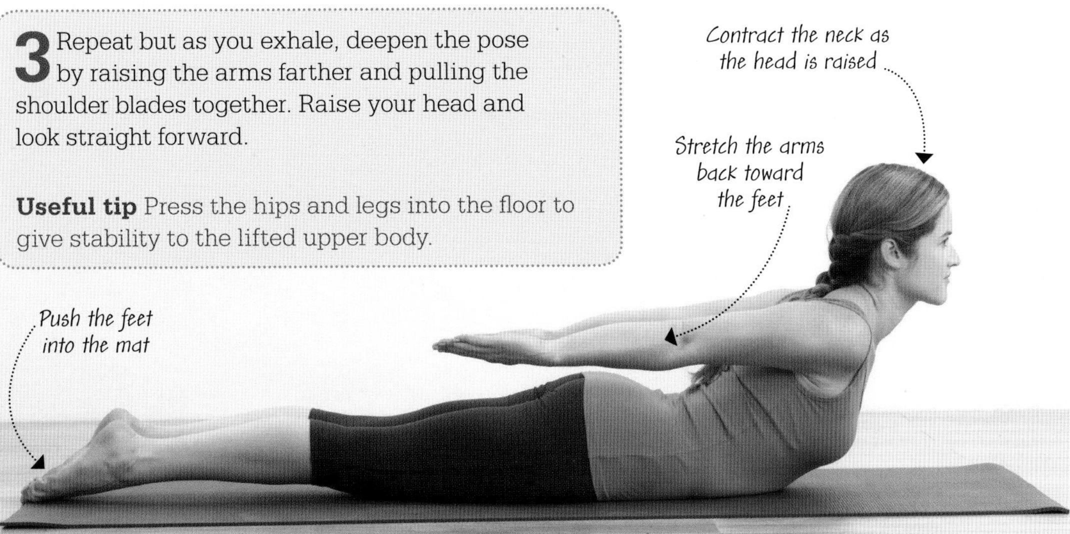
Contract the neck as the head is raised
Stretch the arms back toward the feet
Push the feet into the mat

4 Repeat as before, but this time raise your legs, as well as your arms and upper body, as you exhale. Hold for five to eight breaths, then release as you inhale.

Useful tip If you find it too difficult to raise both legs simultaneously, lift one at a time.

Take care...

This pose involves muscles that are often underdeveloped. If you find that the limbs are shaking, hold for one to two breaths, and repeat the pose.

There is a tendency to bend at the knees as a way of lifting the legs higher. To keep the legs straight, lift to a comfortable height only.

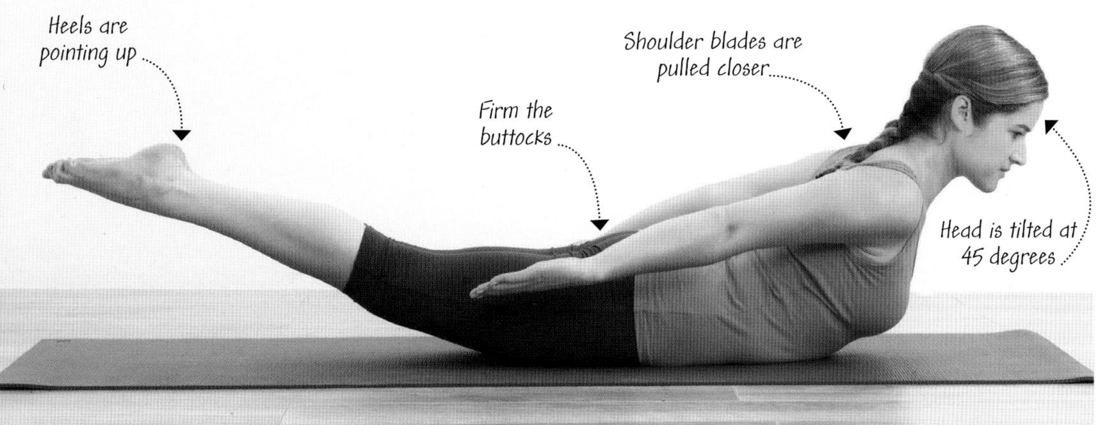
Heels are pointing up
Shoulder blades are pulled closer
Firm the buttocks
Head is tilted at 45 degrees

Half Bow

Strengthen Limbs • **Cleanse** Organs

The Half Bow pose is great for building up core strength. It also benefits key internal organs, stimulating the kidneys, adrenal glands, and reproductive system.

1 Start in a resting position with your feet relaxed, soles upward, and big toes touching. Extend your arms along the sides of your body with your palms facing upward. Rest your head on one cheek, breathing evenly and gently.

Rest on the side of the head

Let the body be fully supported by the floor

Legs are relaxed

3 Change your grip to the outside of your ankle, allowing your leg to partially unbend until your right arm is fully extended. Inhaling, pull your right thigh off the floor. Hold for five to eight breaths. Release on exhalation before repeating on the other side.

Remember Make sure that both your hips are pressed down on the mat and your head and neck are centered.

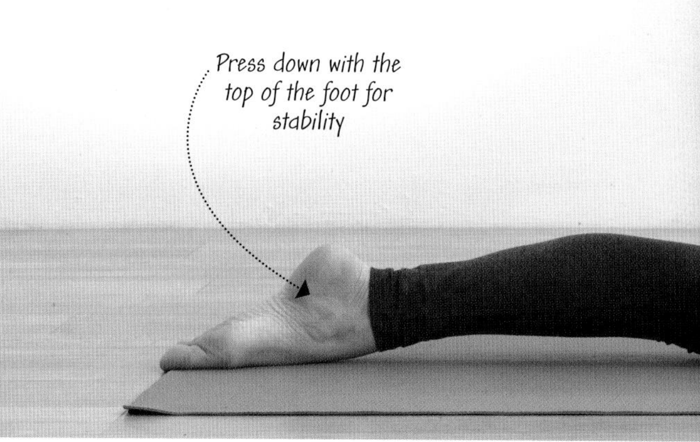

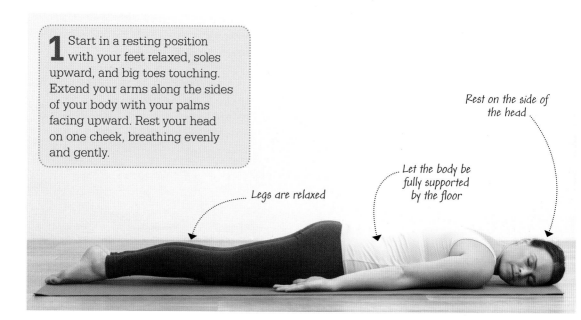
Press down with the top of the foot for stability

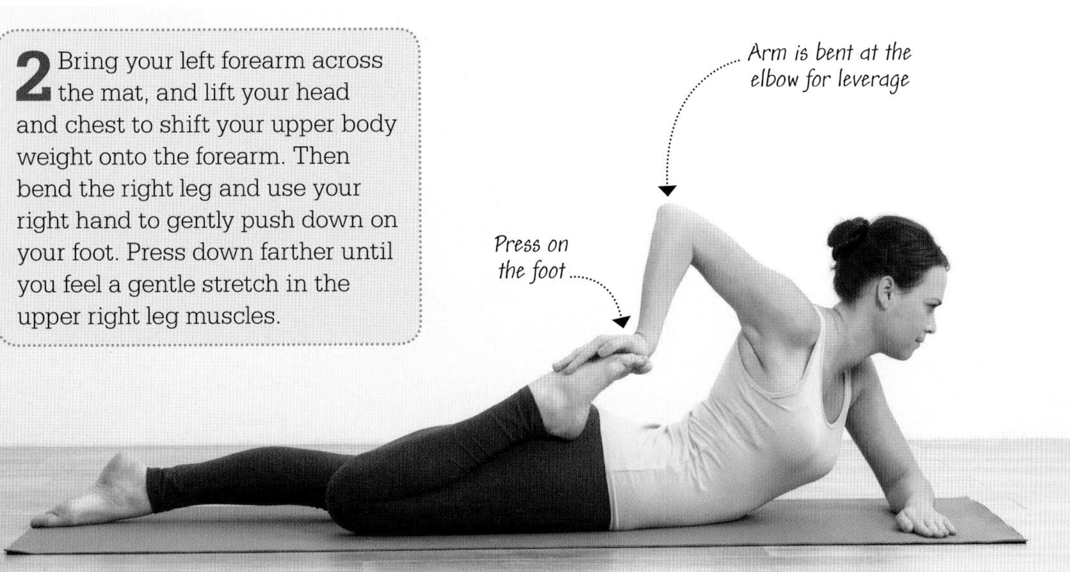
Arm is bent at the elbow for leverage
Press on the foot

2 Bring your left forearm across the mat, and lift your head and chest to shift your upper body weight onto the forearm. Then bend the right leg and use your right hand to gently push down on your foot. Press down farther until you feel a gentle stretch in the upper right leg muscles.

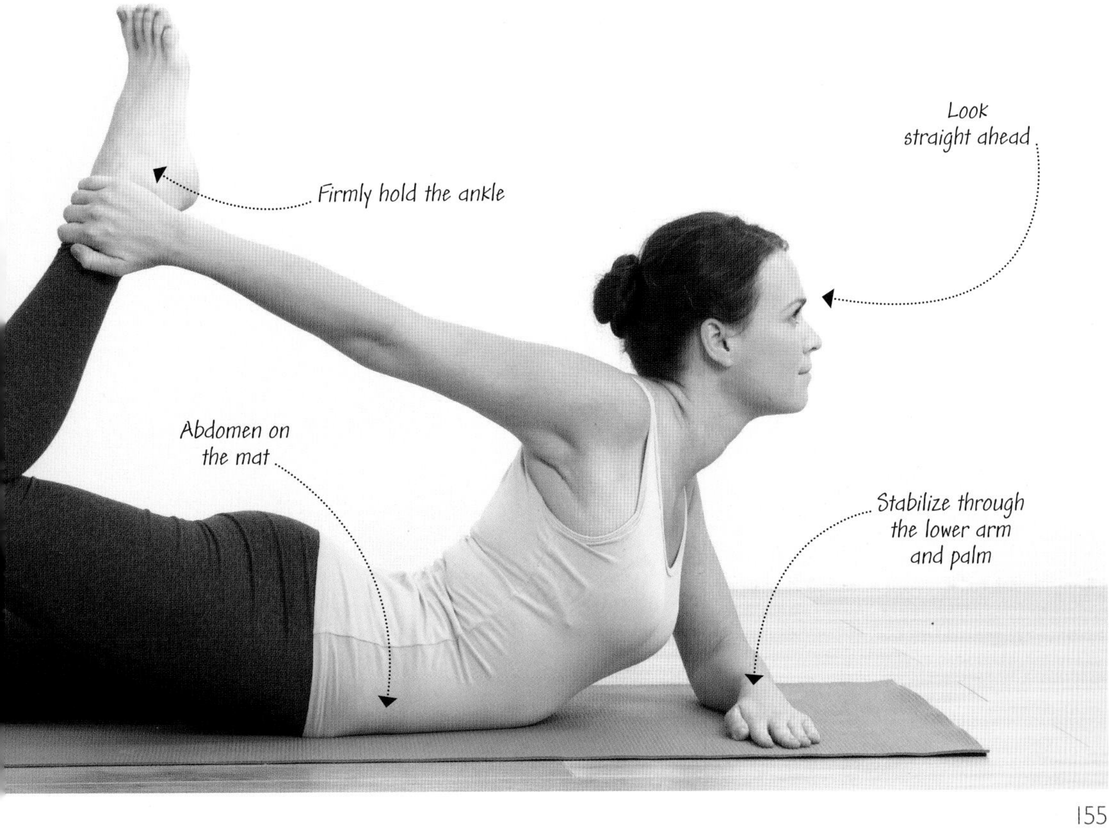

Look straight ahead

Firmly hold the ankle

Abdomen on the mat

Stabilize through the lower arm and palm

Full Bow

Strengthen Spine • **Massage** Abdominal Organs

The Full Bow combines elements of the Cobra and Locust poses to strengthen the back muscles and stimulate the organs of the abdomen.

1 Start by lying prone, forehead on the mat, hands by your sides with your palms turned up. Exhale and bend your knees, bringing your heels as far forward as possible. Reach back and grasp your ankles. Keep your knees hip-width apart.

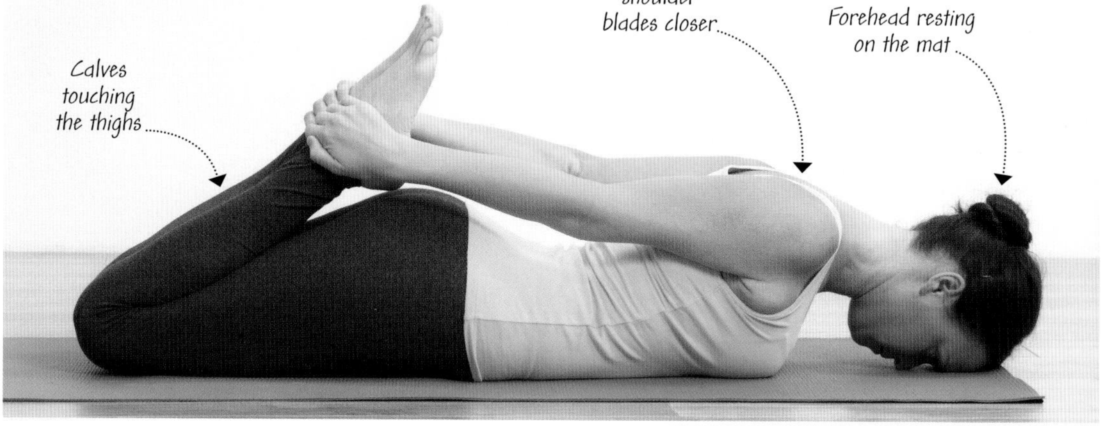

Calves touching the thighs

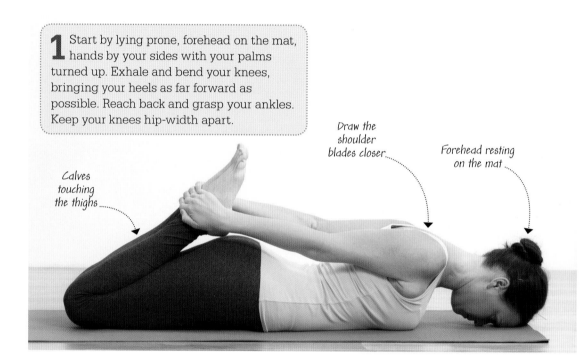

Draw the shoulder blades closer

Forehead resting on the mat

Take care...

Your feet and lower legs should point up toward the ceiling when you are in the full bow pose. Do not hold the feet wide as this causes the lower legs to be pulled downward and the ankles to flex down.

Make sure that your arms are fully extended before you push upward. Keep them extended throughout the posture.

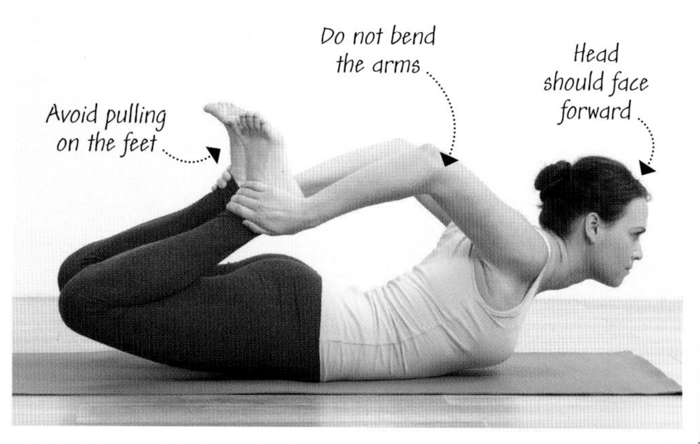
Avoid pulling on the feet
Do not bend the arms
Head should face forward

2 Inhaling, strongly thrust your heels toward your head while also lifting your thighs clear of the floor. This should pull your upper body and head clear of the mat. Contract the neck muscles as you look upward. Hold for several breaths before releasing your feet on exhalation.

Useful tip Place a rolled-up towel under your thighs if it is difficult to lift them.

Make it easier

If you struggle to keep hold of your ankles while raising your thighs, chest, and head, try using a strap. Put the strap around the ankles and hold the ends with both hands.

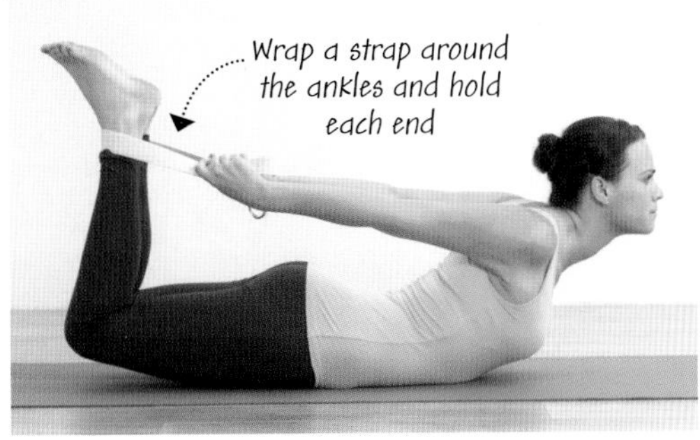
Wrap a strap around the ankles and hold each end

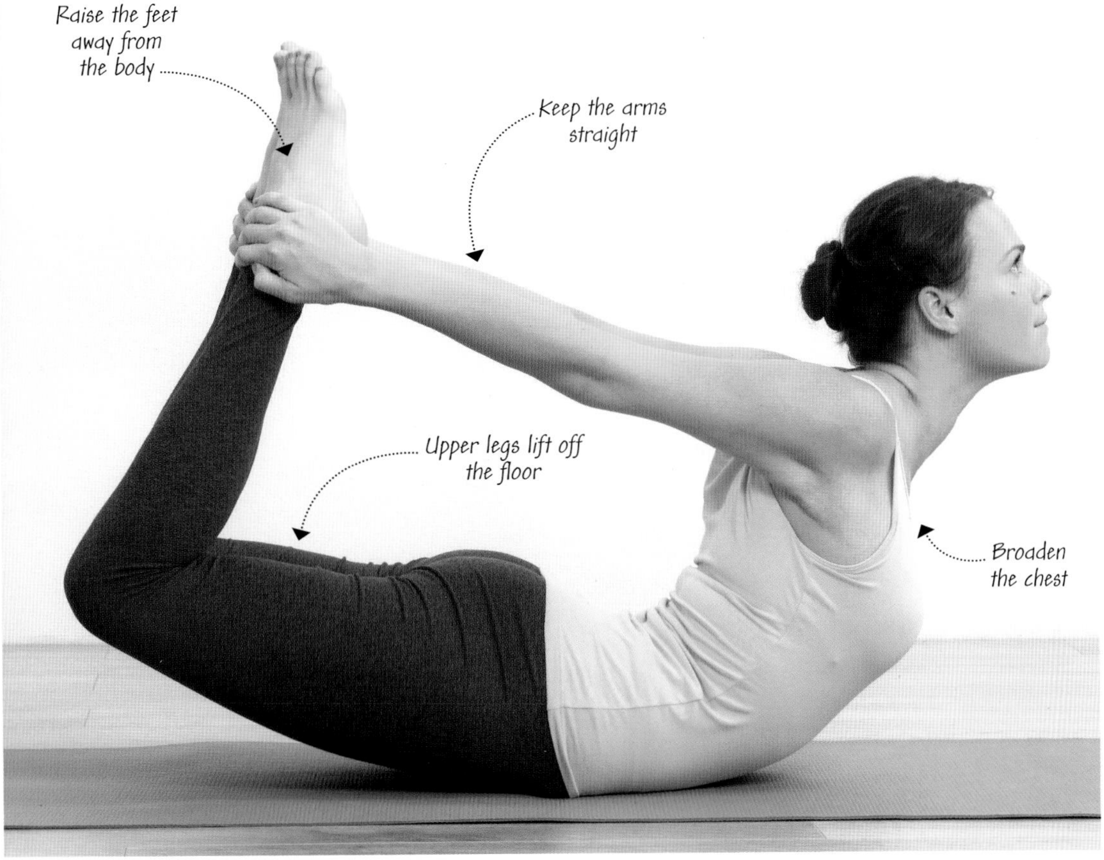

Raise the feet away from the body

Keep the arms straight

Upper legs lift off the floor

Broaden the chest

Seated Forward Bend

Stretch Hamstrings • **Release** Spine

This deceptively simple-looking pose will bring great benefits to the hamstrings and spine, if performed correctly.

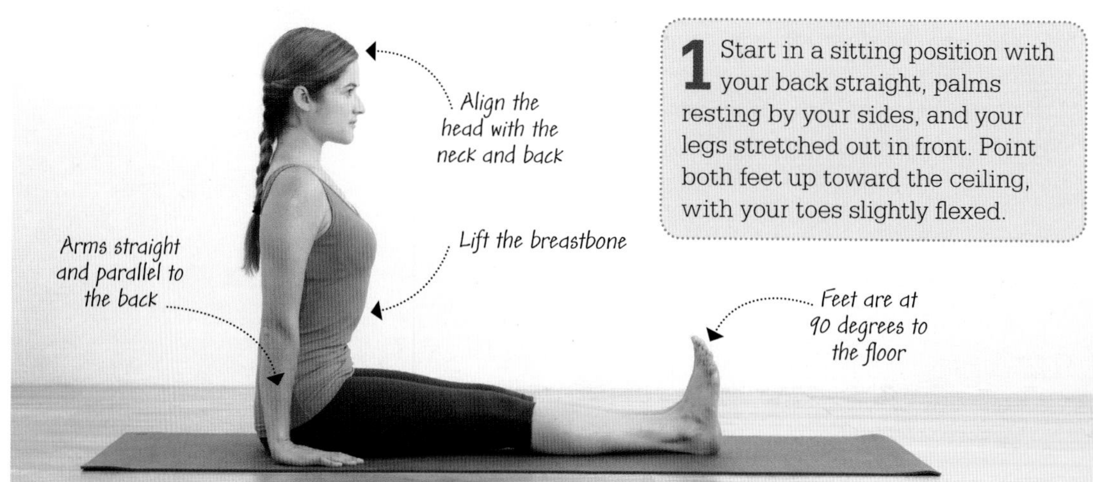
Align the head with the neck and back
Lift the breastbone
Arms straight and parallel to the back
Feet are at 90 degrees to the floor

1 Start in a sitting position with your back straight, palms resting by your sides, and your legs stretched out in front. Point both feet up toward the ceiling, with your toes slightly flexed.

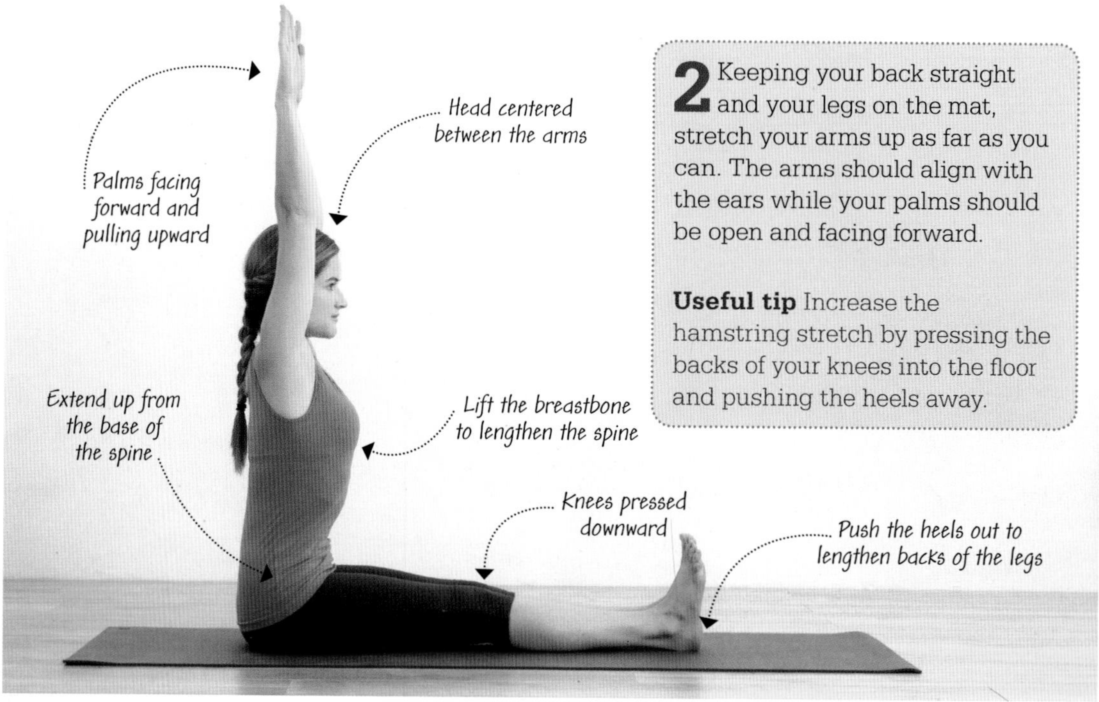

Palms facing forward and pulling upward

Head centered between the arms

Extend up from the base of the spine

Lift the breastbone to lengthen the spine

Knees pressed downward

Push the heels out to lengthen backs of the legs

2 Keeping your back straight and your legs on the mat, stretch your arms up as far as you can. The arms should align with the ears while your palms should be open and facing forward.

Useful tip Increase the hamstring stretch by pressing the backs of your knees into the floor and pushing the heels away.

3 Ensuring your back remains straight, lean forward from the waist and, keeping your arms straight, reach forward toward your ankles.

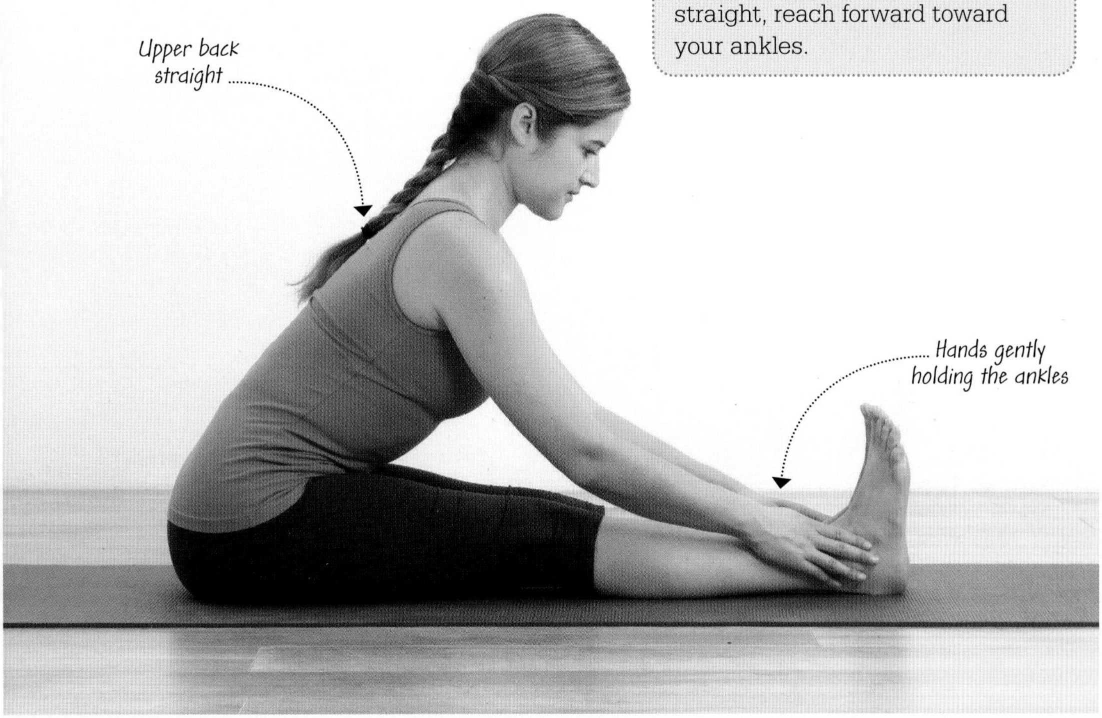

Upper back straight

Hands gently holding the ankles

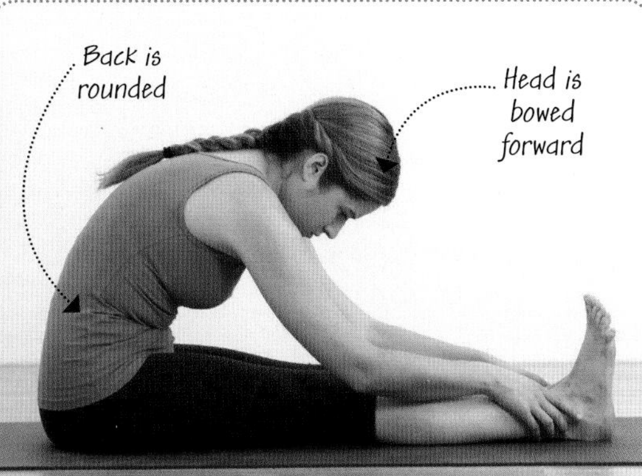
Back is rounded
Head is bowed forward

What not to do

To compensate for stiffness in the lower back, there is a tendency to curve the upper back when bending forward.

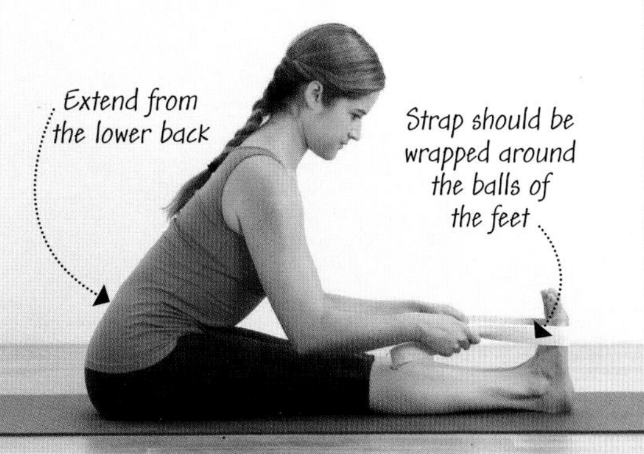
Extend from the lower back
Strap should be wrapped around the balls of the feet

Make it easier

If you cannot hold your ankles, use a strap to connect the hands to the feet and bend forward without rounding the upper back.

Seated Forward Bend Variation

Lengthen Lower Back • **Develop** Body Sense

The forward bend variations with secure hand grips encourage the lengthening of the lower vertebrae and hamstrings.

1 In a sitting position with your legs extended in front of you, exhale as you bend forward, extending your arms and keeping your back straight. Firmly grasp your big toes using the classical foot hold, as shown on the right.

Wrap the index fingers around the big toes and place both thumbs on top of the toes to help secure the limb positions

Position of the hands

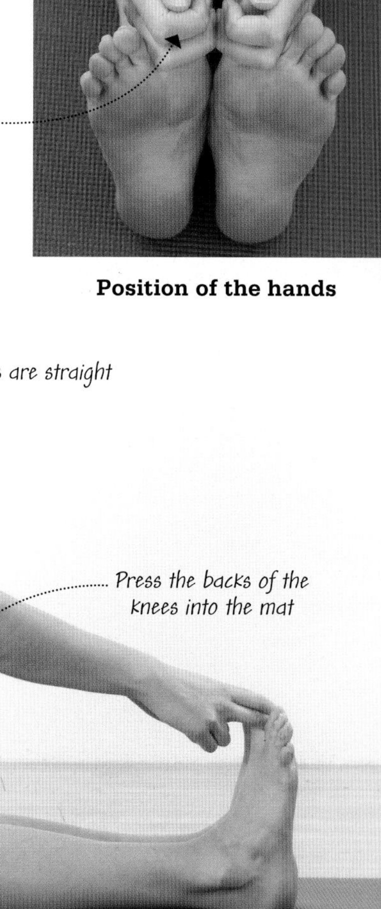

Keep the back, neck, and head aligned

Arms are straight

Lean forward from the hips without curving the back

Press the backs of the knees into the mat

2 On exhalation, bend farther forward so you stretch and lengthen the spine. Bend your elbows, and use your arms to actively assist with the forward movement. Keep your legs straight and continue to hold your toes.

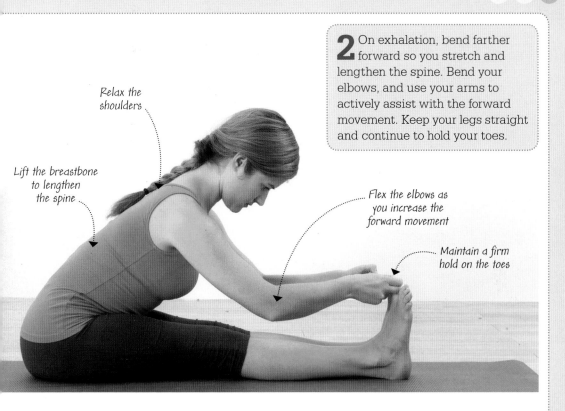

Relax the shoulders

Lift the breastbone to lengthen the spine

Flex the elbows as you increase the forward movement

Maintain a firm hold on the toes

3 Exhale to bend forward until the elbows touch the mat and the abdomen rests on the upper thighs. With each exhalation, extend a fraction more, looking at your toes for focus.

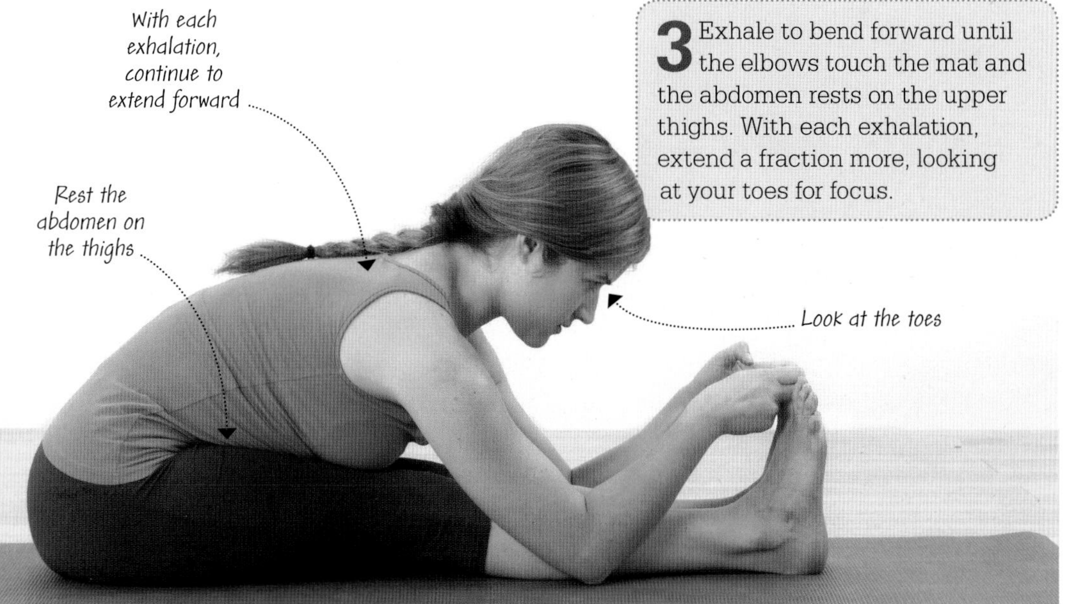
With each exhalation, continue to extend forward
Rest the abdomen on the thighs
Look at the toes

Dolphin

Strengthen Core • **Develop** Confidence

The Dolphin strengthens your abs and arms, preparing you for the more advanced Head Stand and other arm-balance postures, which you might do as you progress.

1 Start in a sitting position with your legs slightly apart and folded under your buttocks. Rest your hands on your thighs.

Useful tip To straighten the back in this sitting position, focus on breathing from the abdomen and lifting the rib cage as you inhale.

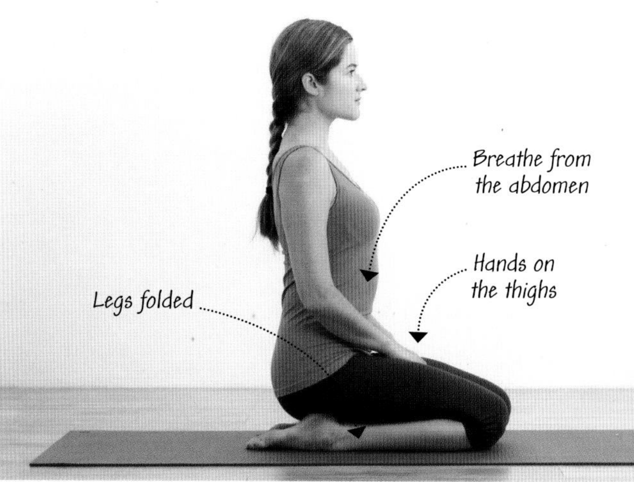
Breathe from the abdomen
Hands on the thighs
Legs folded

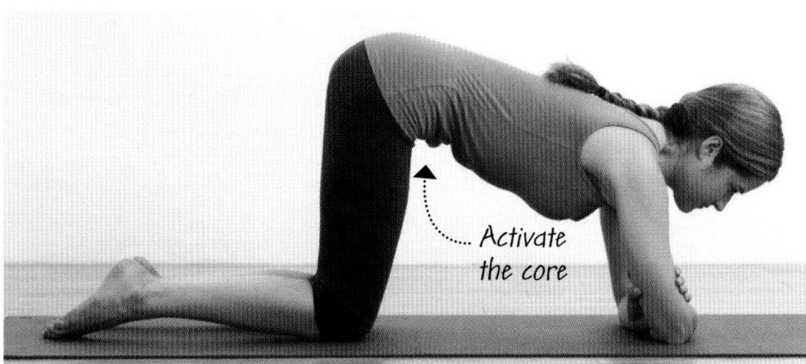
Activate the core

2 Lift your buttocks off your heels, lean forward, and place your forearms on the floor. Hold the elbows with your hands and look downward.

Remember Make sure your knees are aligned with your hips.

3 Keeping your elbows in this position, open your forearms to a 45-degree angle. Interlock the fingers in a triangle shape. Push your shoulders back and down.

Useful tip Align your elbows with your knees.

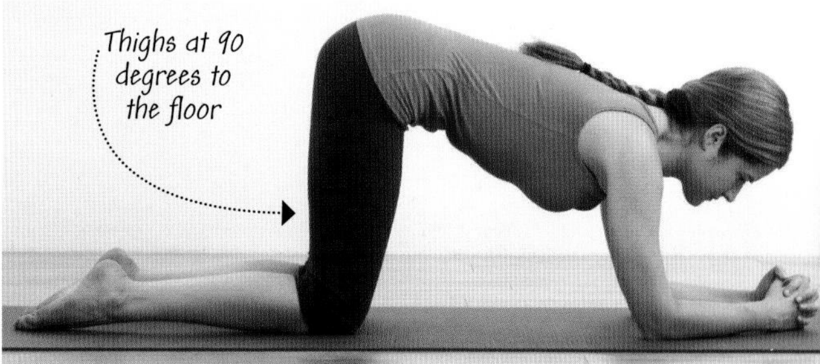
Thighs at 90 degrees to the floor

4 Lower your forehead to the mat. Curl your toes inward to grip as you straighten your legs and lift them upward into an inverted V-shape.

Careful! These steps can be strenuous on the upper body. Rest in the child's pose afterward.

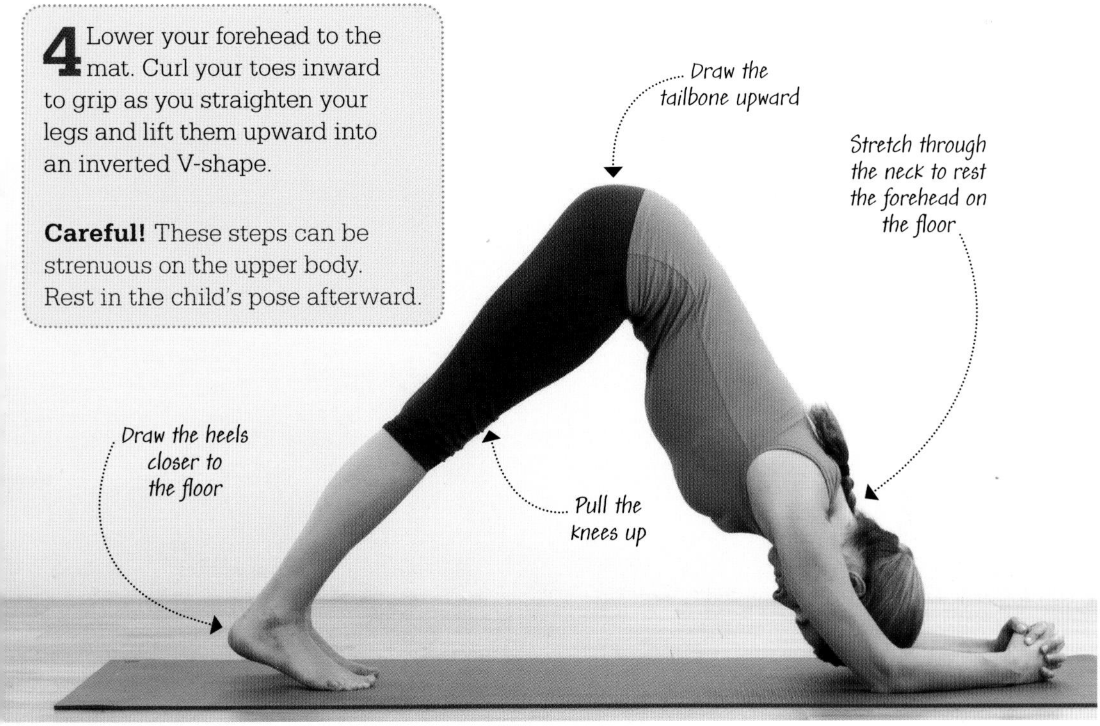

Draw the tailbone upward
Stretch through the neck to rest the forehead on the floor
Draw the heels closer to the floor
Pull the knees up

5 Inhale as you raise your head. Without moving your feet, move your shoulders forward over your hands. As you exhale, revert back to your previous position (step 4). Repeat steps 4 and 5 about five times.

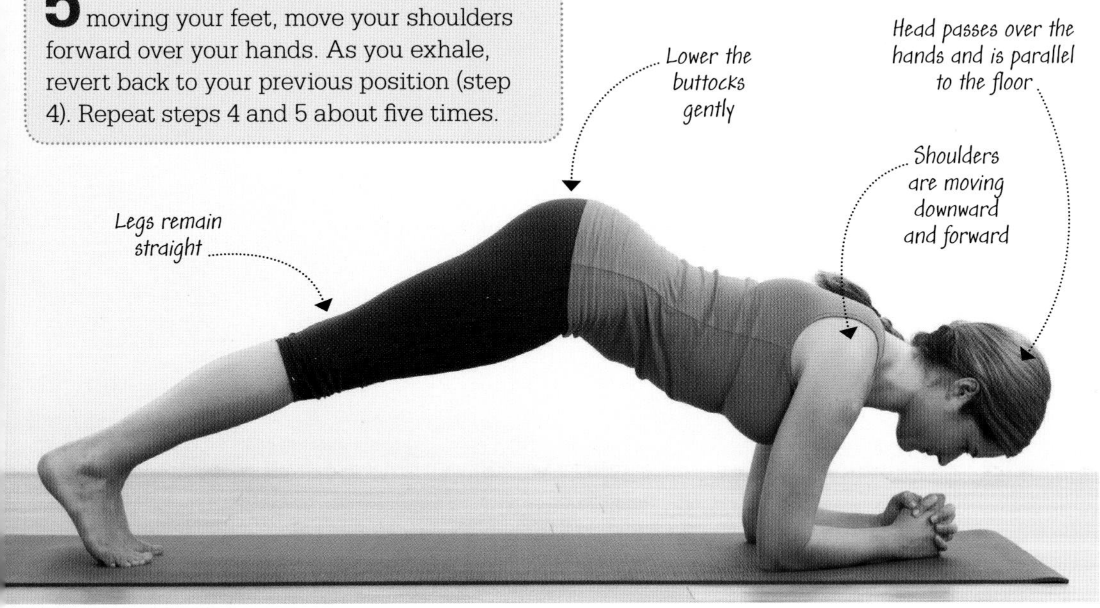

Lower the buttocks gently
Head passes over the hands and is parallel to the floor
Shoulders are moving downward and forward
Legs remain straight

Shoulder Stand

Improve Circulation • **Promote** Youthfulness

Yoga inversions reverse the direction of blood flow, rejuvenating the whole body. Increasing blood flow to the brain also helps to relieve emotional and mental stress.

1 To begin, lie on your back on the mat with your legs together and your arms by your sides. Rest your head with your chin slightly downward and focus on making your breathing regular and even.

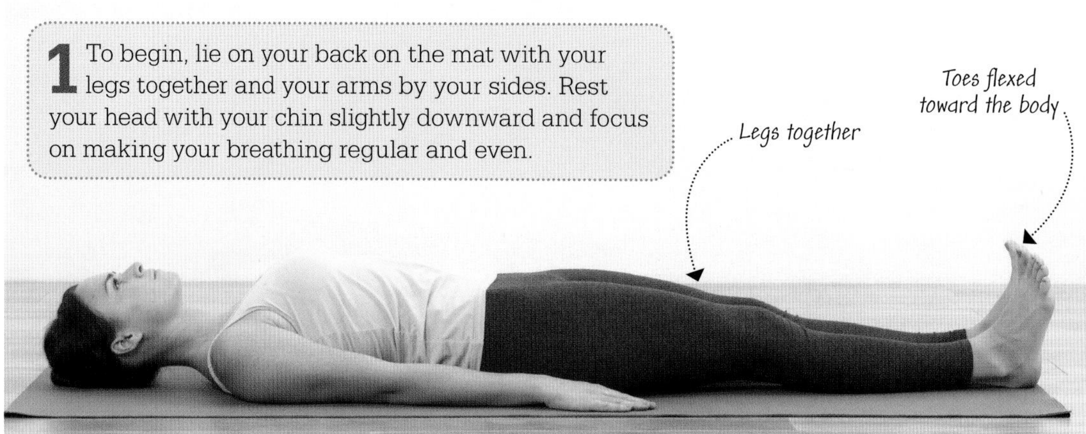

Legs together
Toes flexed toward the body

2 Keeping your palms, arms, shoulders, and head in contact with the mat, inhale as you lift both your legs up with the knees locked, tilting them toward your head.

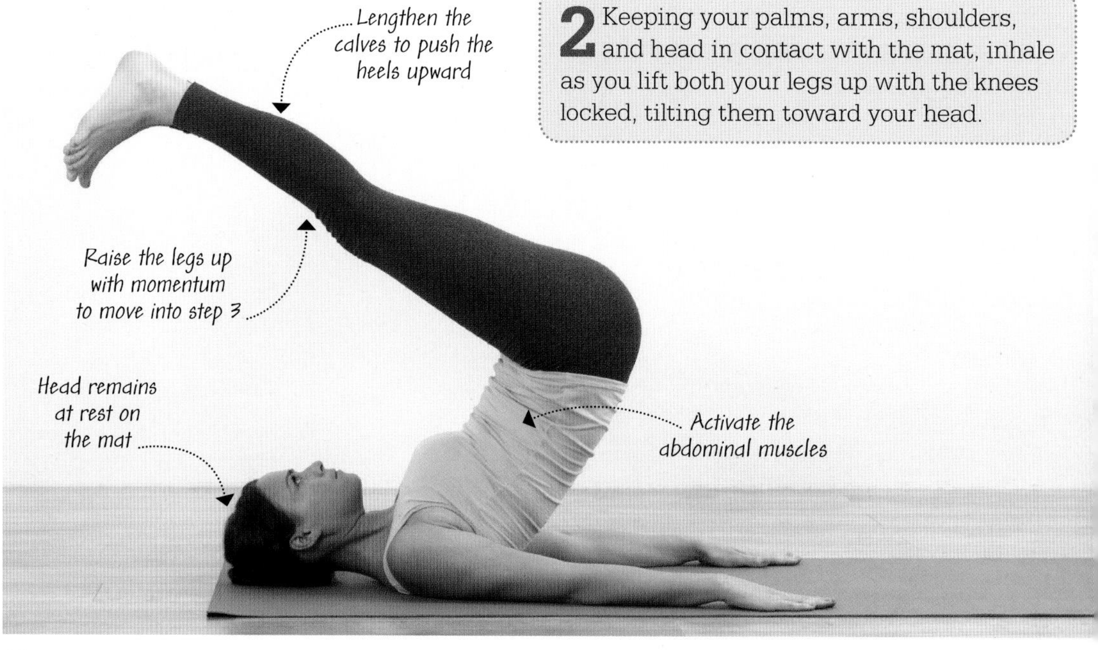

Lengthen the calves to push the heels upward

Raise the legs up with momentum to move into step 3

Head remains at rest on the mat

Activate the abdominal muscles

3 Still using step 2's inhalation, continue raising your legs, bringing your feet over your head and lifting your back off the floor. Bend your elbows to support the lower back with your palms—thumbs outward, palms on either side of the spine.

Remember Work on actively using your arms and hands to straighten your torso and legs.

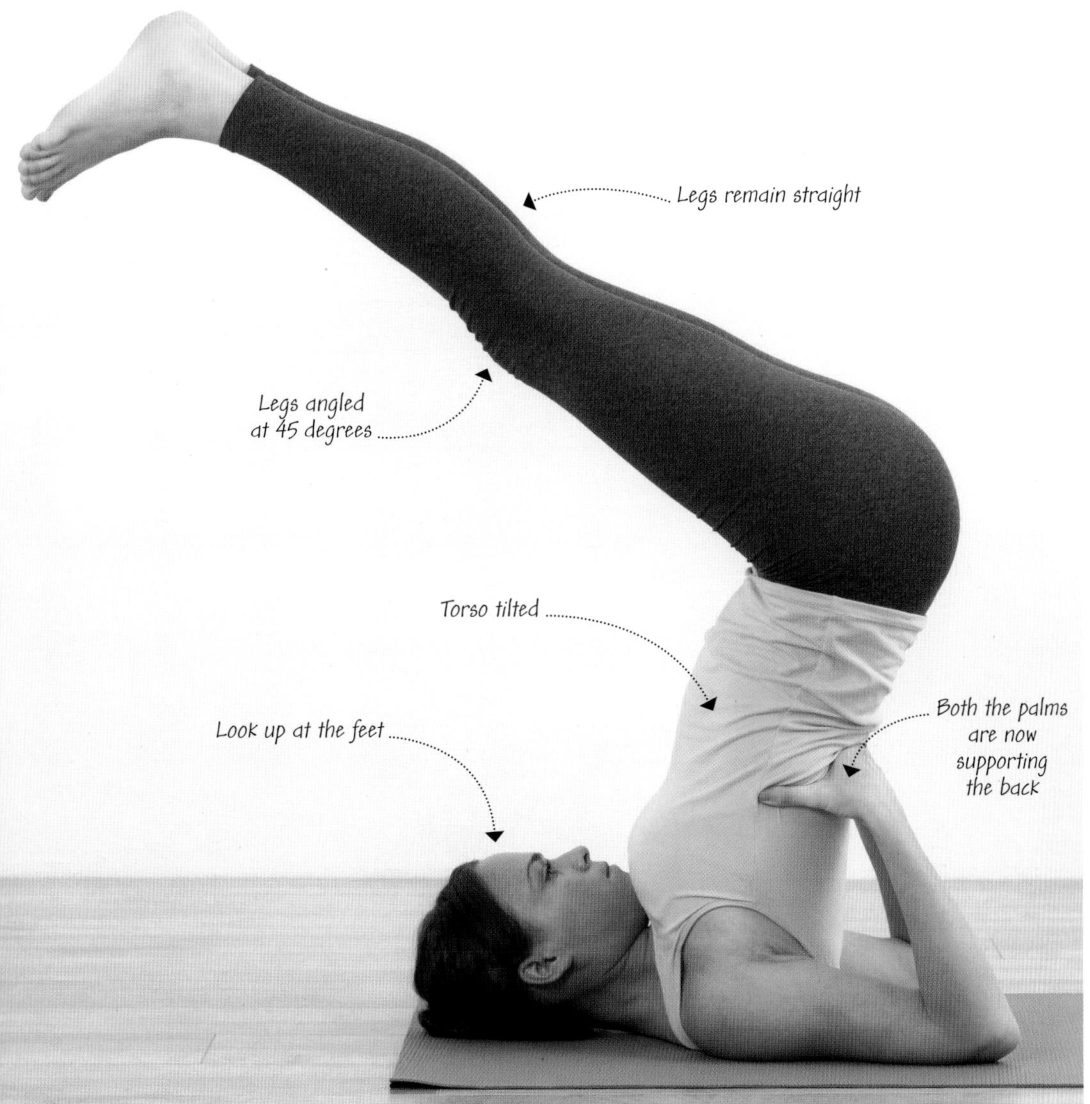
Legs remain straight
Legs angled at 45 degrees
Torso tilted
Look up at the feet
Both the palms are now supporting the back

4 Bring your hands farther up the spine as you raise your legs. Your weight should be on your shoulders and hands as your torso, hips, and knees come into alignment. Hold this pose for 10–15 breaths. Work on extending the torso and legs upward.

Useful tip Narrow the gap between your chest and chin as much as you possibly can.

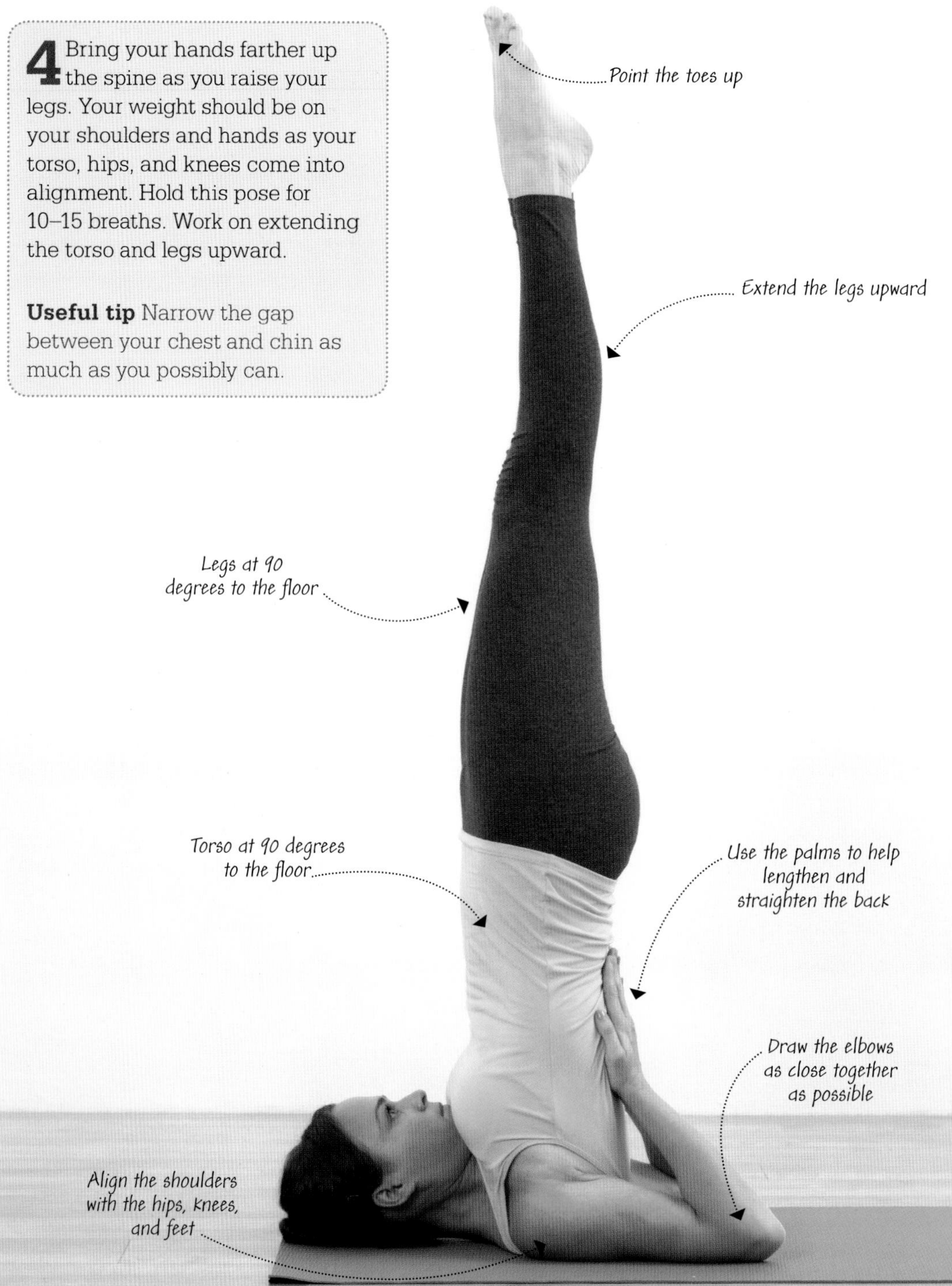
Point the toes up
Extend the legs upward
Legs at 90 degrees to the floor
Torso at 90 degrees to the floor
Use the palms to help lengthen and straighten the back
Draw the elbows as close together as possible
Align the shoulders with the hips, knees, and feet

5 To release, bend your knees and lower them to touch your forehead. Alter your hand position to support your back and roll gently back onto the mat. Toward the end of the roll, place your palms flat on the mat, and allow your whole body to be supported by the floor.

Careful! Use your palms and arms to gradually unbend your spine, one vertebra at a time, until your back is on the mat

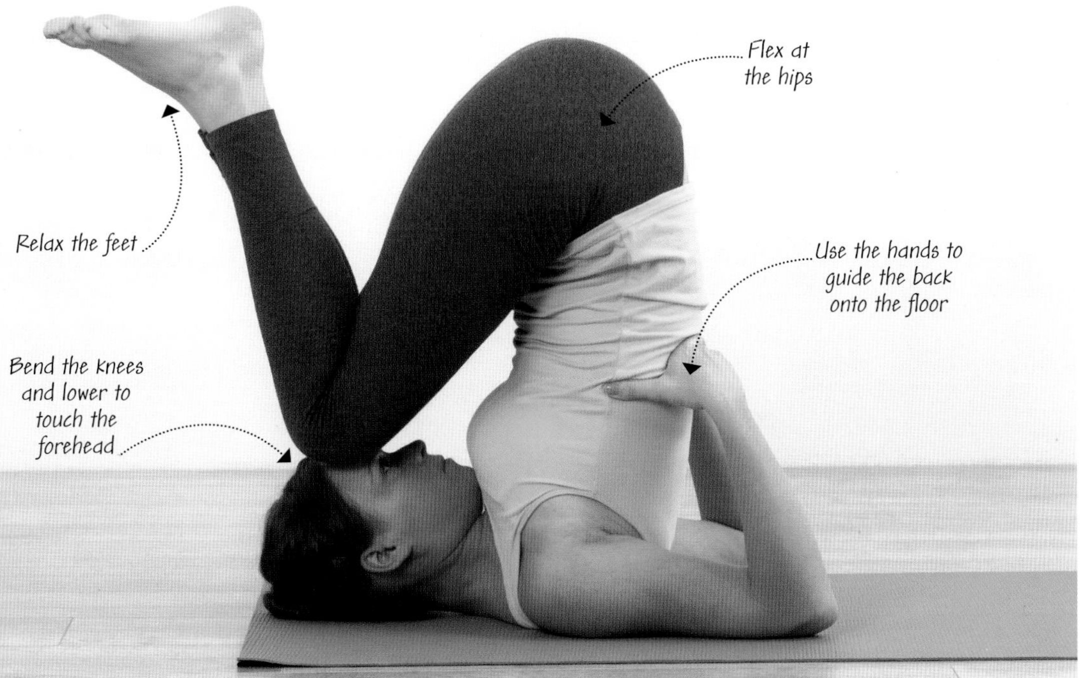

Flex at the hips
Relax the feet
Use the hands to guide the back onto the floor
Bend the knees and lower to touch the forehead

Take care...

Avoid angling the elbows as this can strain the wrists. Adjust your elbows gently to be in line with your shoulders.

Ensure that the feet are together and the toes are pointing upward and assisting in lengthening through the back and spine.

Avoid angling the torso. To straighten the body, use your palms to gently straighten your spine and draw your chest to your chin.

Avoid bending at the knees when your legs are elevated by firming your bottom to align the spine and legs and locking your knees.

Plow

Stretches Back • **Improves** Digestion

The Plow Pose is a natural progression from the Shoulder Stand. It promotes spinal flexibility and good digestion.

1 Start this position by resting with your back flat on the floor, with your palms flat on the ground beside you, and your legs extended. Keep your legs together and your feet relaxed.

Extend the feet with the toes pointing forward

Breathe through the abdomen

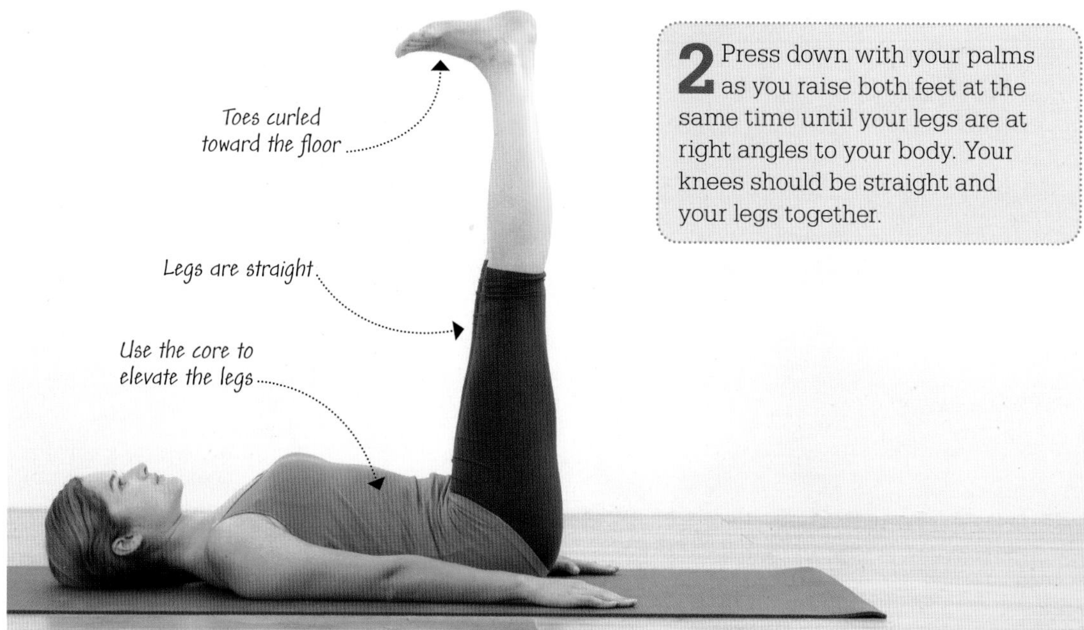
Toes curled toward the floor
Legs are straight
Use the core to elevate the legs

2 Press down with your palms as you raise both feet at the same time until your legs are at right angles to your body. Your knees should be straight and your legs together.

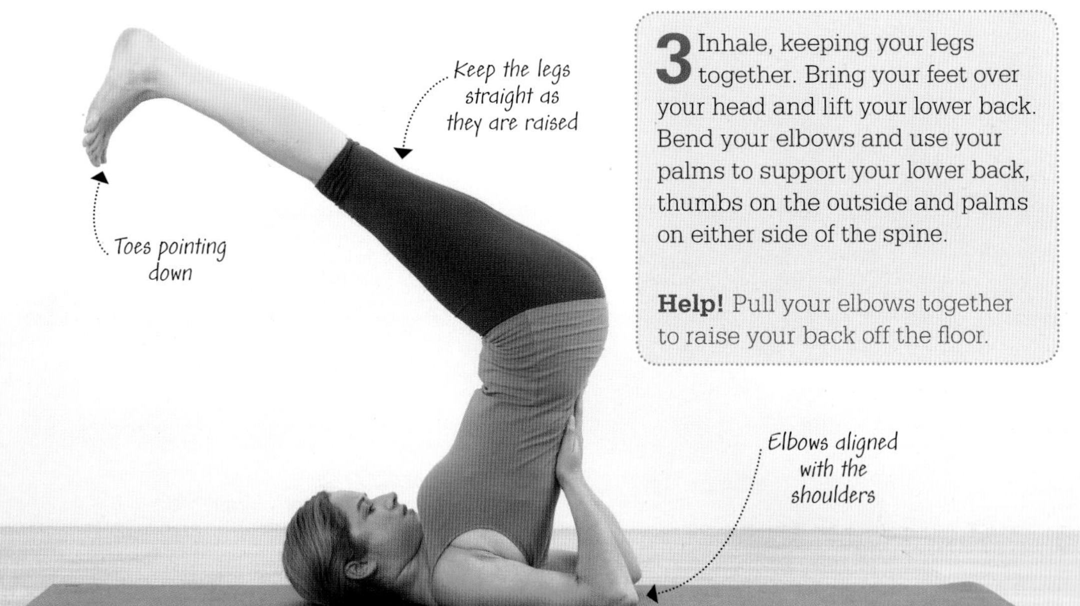

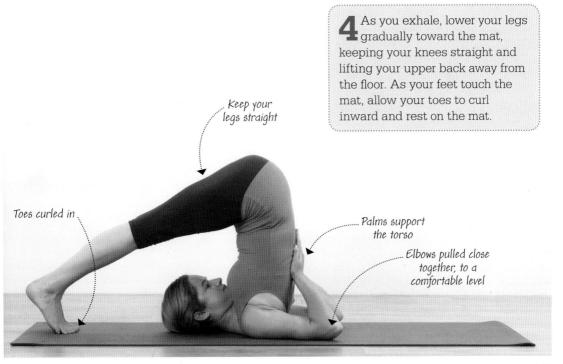
Keep the legs straight as they are raised
Toes pointing down
Elbows aligned with the shoulders

3 Inhale, keeping your legs together. Bring your feet over your head and lift your lower back. Bend your elbows and use your palms to support your lower back, thumbs on the outside and palms on either side of the spine.

Help! Pull your elbows together to raise your back off the floor.

4 As you exhale, lower your legs gradually toward the mat, keeping your knees straight and lifting your upper back away from the floor. As your feet touch the mat, allow your toes to curl inward and rest on the mat.

Keep your legs straight

Toes curled in

Palms support the torso

Elbows pulled close together, to a comfortable level

5 When your torso is upright, release your hands from supporting the lower back. Straighten your arms and lower them until your palms touch the mat.

Careful! Try to keep your arms parallel and in line with your shoulders as you bring them down.

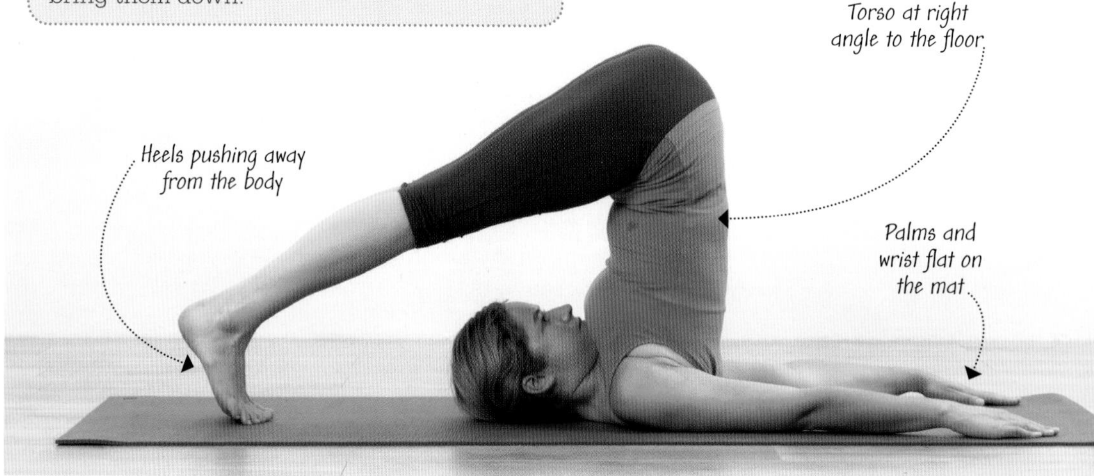
Torso at right angle to the floor
Heels pushing away from the body
Palms and wrist flat on the mat

Variations

Variation 1 Bring your hands together and interlock the fingers. Rest your hands on the mat.

Variation 2 Keeping your legs straight, walk your feet as far apart as possible.

Variation 3 This Plow variation is often called the Ear-closing Pose. The legs are bent with the knees resting on the floor beside the ears. The arms are brought forward and the hands are folded over the bent legs.

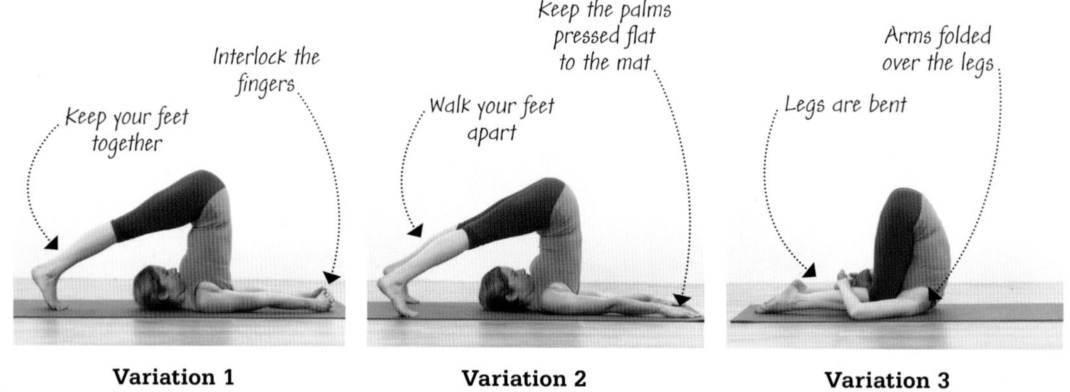
Interlock the fingers
Keep your feet together
Keep the palms pressed flat to the mat
Walk your feet apart
Arms folded over the legs
Legs are bent

Variation 1 **Variation 2** **Variation 3**

6 To release, raise your legs so they are parallel with the ground, then slowly roll your spine back to the floor, followed by your legs.

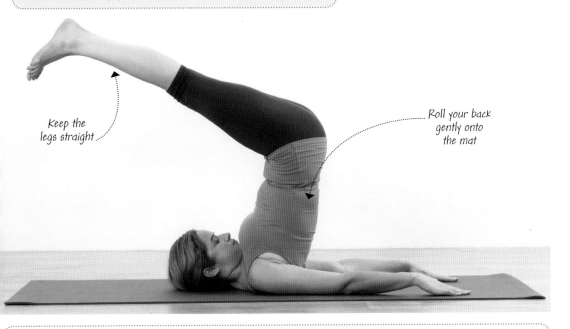
Keep the legs straight
Roll your back gently onto the mat

Take care...

Don't have the shoulders blades apart with the arms stretched wide. Being able to bring your shoulder blades together helps to elevate the back vertically.

Do not float the legs. If you are unable to keep your legs straight with the toes resting on the mat, then bend the knees slightly to allow the feet to rest on the mat.

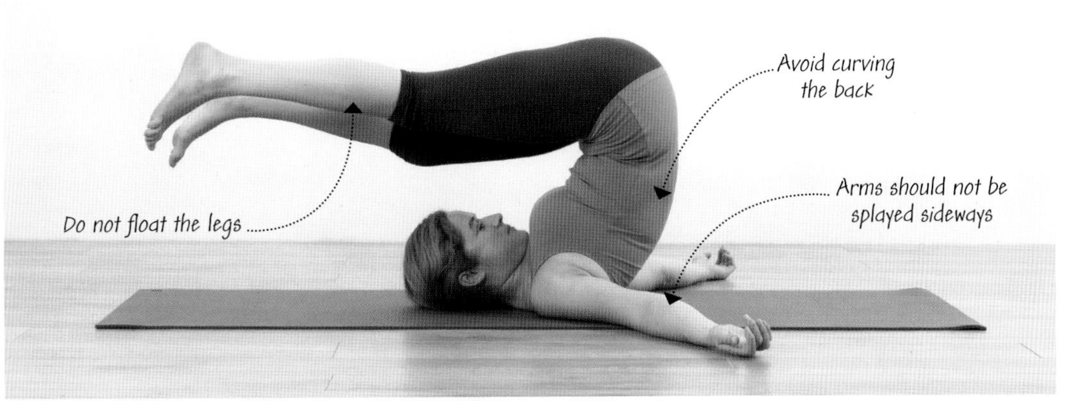
Avoid curving the back
Arms should not be splayed sideways
Do not float the legs

Fish

Increase Chest Capacity • **Relieve** Neck Tension

This pose involves a strong compression of the cervical vertebrae and is a good counter-stretch to the Shoulder Stand and Plow poses.

1 Lie stretched on your back with your legs close together and your arms by your sides. Lift your pelvis to place your palms under your buttocks. Point your toes slightly away from your body. Focus on breathing.

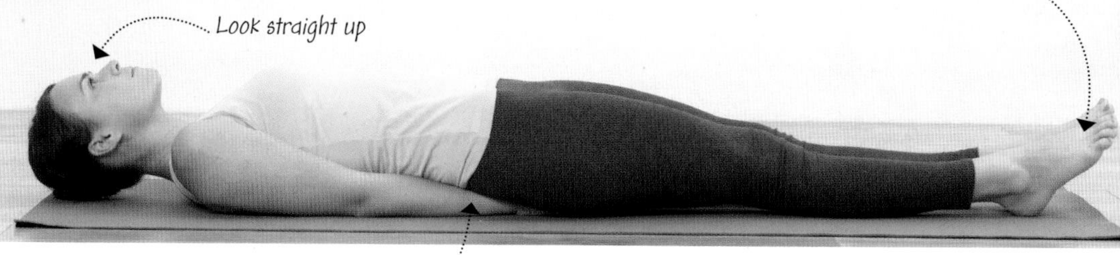
Legs and feet together
Look straight up
Tuck pressed-down palms under the bottom

Take care...

Not tilting the head back far enough will result in weight being borne through the back of the head, rather than the crown. If this happens, try practicing the pose using a firm bolster tucked under the back for support, ensuring that you come to rest on the crown of your head comfortably. Keep the neck soft.

This pose must only be practiced if you are able to bring the crown of your head to rest on the floor.

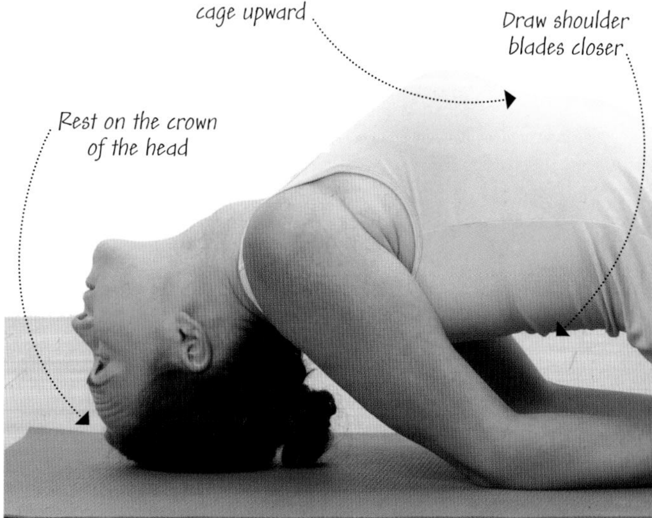
Draw the rib cage upward
Draw shoulder blades closer
Rest on the crown of the head

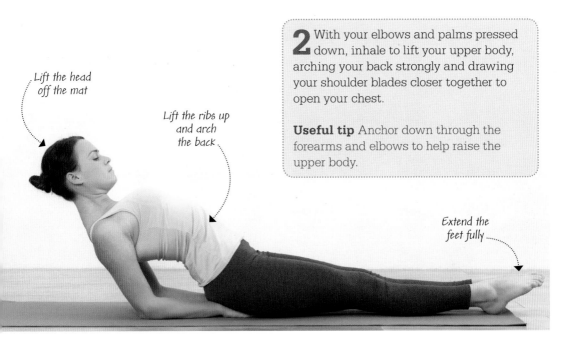

2 With your elbows and palms pressed down, inhale to lift your upper body, arching your back strongly and drawing your shoulder blades closer together to open your chest.

Useful tip Anchor down through the forearms and elbows to help raise the upper body.

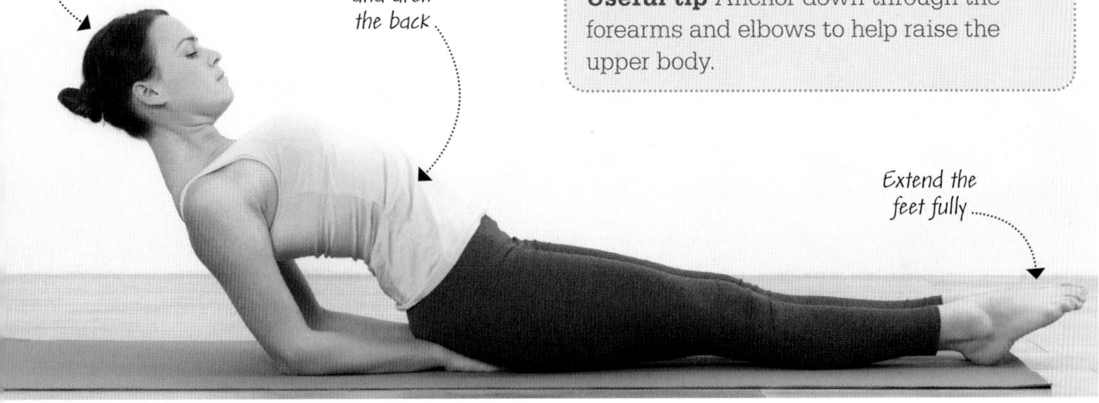

Lift the head off the mat

Lift the ribs up and arch the back

Extend the feet fully

3 Continue the movement, tilting your head as far back as possible, so that the crown of your head comes to rest flat on the floor. Hold the pose for seven to eight breaths, or longer if comfortable. To release from the pose, exhale to lower your torso and head to the mat.

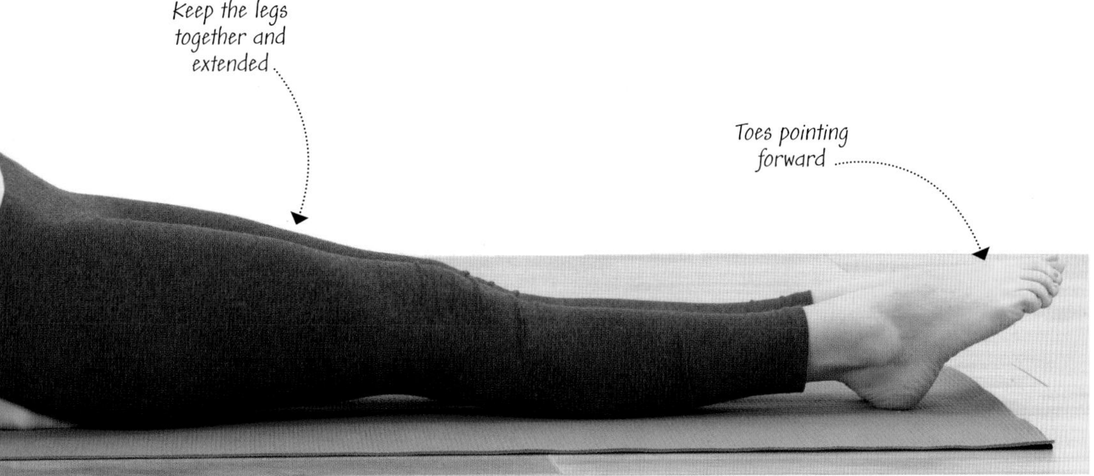
Keep the legs together and extended
Toes pointing forward

15-Minute Back Bend Sequence

1 Mountain Pose
pp.44–45

2 Warrior Lunge
pp.104–105

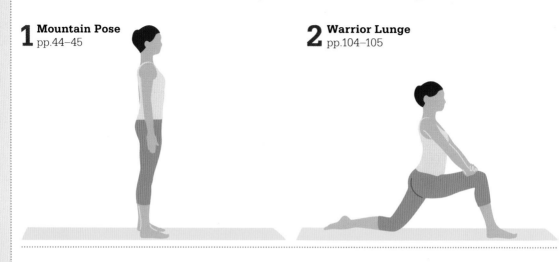

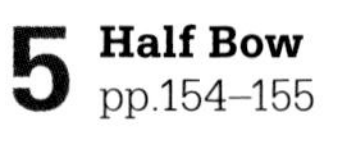

5 Half Bow
pp.154–155

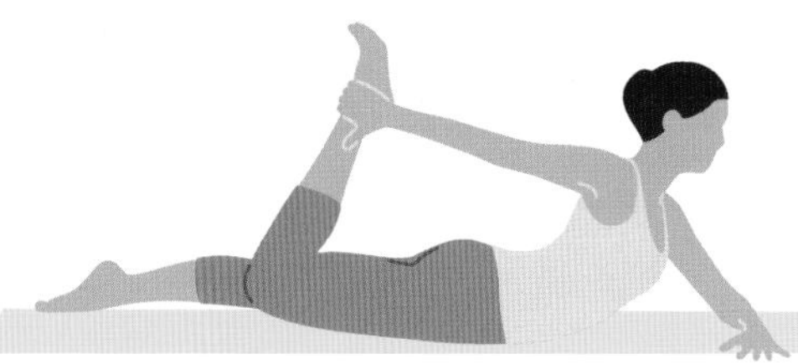

6 Full Bow
pp.156–157

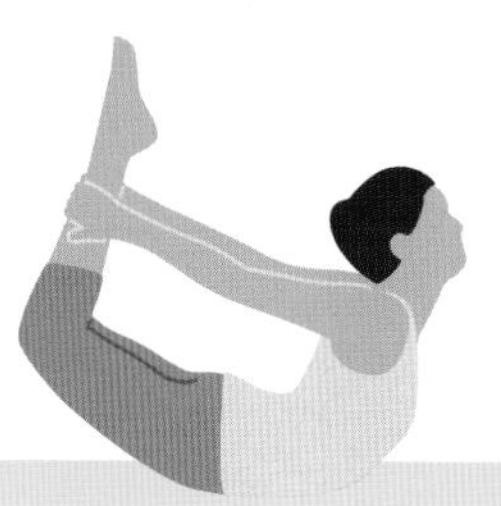

9 Crossed Leg Forward Bend
pp.122–123

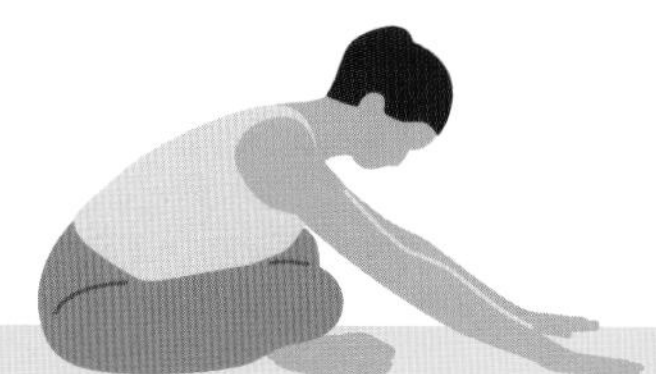

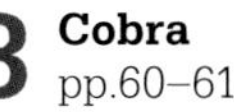

3 Cobra pp.60–61

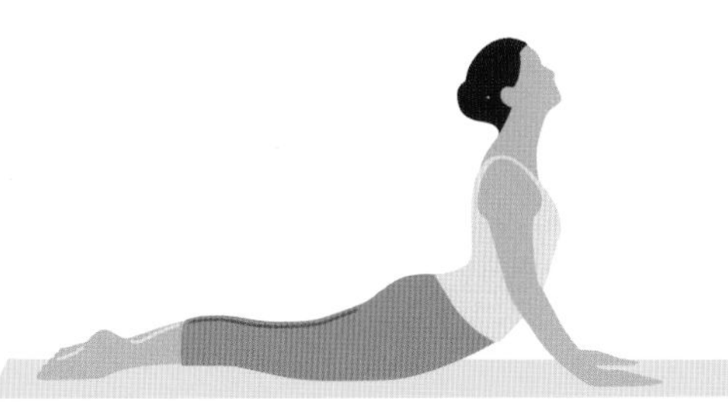

4 Child's Pose pp.62–63

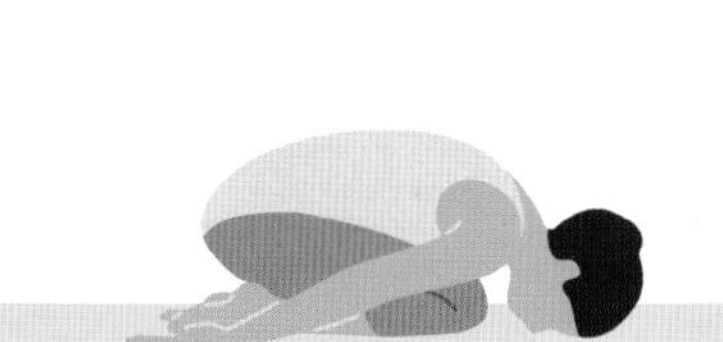

7 Child's Pose pp.62–63

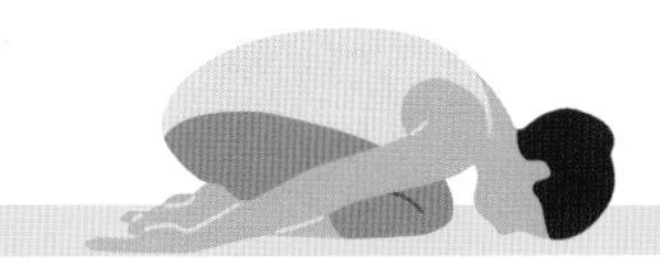

8 Dolphin pp.162–163

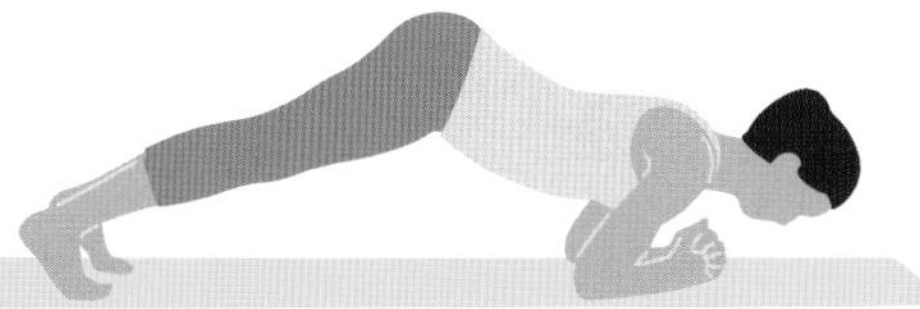

10 Corpse and Final Relaxation pp.78–81

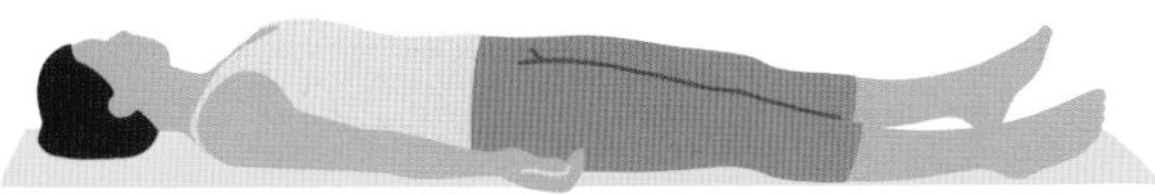

15-Minute Standing Sequence

1 Mountain Pose pp.44–45

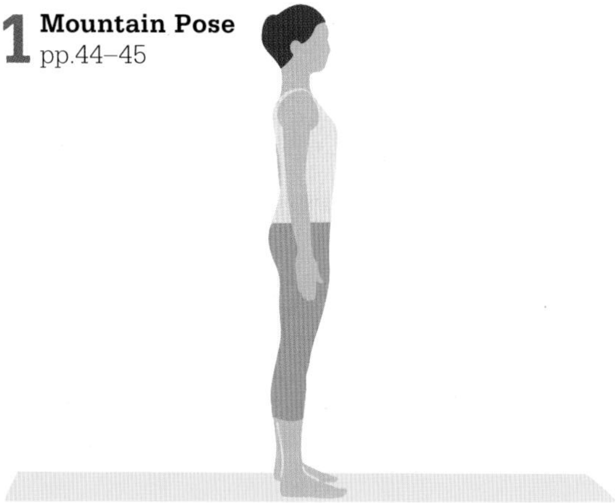

2 Triangle pp.50–51

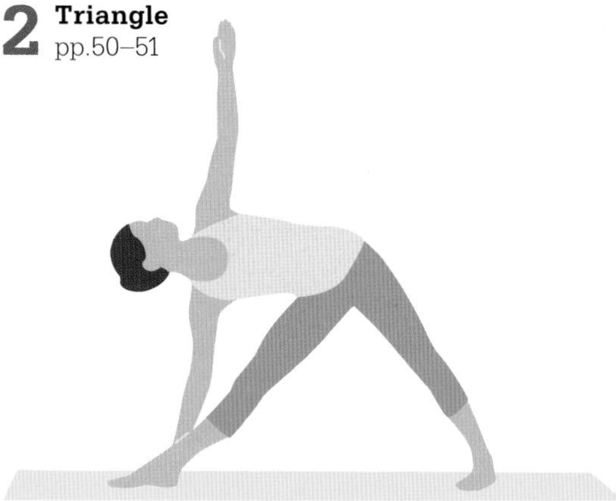

5 Warrior 1 pp.146–147

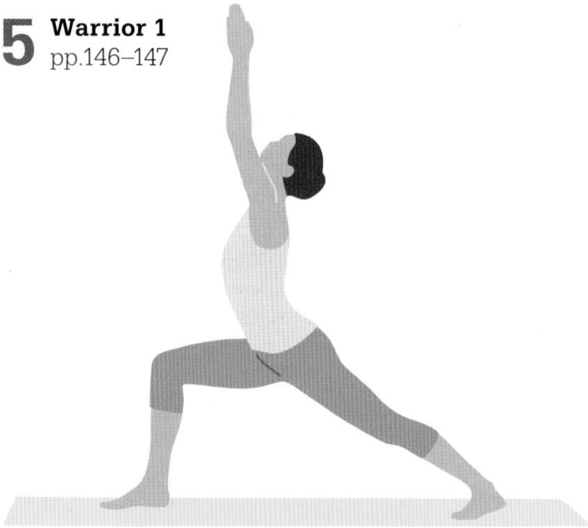

6 Warrior 2 pp.98–99

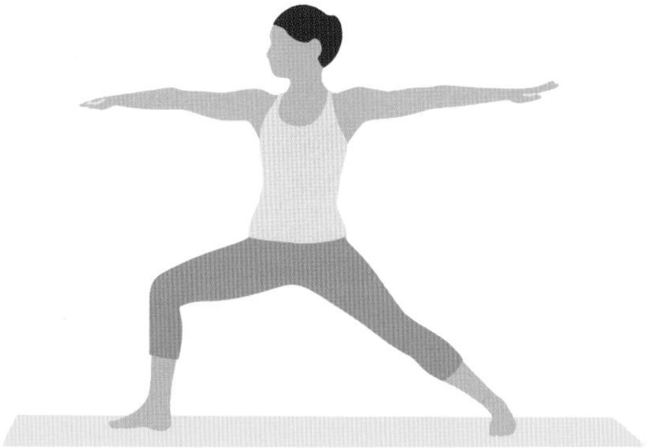

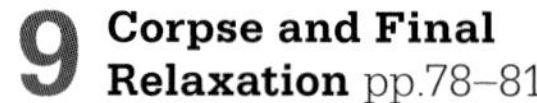
9 Corpse and Final Relaxation pp.78–81

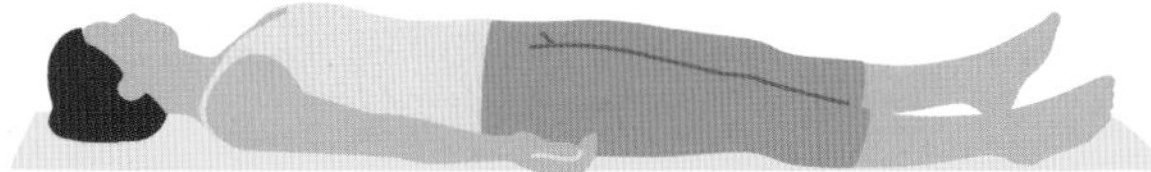

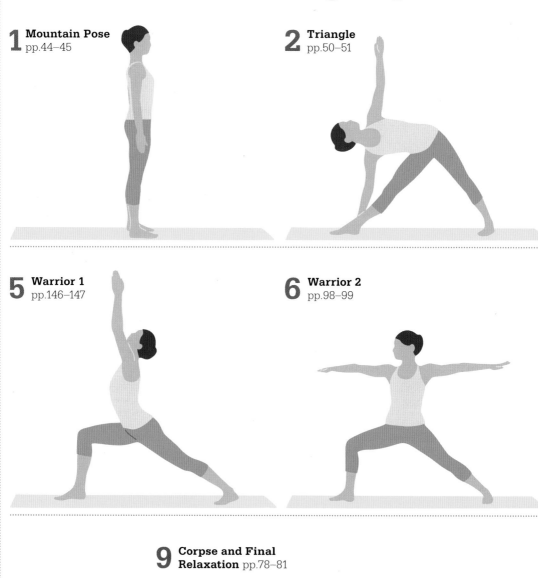

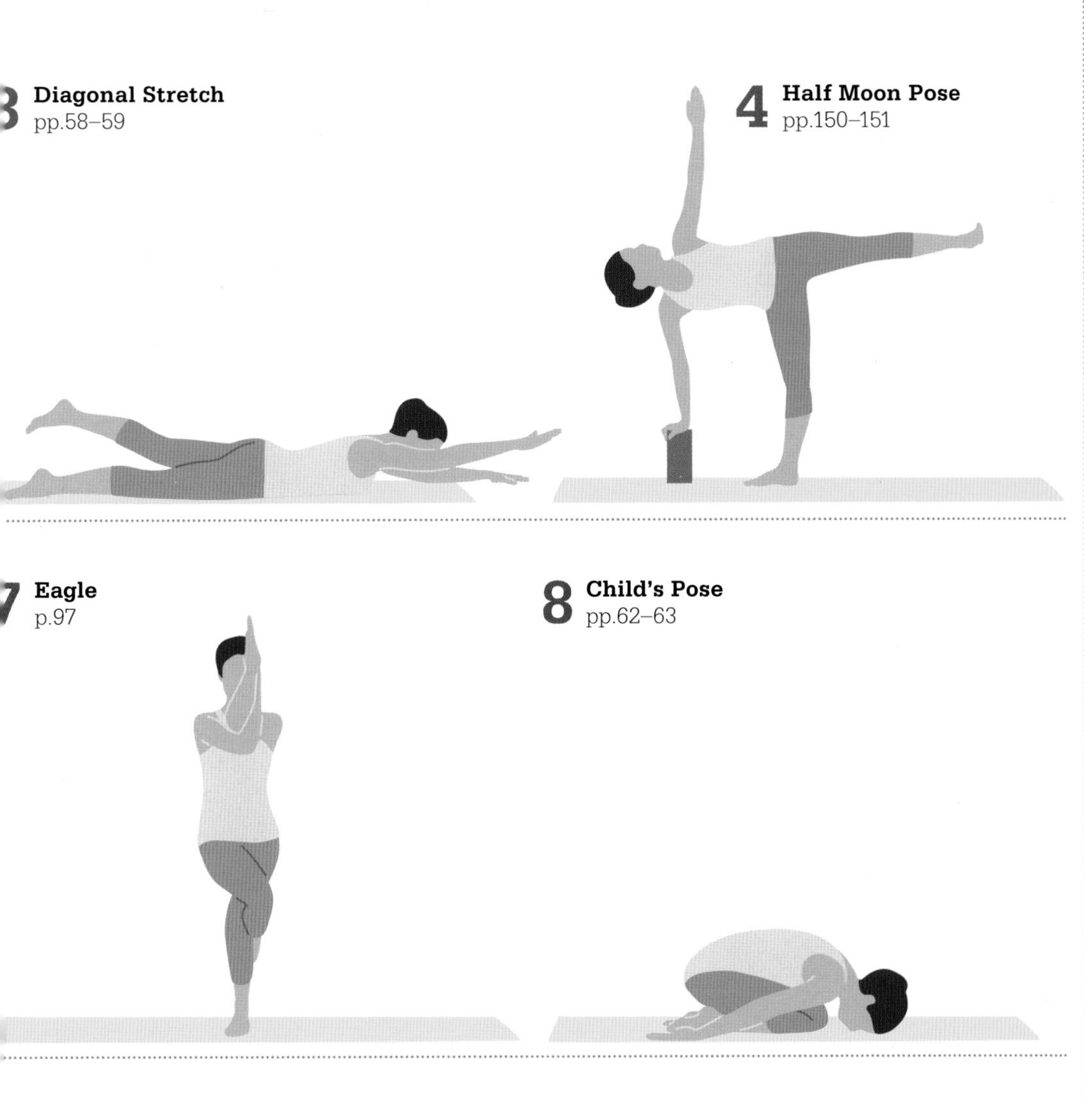
3 Diagonal Stretch
pp.58–59
4 Half Moon Pose
pp.150–151
7 Eagle
p.97
8 Child's Pose
pp.62–63

15-Minute Inversion Sequence

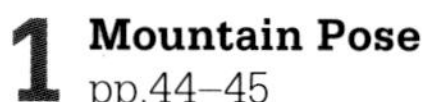

1 Mountain Pose
pp.44–45

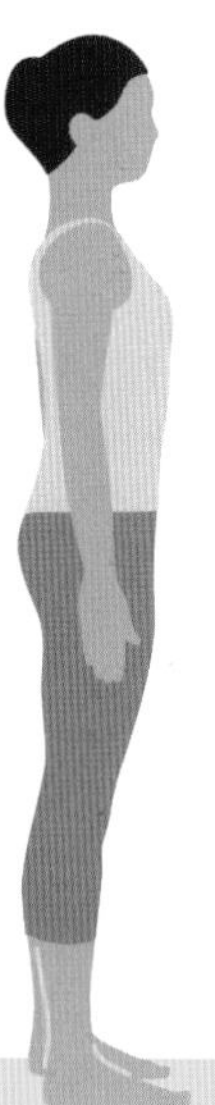

2 Wide Forward Bend
pp.106–107

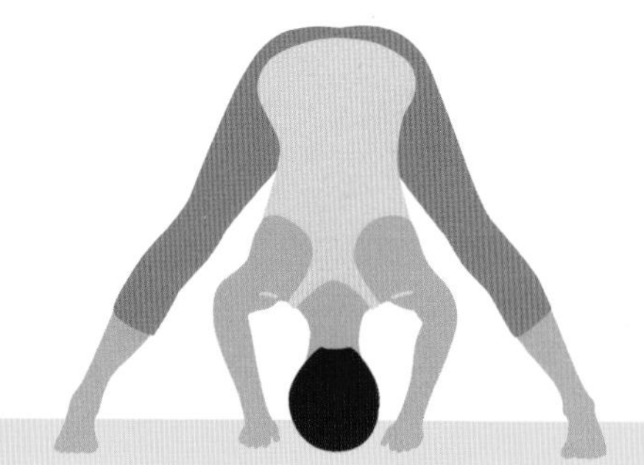

5 Bridge
pp.124–125

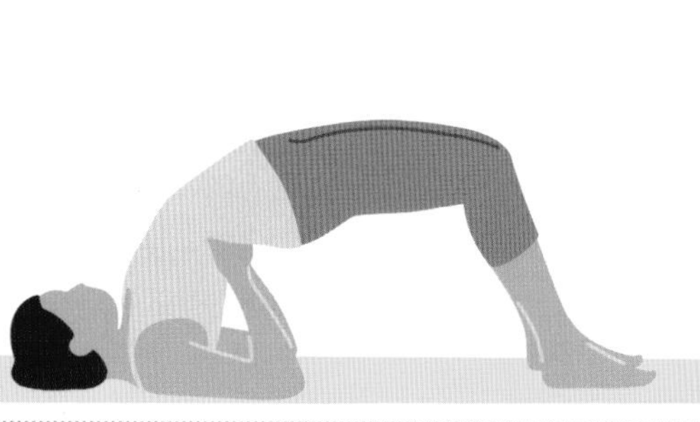

6 Shoulder Stand
pp.164–167

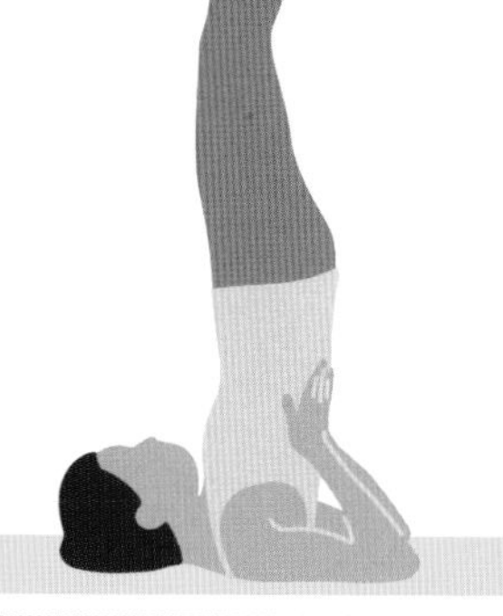

9 Fish
pp.172–173

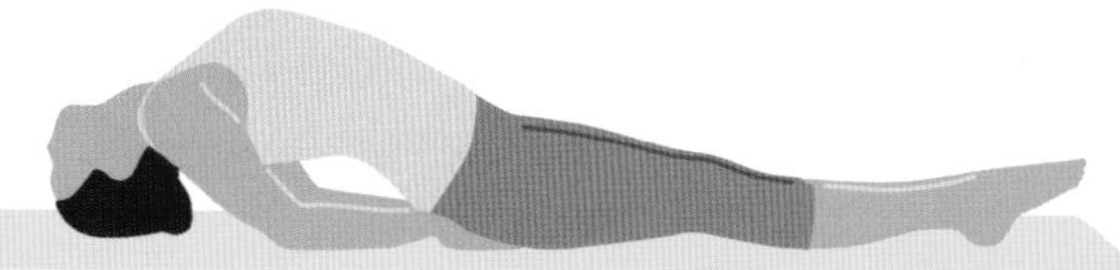

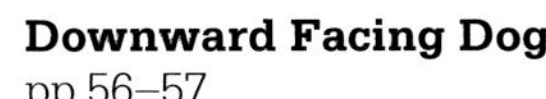

3 Downward Facing Dog
pp.56–57

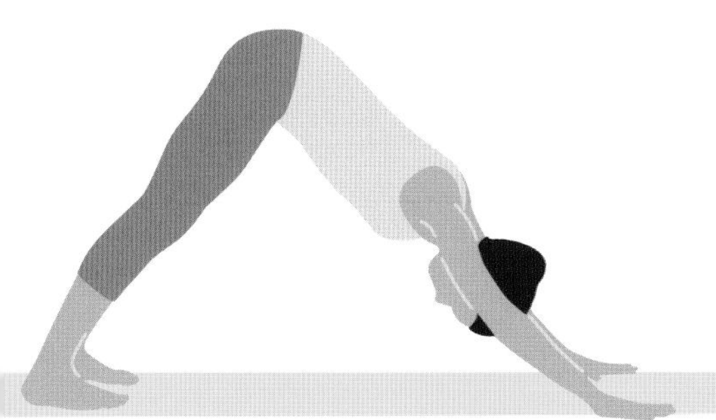

4 Child's Pose
pp.62–63

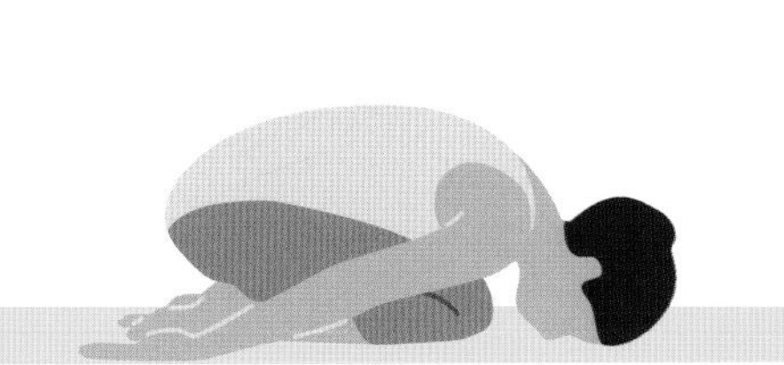

7 Plow
pp.168–171

8 Plow Variation 2
p.170

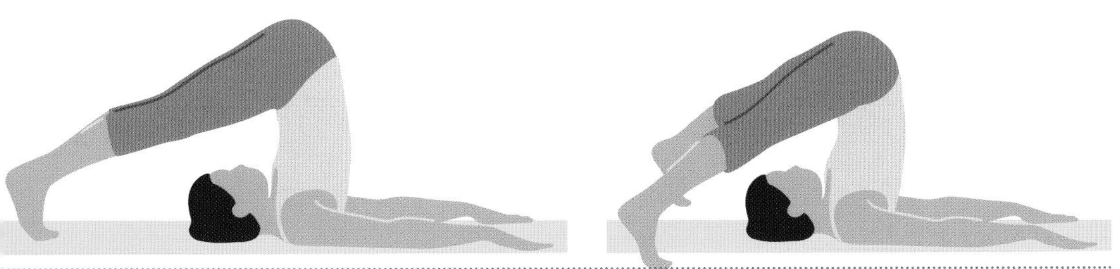

10 Corpse and Final Relaxation
pp.78–81

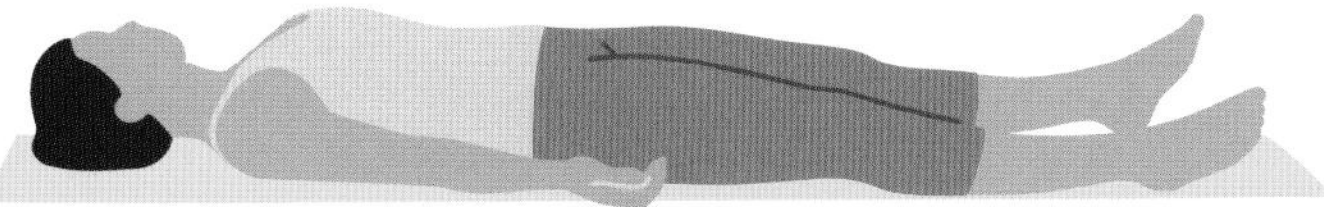

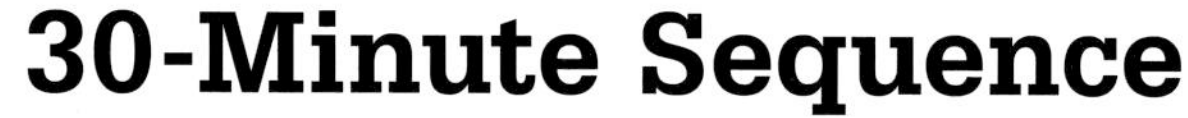
30-Minute Sequence

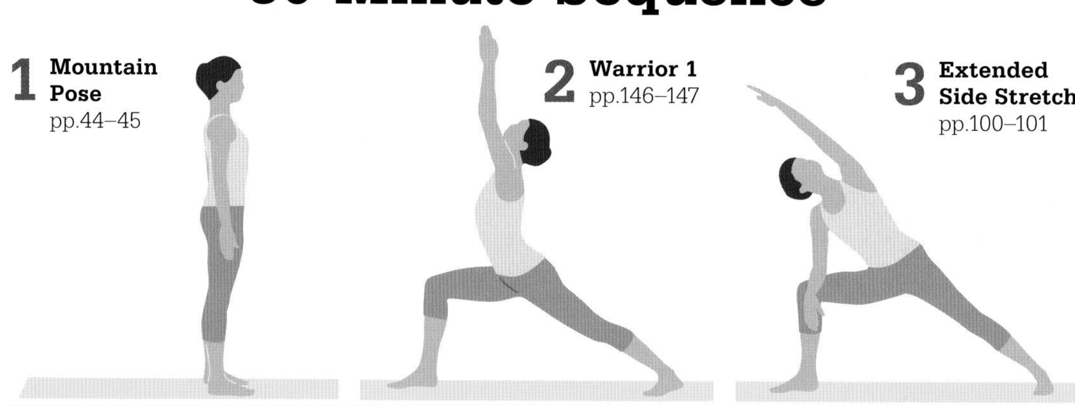
1 Mountain Pose
pp.44–45
2 Warrior 1
pp.146–147
3 Extended Side Stretch
pp.100–101

7 Warrior Lunge
pp.104–105

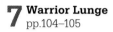

8 Child's Pose
pp.62–63

9 Half Bow
pp.154–155

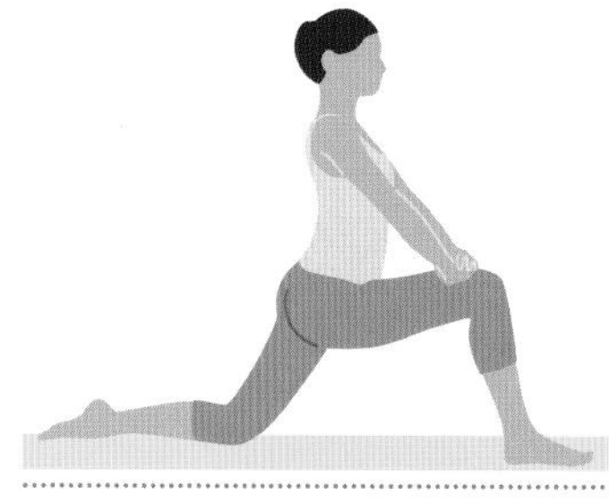

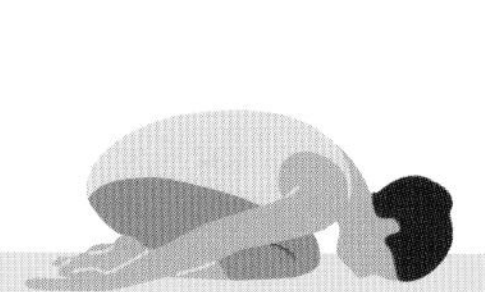

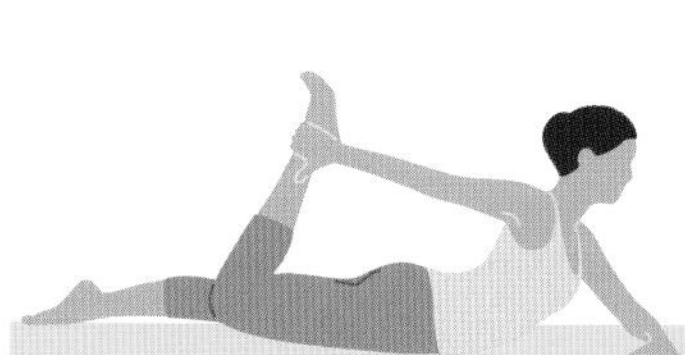

13 Shoulder Stand
pp.164–167

14 Plow
pp.168–171

15 Fish
pp.172–173

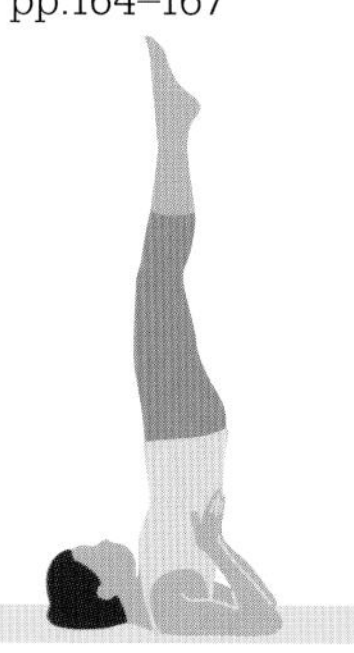

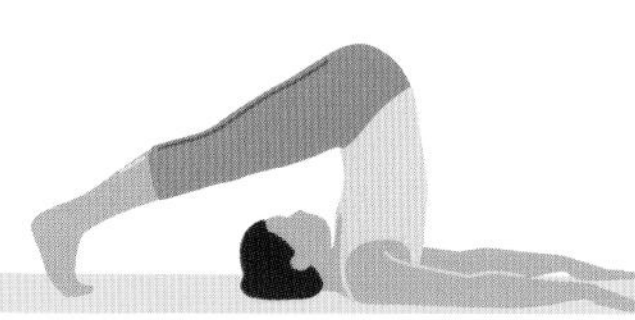

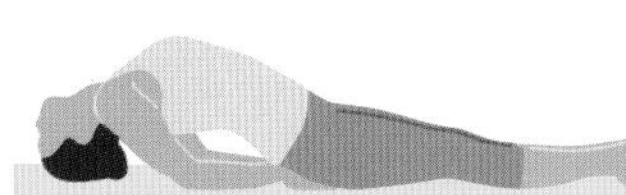

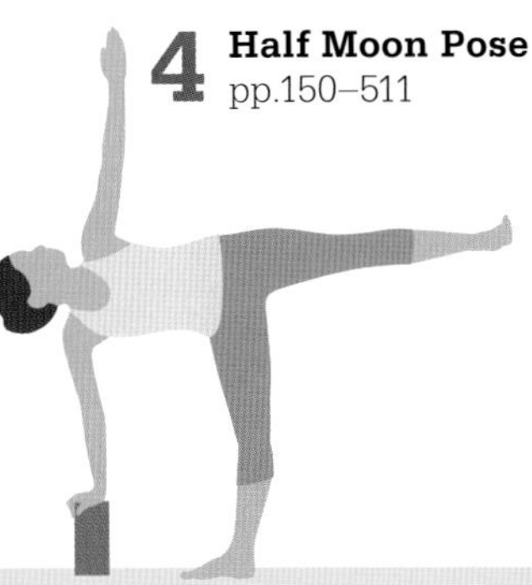

4 Half Moon Pose pp.150–511

5 Downward Facing Dog pp.56–57

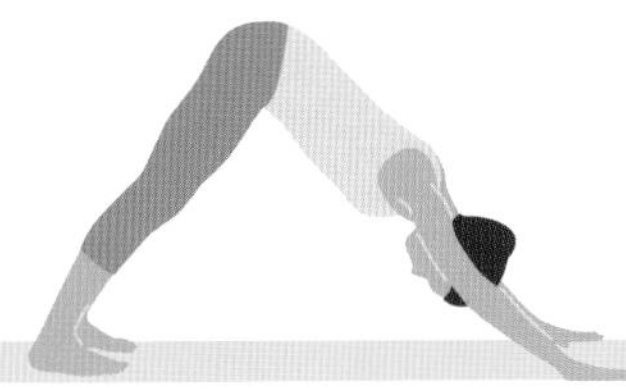

6 Child's Pose pp.62–63

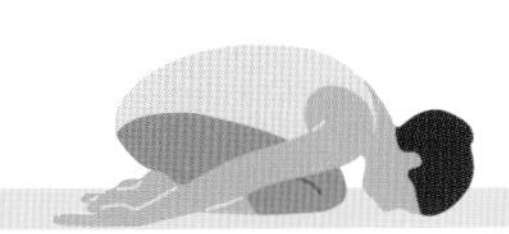

10 Seated Forward Bend pp.158–159

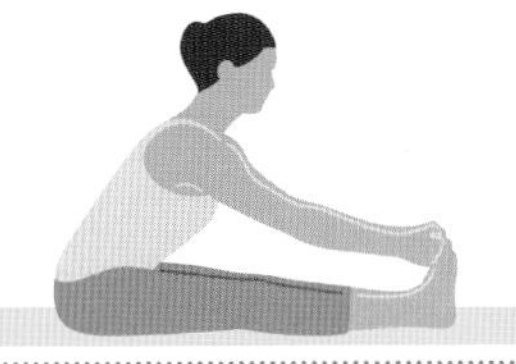

11 Dolphin pp.162–163

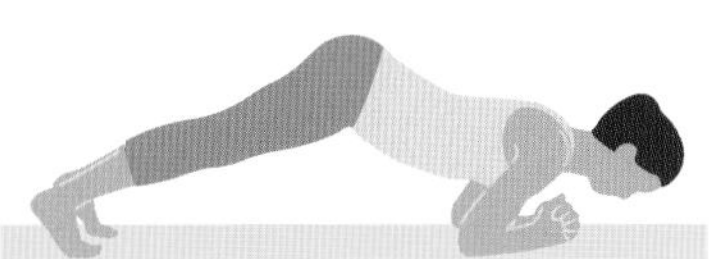

12 Bridge pp.124–125

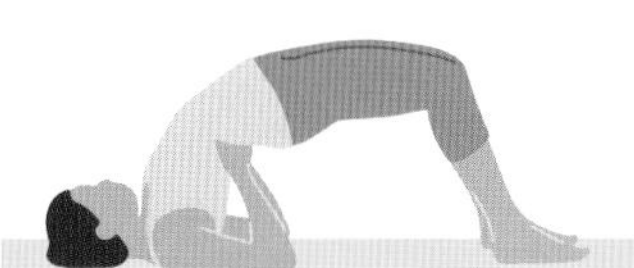

16 Crossed Leg Forward Bend pp.122–123

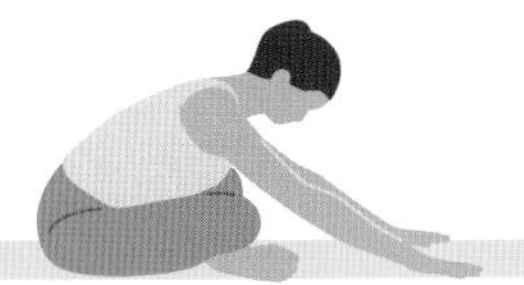

17 Corpse and Final Resolution pp.78–81

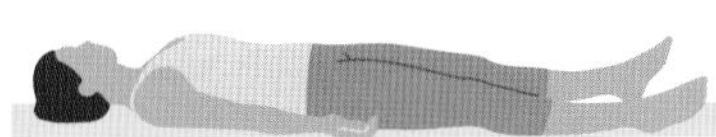

45-Minute Sequence

1 Sun Salutation
pp.64–71

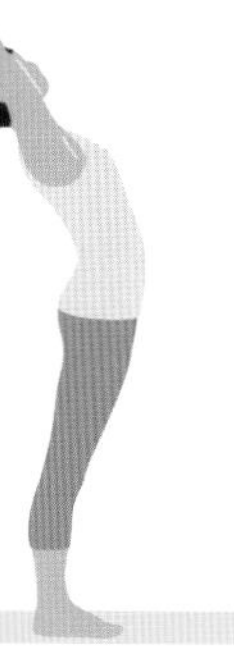

2 Triangle
pp.50–51

3 Half Moon
pp.150–151

7 Wide Forward Bend
pp.106–107

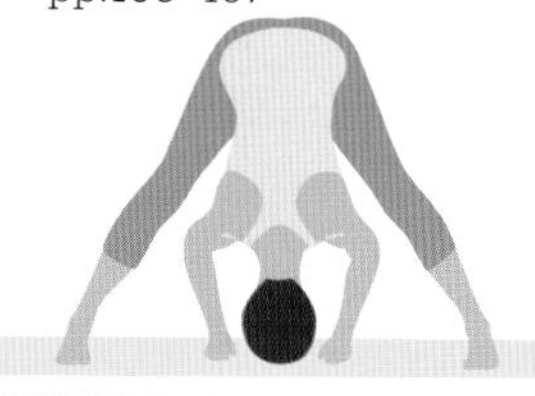

8 Downward Facing Dog
pp.56–57

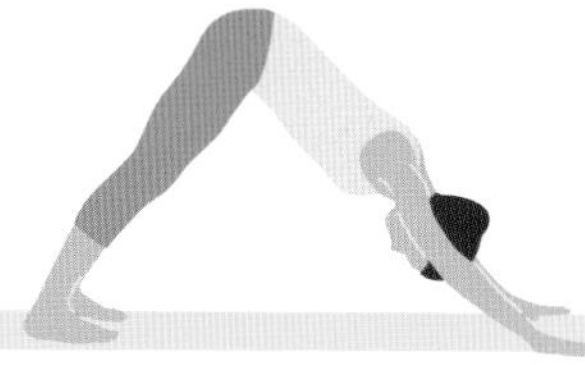

9 Child's Pose
pp.62–63

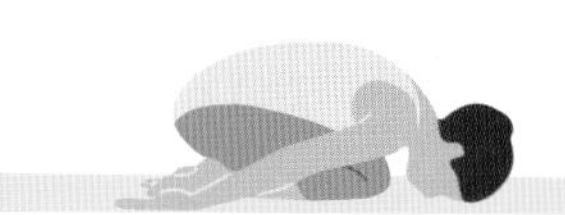

13 Cobbler
pp.74–75

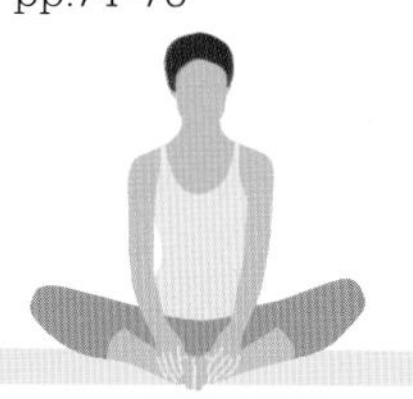

14 Dolphin
pp.162–163

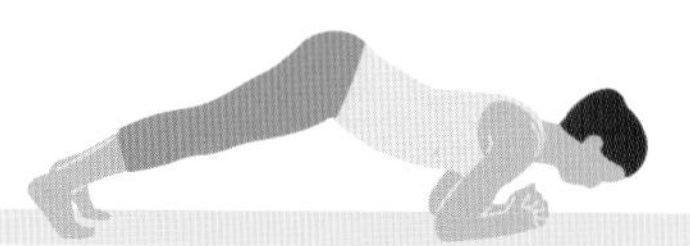

15 Bridge
pp.124–125

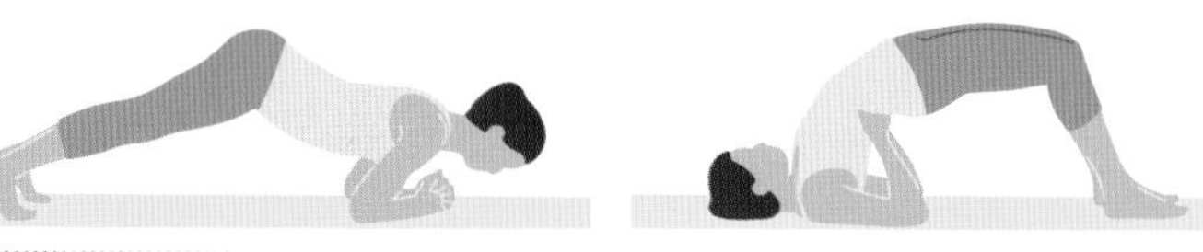

19 Fish
pp.172–173

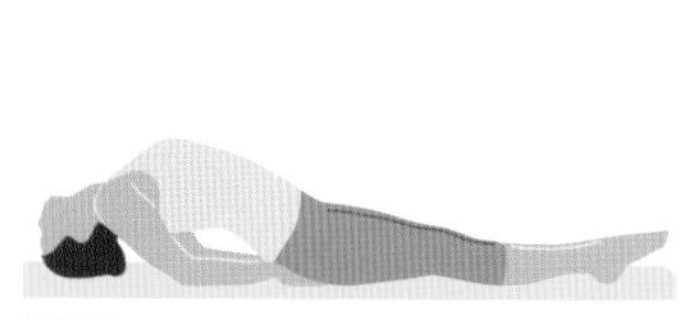

20 Seated Forward Bend
pp.158–159

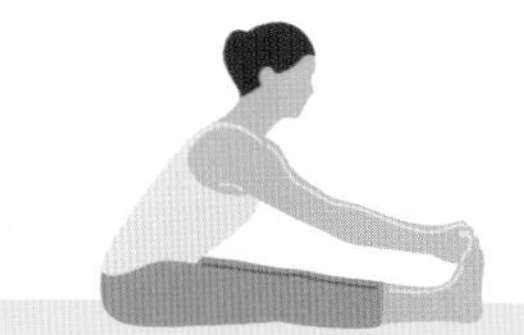

21 Corpse and FInal Relaxation
pp.78–81

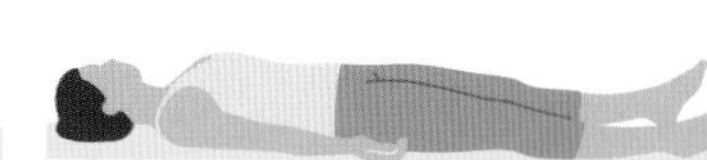

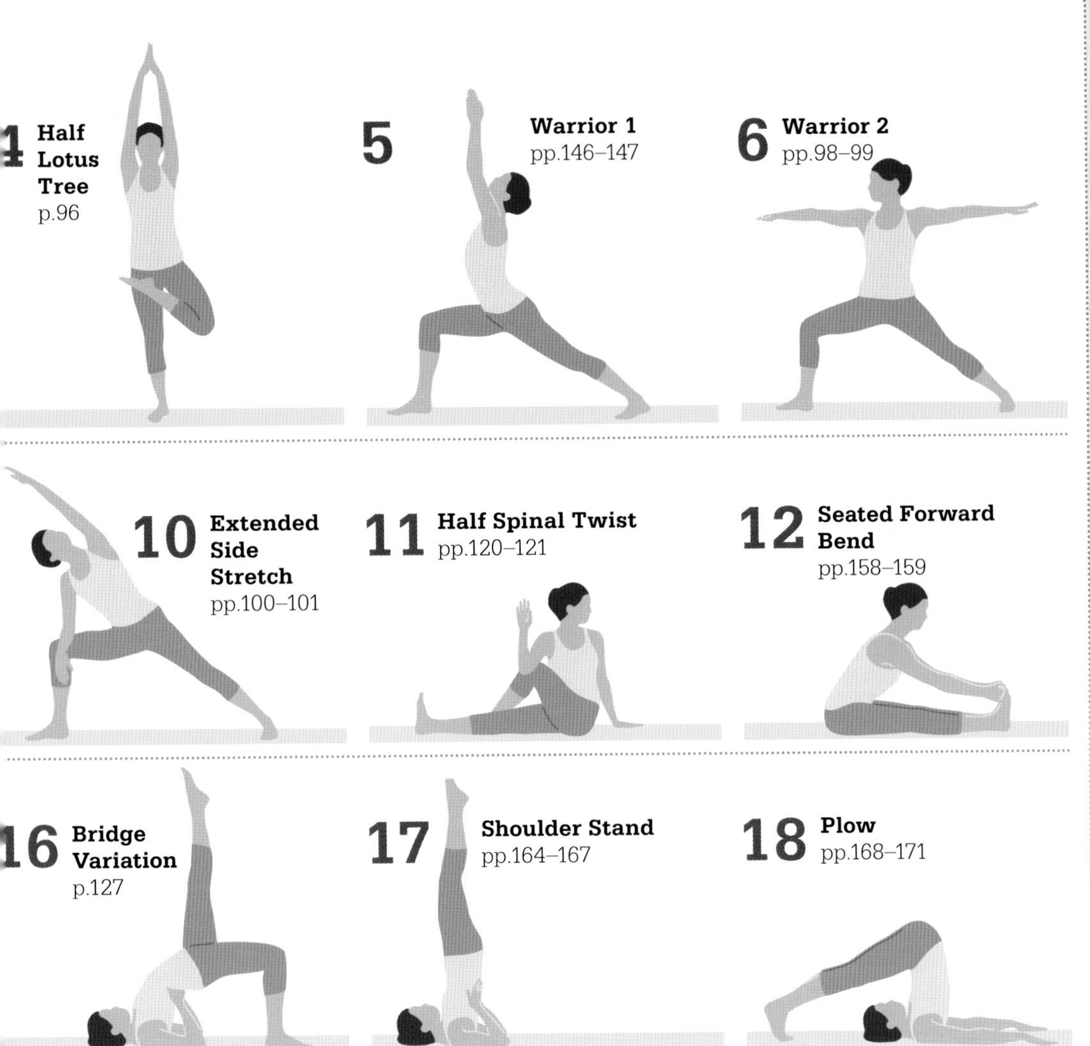
4 Half Lotus Tree p.96
5 Warrior 1 pp.146–147
6 Warrior 2 pp.98–99
10 Extended Side Stretch pp.100–101
11 Half Spinal Twist pp.120–121
12 Seated Forward Bend pp.158–159
16 Bridge Variation p.127
17 Shoulder Stand pp.164–167
18 Plow pp.168–171

Assess your progress

Having worked your way through the book to this point, it's now important to assess your progress. Once you've mastered the basics, it's appropriate to consider how you can adapt your yoga practice to better meet your own particular needs as an individual, both in the short term and the long term. Focusing your practice through applied knowledge is the key to progressing further in yoga.

Focusing your practice

The guidelines on these pages should provide you with a clearer idea of what you might wish to include in a customized practice sequence. For example, you may have a long-term goal of increasing your spinal flexibility and so can adopt a sequence that reflects that. However, you are not limited to that one sequence and, if you are feeling particularly tense after a trying day, then it would make sense to shift the emphasis of your practice to relaxation by modifying or changing your usual routine. Feeling that you are investing in your own wellbeing, rather than following somebody else's prescribed formula, will give you the motivation required to keep practicing.

"What do you enjoy?"

Take some time to think about those elements of your practice you most enjoyed. Is there any posture that you feel has given you particular satisfaction and enjoyment? If so, focusing on this can help you determine the broad direction you wish your practice to take. Some people get greater satisfaction from physical exertion, while others might find that it is the more meditative side of the practice that appeals to them.

"What's not going well?"

You also need to think about those parts of your practice that didn't go well and what elements you didn't enjoy. If you have a great dislike of, or are reluctant to do, a particular pose, this could be indicative of a physical or mental deficiency, which is preventing you from achieving other goals. In this case, you may wish to specifically target that area of weakness in order to be able to eventually correct it.

"What's your emotional and physical state?"

Think about your emotional and physical state at different times of the week—and try to plan accordingly. The yoga you do, for example, after spending the day in your office chair should be different from that done after a day of hard physical exercise. Adopt different plans for your yoga practice according to whether it's a working weekday or a weekend.

"Where can I find out more information?"

For those who wish to study further, there is a tremendous wealth of information available in books and on the internet. Due to the ever-increasing popularity of yoga as a form of exercise and relaxation, there are also many classes and online tutorials available, as well as outlets from which yoga clothing and equipment can be purchased.

"Is your practice working with your lifestyle?"

Most people have to make lifestyle compromises to work around cultural, work, or family commitments, which must be balanced against personal goals and desires. If practicing yoga beyond a certain level requires you to neglect other important aspects of your life, then the practice can become self-defeating. For most people, regularly practicing a sequence they enjoy, which broadly addresses the health issues concerning them, is a perfectly satisfactory way of improving not only their own quality of life, but also that of those with whom they come into contact. There should be no compulsion to keep going beyond what is practical and achievable in your present circumstances.

"What's good to remember?"

Use the knowledge you have gained to balance the sequence. Be aware of including counter-poses where appropriate and allocate sufficient time for both warming up and a proper period relaxation at the end of practice.

"Where do you want to go now?"

Those who do have the time, resources, and inclination to advance their practice should likewise feel free to go ahead and delve deeper into what is truly a diverse and multifaceted body of knowledge. The philosophy that underpins yoga becomes of ever greater relevance to its practice as you explore the subject in greater depth. The more you study, the more it will become apparent that yoga seeks to satisfy human desires by working upon the internal, rather than the materialistic external. The journey of yoga is about finding harmony within, allowing this inner peace to transcend all negative emotions. Yoga and meditation are seen as the means of effecting this change within ourselves. In the same way as basic yoga focuses on the body, practicing advanced yoga means focusing more on controlling the workings of the mind through the practice of meditation.

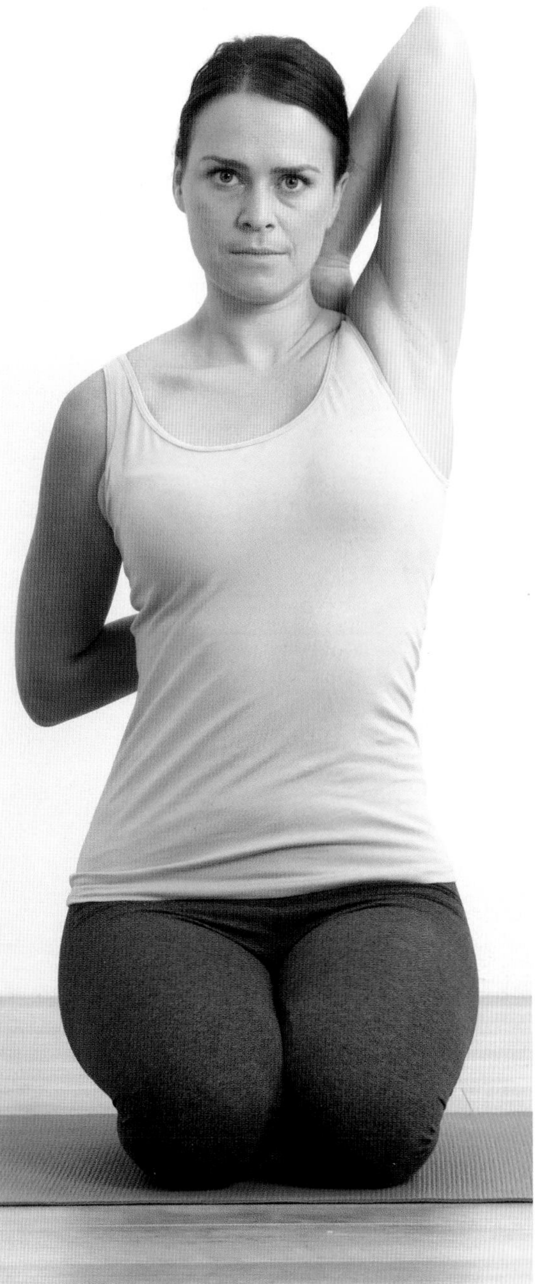

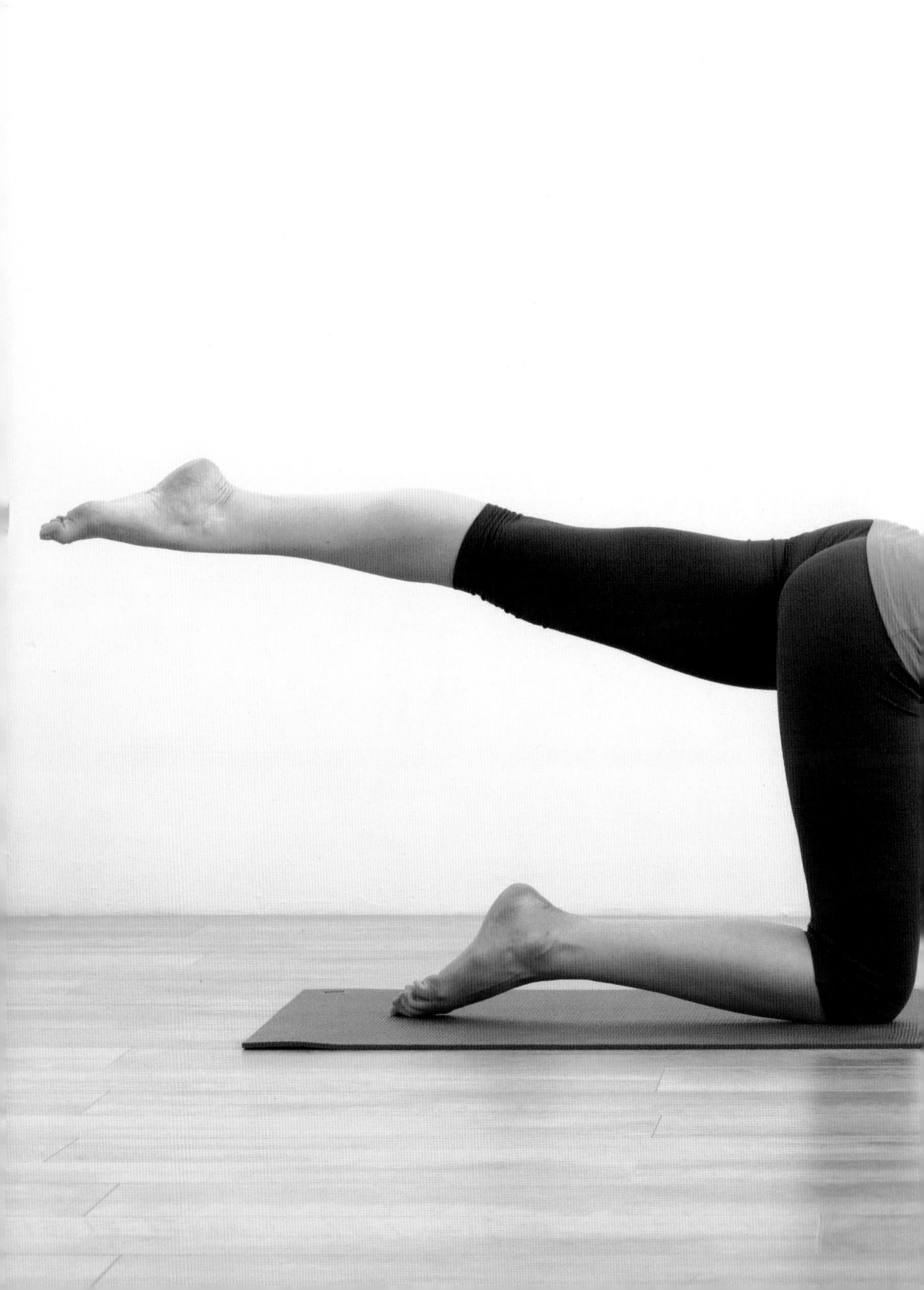

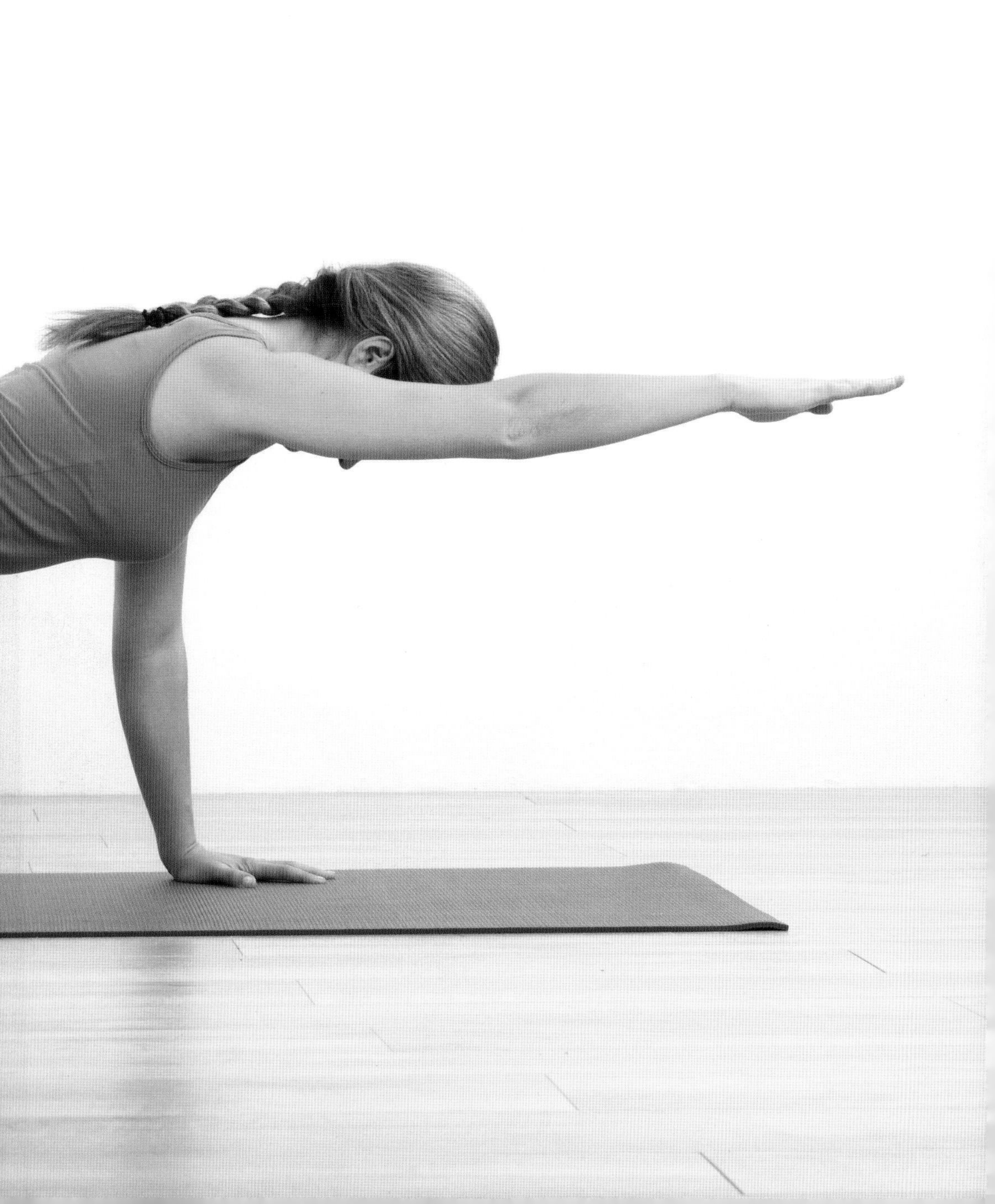

Index

T

UV

WY

About the Author

Nita Patel has been practicing yoga since the age of five and has taught yoga in East London since 1995. She was inspired by the unwavering dedication of B. K. S. Iyengar when she met and worked with him in Pune and has also practiced yoga with Shri K. Pattabhi Jois in Mysore.

Acknowledgments

Photographic Credits

Dorling Kindersley would like to thank **Dave King** for new photography, as well as **Jessica Bentall** and **Joanne King** for modelling.

For further information see www.dkimages.com

Author Acknowledgments

I would like to thank the ancient teacher Patanjali who systemized the school of yoga some millenniums ago and contemporary teachers of yoga for keeping the yoga light alive.

Publisher's Acknowledgments

Many people helped in the making of this book.
Dorling Kindersley would like to thank:

In the UK
Design assistance Vicky Read
Editorial assistance Susannah Marriott, Annelise Evans, Hilary Mandleberg
DK Images Claire Bowers, Freddie Marriage, Emma Shepherd, Romaine Werblow
Indexer Chris Bernstein

At Tall Tree Ltd
Editors Rob Colson, Camilla Hallinan, Deirdre Headon, Catherine Saunders

In India
Senior Editor Garima Sharma
Assistant Art Editor Karan Chaudhary
Design assistance Devan Das, Simran Kaur, Anchal Kaushal, Tanya Mehrotra, Ankita Mukherjee, Anamica Roy, Suzena Sengupta, Vandna Sonkariya, Pooja Verma
DTP Designers Rajesh Singh Adhikari
Deputy Managing Art Editor Priyabrata Roy Chowdhury
Managing Editor Alka Thakur Hazarika